D0699853

Amaurosis Fugax

Eugene F. Bernstein
Editor

Amaurosis Fugax

With 87 Figures, 3 in Full Color

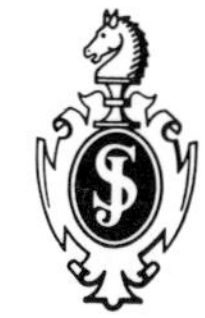

Springer-Verlag
New York Berlin Heidelberg
London Paris Tokyo

Eugene F. Bernstein, M.D., Ph.D.
Division of Vascular and Thoracic Surgery
Scripps Clinic and Research Foundation
10666 North Torrey Pines Road;
Adjunct Professor of Surgery
University of California, San Diego
La Jolla, California 92037, USA

Library of Congress Cataloging-in-Publication Data
Amaurosis fugax.
Includes bibliographies and index.
1. Amaurosis fugax. I. Bernstein, Eugene F., 1930– . [DNLM: 1. Blindness. WW 276 A489]
RE92.5.A43 1987 617.7′12 87-23517
ISBN 0-387-96601-3

Typeset by David E. Seham Associates, Metuchen, New Jersey.
Printed and bound by Arcata Graphics/Halliday, West Hanover, Massachusetts.
Printed in the United States of America.

9 8 7 6 5 4 3 2 1

ISBN 0-387-96601-3 Springer-Verlag New York Berlin Heidelberg
ISBN 3-540-96601-3 Springer-Verlag Berlin Heidelberg New York

Preface

Amaurosis fugax, or "fleeting blindness," has been known as a clinical entity for hundreds of years (1). Since 1859, we also have understood that the phenomenon frequently is related to atheroembolic disease and that it is considered a classic manifestation of ocular transient ischemic attacks and a potential precursor to stroke. However, many questions about this syndrome have remained unanswered until quite recently, when a great deal of new information and thought has been directed to the subject.

Transient monocular blindness (TMB) is only one manifestation of a complicated syndrome of ocular, systemic, and cerebral diseases that may include some degree of monocular blindness. The duration of blindness varies from very brief (seconds) to complete and permanent. The permanent type is referred to as ocular infarction or ocular stroke. Retinal infarction is the most severe degree of monocular blindness and usually is due to embolic occlusion of the central retinal artery or one of its branches. Varying types of arterial emboli have been described, including thrombus, cholesterol, platelets, and fibrin.

More information is now available concerning both ocular stroke from arterial disease and ischemic optic neuropathy as a result of reduced orbital blood flow to the optic nerves. Each of these entities is now known to be quite distinct, with a different underlying pathology and implications for diagnosis and treatment. Recent investigations that span the specialties of ophthalmology, neuro-ophthalmology, neurology, neurosurgery, and vascular surgery have resulted in a further appreciation of the complexities of this syndrome and have opened the doors to new questions.

The purpose of this volume is to collect and organize in a single source not only the contributions to knowledge that recently have been made by the diverse medical specialties involved in the syndrome of TMB but also to place in perspective that knowledge which is uncertain and those questions that remain to be answered. To this end, this work represents an effort at dealing with a number of vexing questions. Why is the blindness episode transient? Why do some patients describe it as the descent of a curtain and others as a blur or a mist or a film? Why is the location of the blind area variable, sometimes originating from the top or the side or the center of the eye? Is the curtain related to the size, location, or composition of emboli? Is the duration of the symptoms important as long as they are completely reversed? Should the word "fleeting" be limited to a particularly short period of blindness?

Other questions deal with specific pathophysiologic aspects of the syndrome. Many patients report repeated episodes in the same eye or the same part of the eye. If the cause is embolic, why do these emboli take the same vascular pathway each time? How much information should we try to obtain about the composition of the emboli in a given patient? Should such information determine the type and degree of suggested treatment? What is the frequency of emboli from the heart, great vessels, carotid bifurcation, or intracranial internal carotid and more distal ophthalmic arterial branches? How can we distinguish between embolic and spastic conditions? Does spasm exist in either the ophthalmic or the retinal arteries? What should be done to distinguish intraocular from extraocular causes for this syndrome?

In addition to these questions about the pathophysiology and mechanism of disease, new information has become available from noninvasive diagnostic laboratory techniques, precise angiographic studies, computerized tomography, magnetic resonance imaging, and positron emission tomography. What is the role of these techniques in the workup of the average patient with TMB? Is there a need for the development of ophthalmic blood flow tests or the use of ophthalmodynamometry? What form of angiographic studies is most appropriate for the workup of these patients? Does it require formal contrast studies or can digital subtraction angiography, either intravenous or intra-arterial, be used? Will the new transcranial Doppler equipment that can be focused accurately on many intracranial vessels be useful in the study of patients with TMB? Does it provide the potential for studying spasm in the ophthalmic artery or for monitoring embolic phenomena? These questions are dealt with in the succeeding chapters of this volume.

Finally, it is most important to try to place in perspective known information about the natural history of this complex condition in comparison with available information about the results of both medical and surgical treatments for the disease. Although data on each of these areas are less complete than we would wish, it is clear that more knowledge than ever before has become available within the last few years on both the untreated and treated patient with various aspects of the amaurosis fugax syndrome. Unfortunately, much of the data from treated patients do not include synchronous controls. Nevertheless, our data base does permit some conclusions to be drawn. Therefore, it seems quite reasonable to collect in a single volume the recent contributions of various investigators who have looked at this syndrome from their own special point of view and to try to synthesize a common approach to the study, diagnosis, and treatment of patients with this disease.

The final chapter in this book is the collaborative work of this entire group of experts, who have attempted to create a Consensus Statement on amaurosis fugax at this time. This "position paper" includes some compromises from the individual points of view of some of the contributors, but it appears to be a reasonable, practical guideline for both clinicians and investigators. It is also an effort to put into perspective those areas in which our current information base is deficient and in which new studies are necessary to help us understand and treat patients with TMB and complete the unraveling of this complex clinical syndrome.

Reference

1. Von Graefe A: Ueber Embolie der Arteria Centralis Retinae als Ursacht plotzlicher Erblindung. *Albrecht von Graefes Arch Klin Exp Ophthalmol* 1859; 5:136–157.

Contents

Contributors

A. Al-Kutoubi, M.D., F.R.C.I., D.M.R.D., Irvine Laboratory for Cardiovascular Investigation and Research, St. Mary's Hospital Medical School, London, UK

Henry J. M. Barnett, M.D., Scientific Director, The John P. Roberts Research Institute, London, Ontario, Canada

Eugene F. Bernstein, M.D., Ph.D., Division of Vascular and Thoracic Surgery, Scripps Clinic and Research Foundation; and Adjunct Professor of Surgery, University of California, San Diego, School of Medicine, La Jolla, California, USA

Allan D. Callow, M.D., Ph.D., Professor, Department of Surgery, Tufts University / New England Medical Center, Boston, Massachusetts, USA

Louis R. Caplan, M.D., Professor and Chairman, Department of Neurology, Tufts University, Boston, Massachusetts, USA

John E. Carter, M.D., Assistant Professor, Division of Neurology and Ophthalmology, The University of Texas, San Antonio, San Antonio, Texas, USA

Daniel P. Connelly, M.D., Department of Surgery, University of California, San Francisco, California, USA

Donald J. Dalessio, M.D., Chairman, Department of Medicine, Scripps Clinic and Research Foundation, La Jolla, California, USA

D. F. S. Deacon, M.D., Irvine Laboratory for Cardiovascular Investigation and Research, St. Mary's Hospital and Medical School, London, UK

Ralph B. Dilley, M.D., Head, Division of Vascular and Thoracic Surgery, Scripps Clinic and Research Foundation, La Jolla, California, USA

J. Donald Easton, M.D., Professor and Chairman, Department of Neurology, Brown University, Providence, Rhode Island, USA

William K. Ehrenfeld, M.D., Professor, Department of Surgery, University of California, San Francisco, San Francisco, California, USA

William S. Fields, M.D., Professor and Chairman, Department of Neuro-Oncology, The University of Texas System Cancer Center, Houston, Texas, USA

Nicolee C. Fode, R.N., M.S., Department of Neurosurgery, Mayo Clinic, Rochester, Minnesota, USA

Mitchell H. Friedlaender, M.D., Division of Ophthalmology, Scripps Clinic and Research Foundation, La Jolla, California, USA

Professeur Jean-Claude Gautier, Professor of Neurology, Chief, Service d'Urgenc'es Cérébrovasculaires, Hôpital de la Salpêtrière, Paris, France

M. Grigg, F.R.A.C.S., Irvine Laboratory for Cardiovascular Investigation and Research, St. Mary's Hospital Medical School, London, UK

Laurence A. Harker, M.D., Director, Roon Research Center for Arteriosclerosis and Thrombosis, Department of Basic and Clinical Research, Scripps Clinic and Research Foundation, La Jolla, California, USA

Michael J.G. Harrison, D.M., F.R.C.P., Francis and Renee Hock Director of Research, The Reta Lila Weston Institute of Neurological Studies, University of London, London, UK

Sohan S. Hayreh, M.D., Ph.D., Professor of Ophthalmology, The University of Iowa Hospitals and Clinics, Iowa City, Iowa, USA

William F. Hoyt, M.D., Professor of Neuro-Ophthalmology, Department of Neurological Surgery, University of California, San Francisco, San Francisco, California, USA

Noreen A. Lemak, M.D., Department of Neuro-Oncology, The University of Texas System Cancer Center, Houston, Texas, USA

Joseph B. Michelson, M.D., Head, Division of Ophthalmology, Scripps Clinic and Research Foundation, La Jolla, California, USA

Jay P. Mohr, M.D., Sciarra Professor of Clinical Neurology, College of Physicians and Surgeons of Columbia University, New York, New York, USA

Andrew N. Nicolaides, M.S., F.R.C.S., Honorary Consultant Cardiovascular Surgeon, Professor of Vascular Surgery, St. Mary's Hospital Medical School, London, UK

K. Papadakis, M.D., Irvine Laboratory for Cardiovascular Investigation and Research, St. Mary's Hospital Medical School, London, UK

Steven Okuhn, M.D., Department of Surgery, University of California, San Francisco, San Francisco, California, USA

Shirley M. Otis, M.D., Head, Division of Neurology, Scripps Clinic and Research Foundation, La Jolla, California, USA

Ralph W. Ross Russell, M.D., F.R.C.P., Professor of Neurology, Consultant Physician, St. Thomas Hospital Medical School, London, UK

Peter J. Savino, M.D., Director, Neuro-Ophthalmology Department, Wills Eye Institute, Philadelphia, Pennsylvania, USA

Marjorie E. Seybold, M.D., Divisions of Ophthalmology and Neurology, Scripps Clinic and Research Foundation, La Jolla, California, USA

Thoralf M. Sundt, Jr., M.D., Professor and Chairman, Department of Neurologic Surgery, Mayo Clinic, Rochester, Minnesota, USA

James F. Toole, M.D., Teagle Professor of Neurology, Wake Forest University, Winston-Salem, North Carolina, USA

M. A. Williams, F.R.C.S., Irvine Laboratory for Cardiovascular Investigation and Research, St. Mary's Hospital Medical School, London, UK

Shirley H. Wray, M.D., Ph.D., Associate Professor, Department of Neurology, Harvard Medical School, and Director, Neurovisual Unit, Massachusetts General Hospital, Boston, Massachusetts, USA

Color Plate

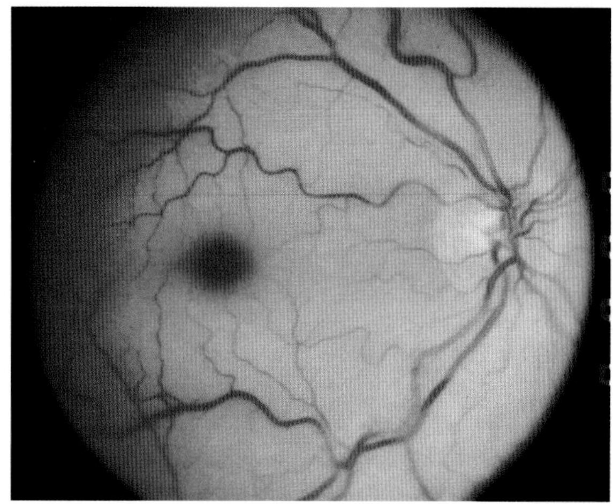

FIGURE 6–1. Opacification of the retina and macula cherry red spot following occlusion of the central retinal artery.

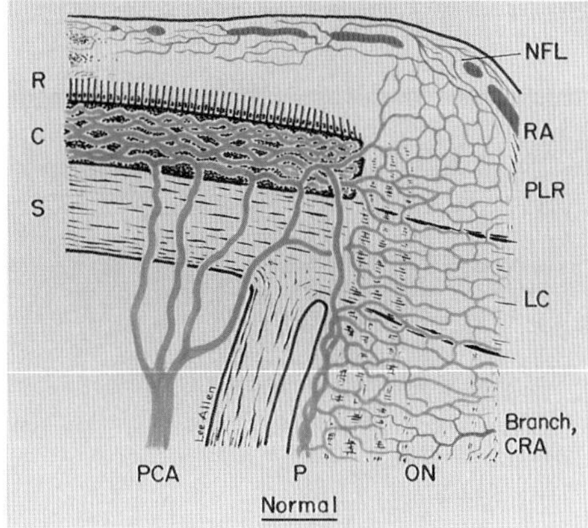

FIGURE 8–2. Blood supply of the optic nerve head and retrolaminar optic nerve. For details, see p. 95.

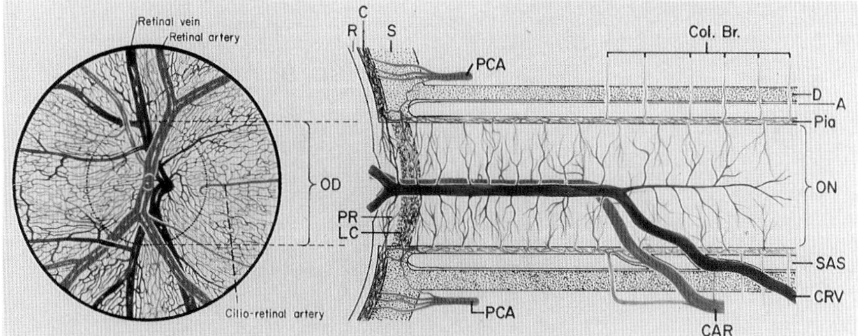

FIGURE 8–3. Blood supply of the optic nerve head and intraorbital optic nerve *(right)* and blood vessels on the surface of the optic disk and adjacent retina *(left)*. For details, see p. 97.

CHAPTER 1

Arterial Blood Supply of the Eye

Sohan Singh Hayreh

The eyeball and the optic nerve are supplied by the ophthalmic artery and its various branches; these include the central artery of the retina, anterior and posterior ciliary arteries (ACAs, PCAs), and collateral branches to the optic nerve. My anatomic studies on the ophthalmic artery and its branches in man have revealed gross inaccuracies in the classical, prevalent textbook descriptions of these arteries (1–8). That was a quarter of a century ago, but the textbooks still continue to propagate the old erroneous descriptions.

The Ophthalmic Artery

Origin

The ophthalmic artery arises as the first major branch of the internal carotid artery (ICA). It originates after the ICA emerges out of the cavernous sinus to lie under the optic nerve in 91.5% (Figs. 1–1 and 1–2) and from the intracavernous part of the ICA in 7.5% (Fig. 1–3). However, this is not invariable. The ophthalmic artery may have the following abnormal origins, which are discussed in detail elsewhere (4,5):

1. *From the middle meningeal artery*. The blood supply to the orbit may come partially or totally from the middle meningeal artery (Fig. 1–4). In my study (5), in six of 170 specimens, the ophthalmic artery arose from the middle meningeal artery because of an abnormal development of the normally existing anastomosis between the middle meningeal artery and the lacrimal artery through the superior orbital fissure (Fig. 1–4, part 1). This anastomosis represents a prominent fetal connection (3). In four of these, a big trunk arose from the middle meningeal artery and a small one from the ICA, and these two trunks communicated with each other in the orbit (Fig. 1–4, parts 2 and 3). The ocular branches, especially the central retinal artery (CRA), arose from the trunk arising from the ICA. Chanmugam (9) reported a case in which the two

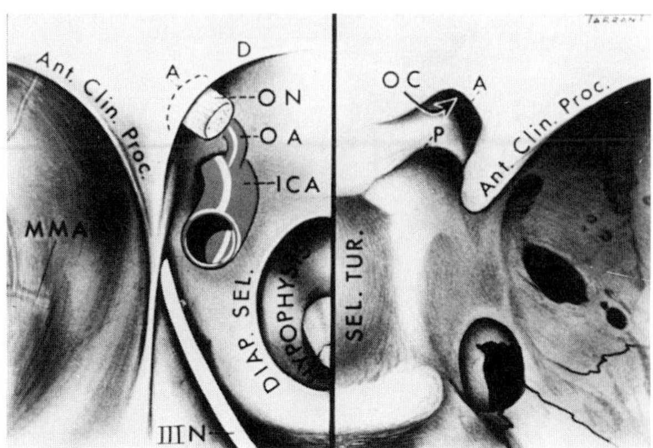

FIGURE 1–1. Right half shows cranial opening of the optic canal and surrounding bony landmarks, as seen at the base of the skull. Left half shows cranial opening of the optic canal with dural margin intact, optic nerve, ophthalmic artery, internal carotid artery, hypophysis, and diaphragma sellae, as seen after removal of the brain. Reproduced from Hayreh SS, 1963 (3). (Consult key on pp. 21, 22 for abbreviations used in Figs. 1–1 to 1–8.)

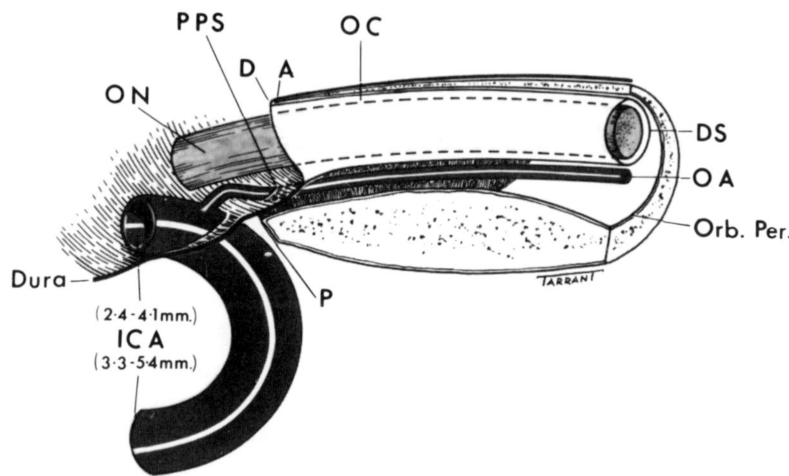

FIGURE 1–2. Lateral view of the optic canal and cavernous and intracranial part of the internal carotid artery shows details of origin and intracranial and intracanalicular course of the ophthalmic artery. The diameters of the lumen of the internal carotid artery before and after the origin of the ophthalmic artery are shown. Reproduced from Hayreh SS, 1963 (3).

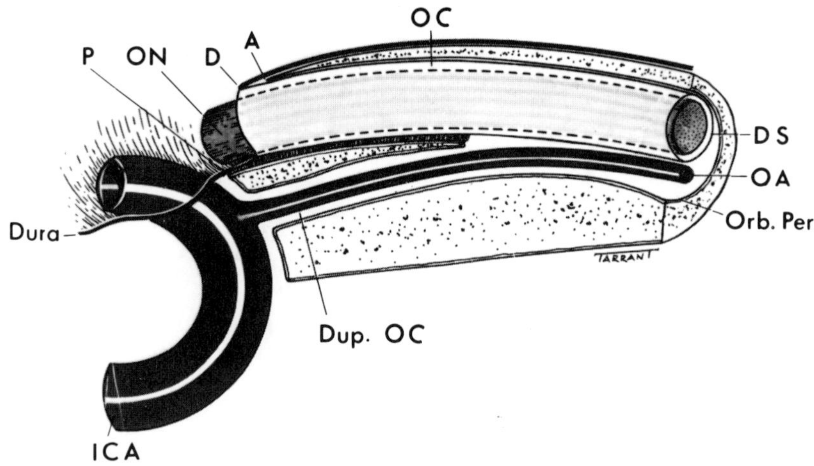

FIGURE 1–3. Same as in Fig. 1–2, but shows an extradural origin of the ophthalmic artery and its course through duplicate optic canal. Reproduced from Hayreh SS, 1963 (3).

trunks did not communicate with each other, an arrangement usually seen at the 18-mm stage of fetal life. In two of my specimens (5) the trunk from the ICA had either disappeared (Fig. 1–4, part 4) or atrophied so that the blood supply to the entire ophthalmic arterial bed came only from the middle meningeal artery.

2. *From the middle cerebral artery*. When the ipsilateral ICA is absent, the ophthalmic artery may arise from the middle cerebral artery, a branch of the circle of Willis (10,11).
3. *From the posterior communicating artery*. In one case with bilateral absence of the ICA, the ophthalmic artery arose from the posterior communicating artery (12).
4. *From the maxillary artery*. In one reported case (13), the ICA was replaced by two branches of the maxillary artery, which entered the skull through the foramen ovale and foramen rotundum and joined to form a single vessel. This vessel gave off the ophthalmic artery and other intracranial branches of the ICA, an arrangement regularly found in the ruminants.

Course

The ophthalmic artery has an intracranial, an intracanalicular, and an intraorbital course (Figs. 1–5, 1–6). At its origin, the ophthalmic artery usually lies in the subdural space, under the medial or central part of the optic nerve. Usually the rest of the intracranial course is related intimately

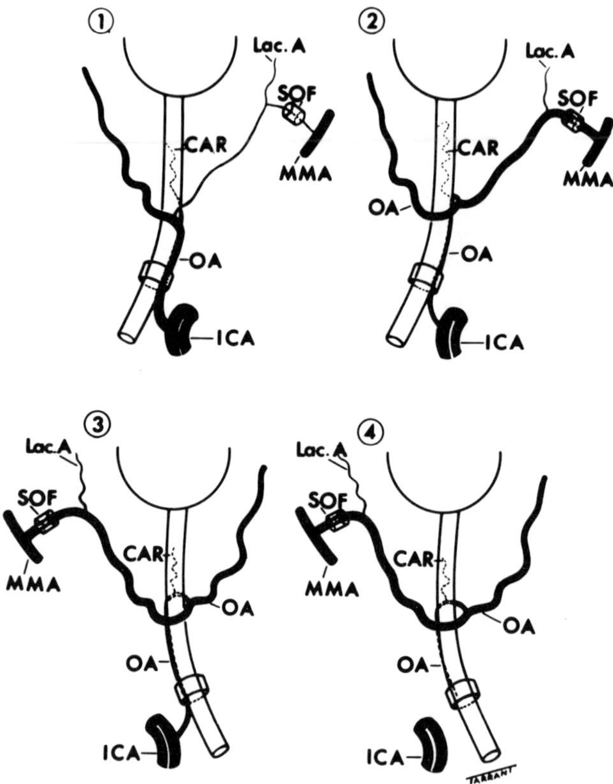

FIGURE 1–4. Variations in origin and intraorbital course of the ophthalmic artery. *(1)* - Normal pattern. *(2,3)* - The ophthalmic artery arises from the internal carotid artery as usual, but the major contribution comes from the middle meningeal artery. *(4)* - The only source is the middle meningeal artery. Reproduced from Hayreh SS, 1963 (3).

to the inferolateral part of the optic nerve. A detailed account of these has been reported elsewhere (5). Briefly, the intracanalicular part lies mostly in the optic canal between the two layers of the dura mater and under the optic nerve (Fig. 1–5), but in 3% it may be by itself in a separate duplicate bony optic canal (Fig. 1–3), or, very rarely, may enter the orbit through the superior orbital fissure.

For descriptive purposes, the intraorbital course can be divided into three parts (Fig. 1–6) (6): The first part extends from the point of entrance of the artery into the orbit to the point where it bends to become the second part. The first part of the artery usually is related closely to the inferolateral aspect of the optic nerve and attached to the nerve by loose connective tissue. During the second part, the artery crosses medially

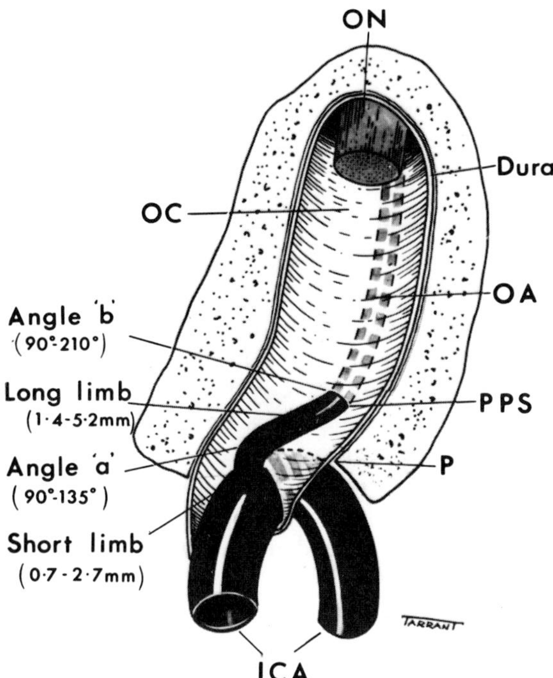

FIGURE 1–5. Origin and intracranial and intracanalicular course of the ophthalmic artery and its subdivisions as seen on opening the optic canal. Reproduced from Hayreh SS, 1963 (3).

over (in 82.6%) or under (in 17.4%) the optic nerve to lie on the superomedial aspect of the nerve. The artery is loosely attached to the nerve in this section. The third part extends from the end of the second part to the termination of the artery at the superomedial angle of the orbital opening. This is the only part of the ophthalmic artery that is not related intimately to the optic nerve, and it is usually markedly tortuous.

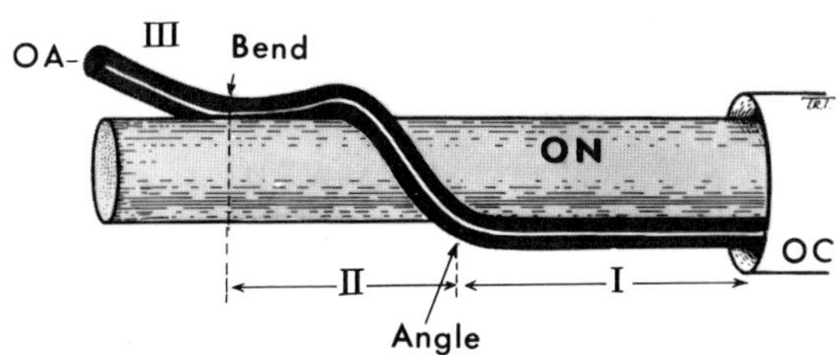

FIGURE 1–6. Intraorbital course of the ophthalmic artery as seen from the lateral side of the optic nerve. Reproduced from Hayreh SS, 1963 (3).

The "angle" between the first and second parts of the ophthalmic artery is well defined, whereas the "bend" between the second and third parts is not (Fig. 1–6).

Branches

My studies revealed that most textbook descriptions of the branches of the ophthalmic artery do not describe their pattern accurately (2). It must be stressed that there is such marked variation in the order of origin of the various branches from the ophthalmic artery that no two specimens, not even from the same person, show an identical pattern. However, certain broad generalizations can be made. Whether the ophthalmic artery crosses over or under the optic nerve in the second part makes an evident difference in the order of its branches up to the origin of the anterior ethmoid artery. The usual order of the origin of the various branches of the ophthalmic artery is summarized in Table 1–1 and shown diagrammatically in Fig. 1–7. A detailed account of each branch of the ophthalmic artery, including its developmental derivation and genesis of order of origin has been presented elsewhere (2,3).

TABLE 1–1. Order of origin of various branches of the ophthalmic artery.

	Ophthalmic Artery Crossed	
Order of origin	Over optic nerve (Fig 1–7, part 2)	Under optic nerve (Fig 1–7, part 1)
1	Central retinal + medial posterior ciliary	Lateral posterior ciliary
2	Lateral posterior ciliary	Central retinal
3	Lacrimal	Medial muscular
4	Muscular to superior rectus and/or levator	Medial posterior ciliary
5	Posterior ethmoid and supraorbital, jointly or separately	Lacrimal
6	Medial posterior ciliary	Muscular to superior rectus and levator
7	Medial muscular	Posterior ethmoid and supraorbital, jointly or separately
8	Muscular to superior oblique and/or medial rectus	Muscular to superior oblique and/or medial rectus
9	To areolar tissue	Anterior ethmoid
10	Anterior ethmoid	To areolar tissue
11	Medial palpebral or inferior medial palpebral	Medial palpebral or inferior medial palpebral
12	Superior medial palpebral	Superior medial palpebral
Terminal	i Dorsal nasal ii Supratrochlear	i Dorsal nasal ii Supratrochlear

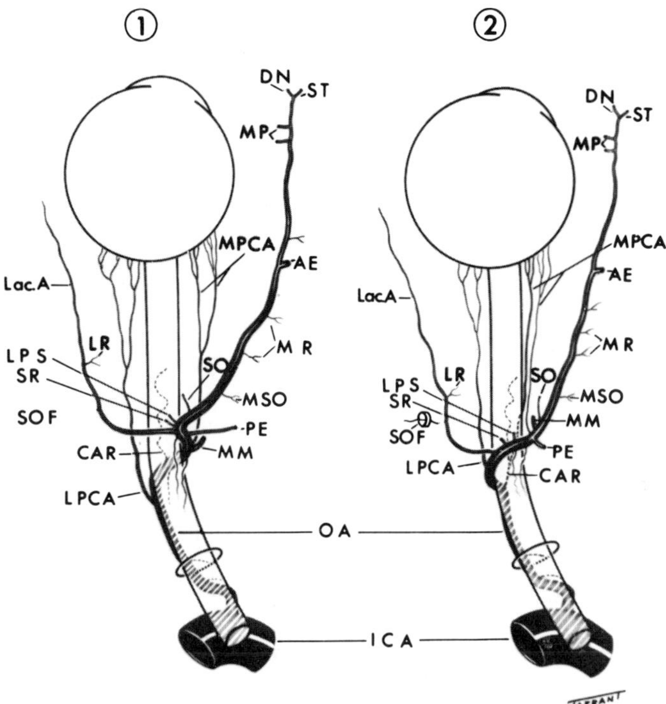

FIGURE 1–7. The pattern of the branches of the ophthalmic artery when it crosses *(1)* under and *(2)* over the optic nerve. Reproduced from Hayreh SS, 1963 (3).

Anastomoses

With the more frequent recognition of occlusion of the ICA, an understanding of the collateral circulation of the brain and the eye has assumed great significance. In such cases, three collateral channels maintain the blood supply to the brain: (1) the circle of Willis; (2) anastomoses between the anterior, middle, and posterior cerebral arteries; and (3) anastomoses between the external and internal carotid arteries. In the last group, anastomoses by way of the ophthalmic artery are one of the important potential anastomoses to be considered. Figure 1–8 shows the various anastomoses between the branches of the ophthalmic artery and those of the external carotid artery (3).

Calibers

The caliber of the ophthalmic artery in the intracranial part varies from 0.7 to 1.4 mm (median, 1.1; mean 1.1±0.2). The caliber of the ICA immediately before and after the origin of the ophthalmic artery is 3.3 to 5.4

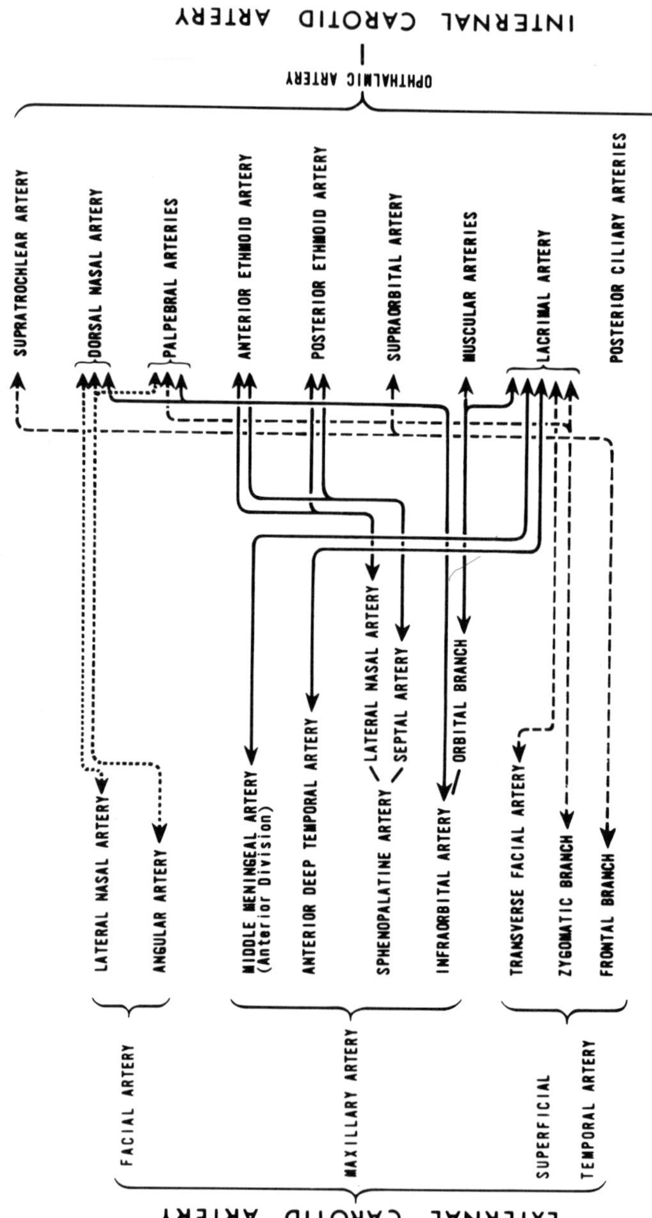

FIGURE 1–8. Diagrammatic representation of anastomoses of the ophthalmic artery with various branches of the external carotid artery. Reproduced from Hayreh SS, 1963 (3).

mm (median, 4.1; mean, 4.2±0.5) and 2.4 to 4.1 mm (median, 3.5; mean, 3.5±0.4), respectively (Fig. 1–2) (5). In my study, in a number of specimens of the ophthalmic artery (5), although the lumen of the ICA was wide open, with marked atherosclerotic changes in the wall, the lumen of the ophthalmic artery at the point of its origin from the ICA was so narrow that a fine needle would hardly go through it. The ophthalmic artery and the ICA showed no significant variation in caliber with age, although in one 4-year-old child the ICAs were smaller than in adults, and the lumens of the ophthalmic arteries were almost the size seen in adults (5).

Ophthalmic Artery Pressure

Ophthalmic artery pressure (OAP) usually reflects indirectly the blood pressure of the ICA. It is measured by ophthalmodynamometry or other methods based on the same principle; these, unfortunately, have limitations in reliability and reproducibility. I feel that the main value of ophthalmodynamometry is in comparing pressures on the two sides of an individual, rather than in measuring the exact pressure. In healthy rhesus monkeys, we cannulated the ophthalmic artery and aorta to measure simultaneously OAP and systemic arterial pressure (14). The following formulas were derived to deduce the OAP from the systemic blood pressure (BP) in normal subjects:

$$\text{Systolic OAP} = 0.80 \times \text{systolic BP} - 8.63\text{ mm Hg} \pm 3.8\text{ mm Hg}$$

$$\text{Diastolic OAP} = 0.80 \times \text{diastolic BP} + 6.95\text{ mm Hg} \pm 3.4\text{ mm Hg}$$

Ocular Arteries

The eyeball is supplied by the central retinal artery and the anterior and posterior ciliary arteries.

Central Retinal Artery

A detailed account of various aspects of the anatomy of the CRA has been given elsewhere (1,7,8). The following is a brief summary.

Origin

The site, order, and mode of origin of the CRA from the ophthalmic artery, as seen in my 102 human specimens, are shown in Table 1–2. The CRA may arise as the first, second, or third branch of the ophthalmic artery, from its first or second parts, or from the angle between the first and second parts. It may arise as an independent branch or in common with other branches of the ophthalmic artery. Two specimens had double CRAs that arose independently from the ophthalmic artery.

TABLE 1–2. Site, order, and mode of origin of the central retinal artery.

	Origin	Total (%)	Ophthalmic artery crosses: Over optic nerve (%)	Ophthalmic artery crosses: Under optic nerve (%)
Site	From first part of ophthalmic artery	22	25	9
	From angle of ophthalmic artery	58	66	27
	From second part of ophthalmic artery	18	6	64
	From third part of ophthalmic artery	2	3	0
Order	As first branch of ophthalmic artery	77	95	14
	As second branch of ophthalmic artery	19	4	73
	As third branch of ophthalmic artery	4	1	14
Mode	As independent branch	37	26	77
	With medial posterior ciliary artery	38	43	18
	With lateral posterior ciliary artery	12	15	0
	With MPCA, LPCA and muscular arteries	2	2	0
	With MPCA and LPCA	5	6	0
	With MPCA and muscular artery	3	2	5
	With muscular artery	3	4	0
	With lacrimal artery and LPCA	1	1	0
Total number of specimens examined		102	80	22

MPCA = medial posterior ciliary artery; LPCA = lateral posterior ciliary artery.

Course

The course of the CRA can be divided for descriptive purposes into three parts: intraorbital (from origin to its entry into the dural sheath of the optic nerve), intravaginal (in the space between the optic nerve and dural sheath), and intraneural (within the optic nerve substance). The CRA penetrates the dural sheath 5.0 to 15.5 mm (median, 10.0; mean, 9.8 ± 1.8) behind the eyeball, usually at the inferomedial aspect of the optic nerve.

Branches

In 97% of specimens, the CRA before its terminal divisions at the optic disc supplies several branches of various sizes from one or another part, with no constant pattern of origin. Table 1–3 summarizes the number of branches seen from the various parts of the CRA. I saw no branches in the lamina cribrosa region. Intraorbital branches supply a variable area of the dural sheath and the optic nerve, extending from the eyeball to the intracanalicular part. The branches from the intravaginal part ramify on the pia and supply the optic nerve anterior to the point of entry of the artery into the nerve and, in about half the cases, also supply branches posterior to this point. The intraneural branches almost invariably supply

TABLE 1–3. Number of branches from various parts of the central retinal artery.

No. of branches observed	Incidence of branches from various parts (%)		
	Intraorbital	Intravaginal	Intraneural
0	48	5	25
1	33	49	27
2	13	35	20
3	2	7	11
4	2	0	11
5	1	0	0
6	0	0	2
7	0	0	0
8	0	0	2
Uncertain	1	4	3
Total no. of specimens examined	92	76	64

the anterior part of the optic nerve. Thus, the CRA plays an important role in the blood supply of the optic nerve.

Anastomoses

The extraocular branches of the CRA establish numerous anastomoses with other branches of the ophthalmic artery, mostly between the pial branches from the CRA (arising from all the three parts—invariably from the intravaginal part and much less frequently from the others) and pial branches from other sources. The following types of anastomoses can be established by the CRA:

1. Anastomoses between the CRA and the recurrent pial branches from the peripapillary choroid (sometimes from the circle of Zinn and Haller). These anastomoses are seen most frequently and are located on the pia of the retrobulbar part of the optic nerve.
2. Anastomoses between the CRA and pial branches from the collateral branches of the orbital arteries. These are the second most common anastomoses of the CRA.
3. Anastomoses between pial branches from different parts of the CRA.

In my study the anastomoses were sufficiently large to allow the injection fluid (liquid latex) to pass easily from one channel to another (1,8).

Thus, the CRA participates in many anastomoses, which usually are large enough to allow collateral circulation and may be of considerable physiologic significance.

Posterior Ciliary Arteries

There is a good deal of confusion as to nomenclature, number, origin, and distribution of the PCAs in man. Based on my anatomical studies in man, I have described the subject in detail elsewhere (2), and, briefly, it is as follows:

Nomenclature

The PCAs have been named by me according to their relation to the optic nerve near their site of entry into the eyeball. The lateral PCA lies lateral to the optic nerve. Humans may have one (in about 75%) two (in about 20%), or none (in about 3%). The medial PCA lies medial to the optic nerve. Humans may have one (in about 70%) or two (in about 30%). The superior PCA is seen in only 9%, and there may be one (in 7%) or two (in 2%); these are usually small.

The various PCAs run forward, divide into a large number of small branches, and pierce the sclera near the optic nerve. Out of these branches of the PCAs, one on the medial and another one on the lateral side form the long PCAs; the rest are called the short PCAs. The number of short PCAs piercing the sclera varies from about 10 to 20, depending upon the number of times the PCAs have subdivided before reaching the sclera. Thus, there are three types of PCAs. The main PCAs arise from the ophthalmic artery and are usually two or three (medial and lateral PCAs). There are two long PCAs, one medial and the other lateral. Erroneously, the main PCAs have been designated as "long" PCAs right from their origin from the ophthalmic artery. The long PCAs do not arise directly from the ophthalmic artery. The third type, the 10 to 20 short PCAs, also do not arise directly from the ophthalmic artery.

TABLE 1–4. Mode of origin of various PCAs from the ophthalmic artery.

Mode of origin	Lateral PCA %	Medial PCA %	Superior PCA %
Independent branch	73	58	3.5
In common with other orbital arteries:			
CRA	8.5	36	0
Muscular	5	22	3.5
CRA + muscular	0	5	0
Muscular + lacrimal	2	0	0
LPCA + MPCA + CRA + muscular	2	2	0
LPCA + MPCA + CRA	2	2	0
MPCA + LPCA	2	2	0
Lacrimal	19	2	0
LPCA + superior PCA	2	0	2

PCA = posterior ciliary artery; CRA = central retinal artery; LPCA = Lateral posterior ciliary artery; MPCA = medial posterior ciliary artery.

I want to stress very strongly that unless this terminology is clearly understood and adhered to, there may be tremendous confusion, as is the case in the textbooks.

Number of PCAs

The ophthalmic artery in humans gives out one (in 3%), two (in 48%), three (in 39%), four (in 8%), or five (in 2%) PCAs. When there are more than three PCAs, the additional arteries are usually small.

Origin

The PCAs may arise from the ophthalmic artery as independent branches or in common with other branches of the ophthalmic artery (Table 1–4). They may arise from different parts of the ophthalmic artery (Table 1–5).

Distribution

The short PCAs supply the following: (a) The choroid as far as the equator. (b) The Retina: The choroid supplies the overlying retina to a depth of about 130 μm including the retinal pigment epithelium and adjacent outer layers of the retina up to the outer part of the inner nuclear layer. If a cilioretinal artery is present, then the entire thickness of the retina is supplied in the distribution of the cilioretinal artery.

(c) Anterior part of the optic nerve: The PCA circulation is the main source of blood supply to the optic nerve head and the adjacent retrolaminar part of the optic nerve (15–17).

The long PCAs supply a sector of the choroid, starting almost immediately from the point where it joins the choroid temporal to the macular

TABLE 1–5. Site of origin of various PCAs from the ophthalmic artery.

	Ophthalmic artery crosses			
	Over optic nerve		Under optic nerve	
Part of ophthalmic artery	Type of PCA	Prevalence %	Type of PCA	Prevalence %
First part	MPCA	20.5	MPCA	0
	LPCA	9	LPCA	80.5
Angle between first and second parts	MPCA	36.5	MPCA	20
	LPCA	36.5	LPCA	27
Second part	MPCA	9	MPCA	87
	LPCA	77	LPCA	0
Bend between second and third parts	MPCA	36	MPCA	27
	LPCA	2	LPCA	13
Third part	MPCA	25	MPCA	0
	LPCA	0	LPCA	0

PCA = posterior ciliary artery; LPCA = lateral posterior ciliary artery; MPCA = medial posterior ciliary artery.

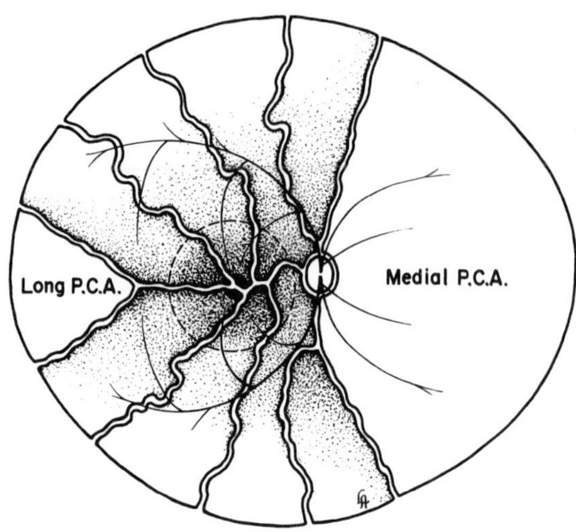

FIGURE 1–9. Diagrammatic representation of distribution by various temporal short PCAs and their watershed zones in posterior part of fundus. Dotted circle in region of distribution of temporal short PCAs represents macular region. Areas of supply by medial PCA and temporal long PCA are shown also. Reproduced from Hayreh SS, 1974 (31).

region after having pierced the sclera and extending forward (Fig. 1–9) (18,19). They also supply the corresponding segment of the anterior uvea.

Discrepancies Between Postmortem Injection and In Vivo Physiologic and Anatomic Studies of the PCA Circulation

Postmortem anatomic studies (19–26) of the PCA circulation (ie, the choroidal vascular bed), after injection of the vessels with latex or similar materials, invariably have shown extensive anastomoses between the various branches of the short PCAs and between the short PCAs and ACAs, with the choriocapillaris forming a continuous anastomotic network over the entire choroid. However, it is well known that inflammatory, metastatic, ischemic, and degenerative lesions in the PCA circulation usually are localized. The advent of fluorescein angiography has permitted studies of not only the blood flow but also the physiologic anatomy in vivo, and the findings have led to a revision of the concept of the PCA circulation in vivo.

Physiologic Anatomy: The in vivo clinical and experimental fluorescein angiographic studies (27,28) have clearly shown that the PCA circulation is segmental, almost like that in the retinal vasculature. The lateral and medial PCAs supply the corresponding half of the choroid. In humans the border between the choroid supplied by the lateral and medial PCAs may be located anywhere between the fovea and nasal border of the optic disk (Fig. 1–10). The position of the watershed zone between the lateral and

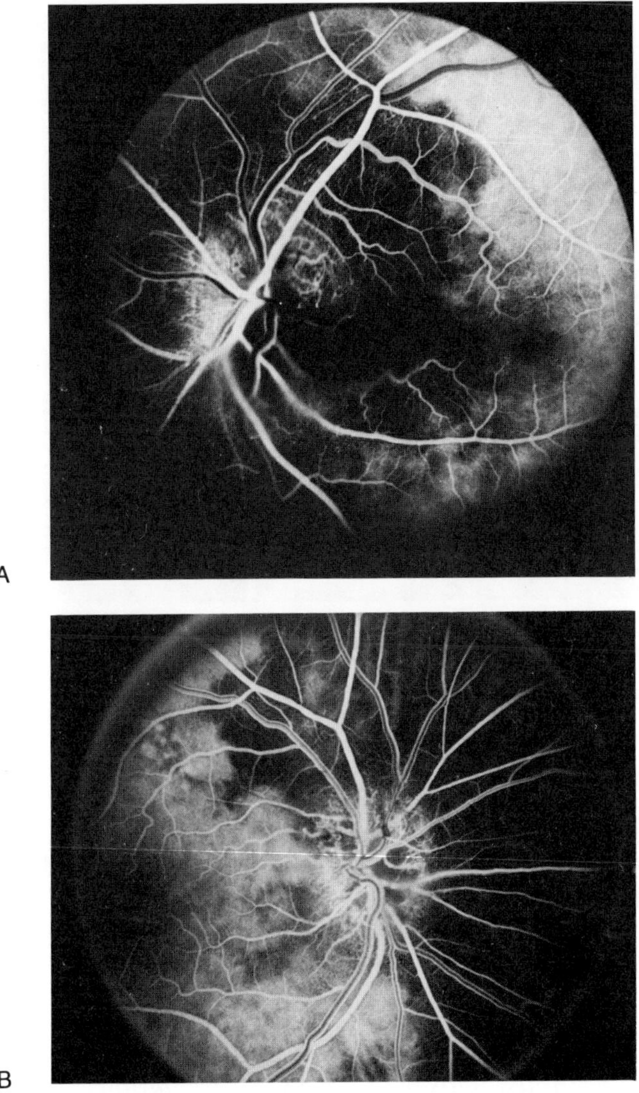

FIGURE 1–10. Fluorescein fundus angiograms of two human eyes (A, left eye; B, right eye) show variations in the areas of the choroid supplied by the medial and lateral PCAs. Reproduced from Hayreh SS, 1983 (28).

medial PCAs (Figs. 1–11, 1–12) is of great clinical significance since it determines the extent of involvement of the optic nerve head in acute ischemia through occlusion of one of the two main PCAs (29,30). The short PCAs supply segments of the choroid extending radially from the posterior pole to the equator. Each segment varies greatly in shape, size, and location and has irregular borders (Fig. 1–9) (27,31). Smaller subdi-

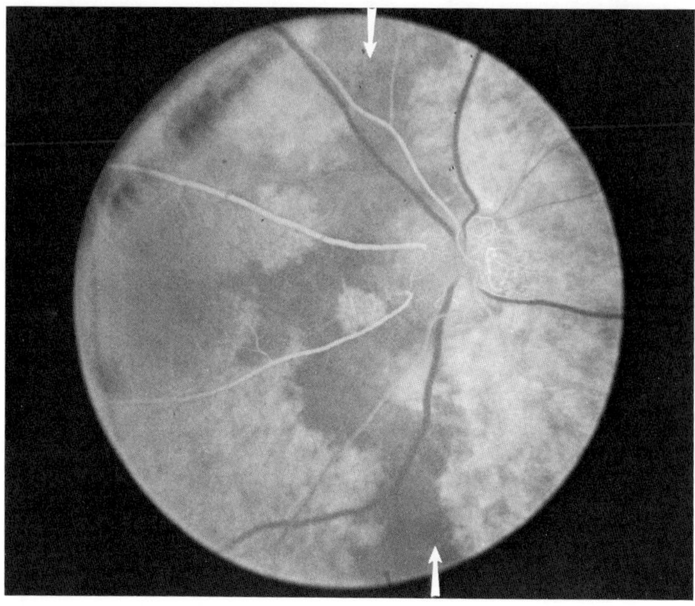

FIGURE 1–11. Fluorescein fundus angiogram of a right human eye shows the location of the watershed zone (arrows) between medial and lateral PCAs. Reproduced from Hayreh SS, 1975 (27).

visions of the short PCAs supply smaller segments of irregular shape and size, having a geographic pattern. Ultimately, each terminal choroidal arteriole supplies a lobule of choriocapillaris. Each lobule of the choriocapillaris is an independent segment, with its own feeding arteriole and draining venule (27,32). The long PCAs supply a sector of the choroid extending radially and temporally from the temporal border of the macular region (Fig. 1–9) (18).

Anastomoses in the PCA Circulation

In vivo experimental and clinical studies (27) on acute occlusion of the PCAs or their smaller divisions have shown that there are no anastomoses among the various branches. These studies indicated that the PCAs and their branches, right down to the terminal choroidal arterioles and choriocapillaris, have a segmental distribution and that PCAs and choroidal arteries are end arteries. The reason for the significant disparity between the postmortem anatomy (based on study of injection casts) and physiologic anatomy (based on in vivo fluorescein angiographic studies) is that the former gives information about the morphologic channels only, whereas the latter show the pattern of actual blood flow in those channels. The physiologic anatomy is the one of real clinical significance.

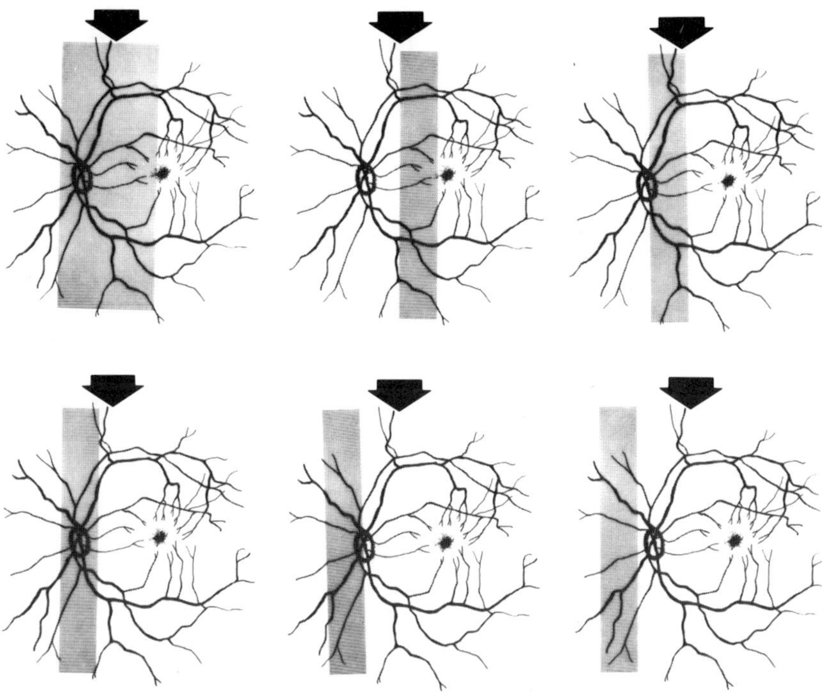

FIGURE 1–12. Diagrammatic representation of the locations of the watershed zone (arrows and shaded areas) between the medial and lateral PCAs in human eyes. In the **upper left illustration,** the shaded area represents the location where the watershed zone may be situated anywhere within this area. The **remaining five illustrations** are examples of the variations in the location.

Watershed or Boundary Zones in the PCA Circulation

Because the arteries in the PCA circulation do not form anastomoses with one another in vivo, the border between the areas of supply of any two adjacent vessels, from the main PCAs to the terminal choroidal arterioles, forms a watershed zone. The watershed zones between the various parts of the PCA circulation are arranged as follows. The arrangement of watershed zones between lateral and medial PCAs (main PCAs) is as described previously (Figs. 1–11, 1–12). The watershed zones between the temporal short PCAs are arranged somewhat radially, radiating from the macular region, so that these watershed zones meet in the macular region (Fig. 1–9) (31). The watershed zone between the PCAs and ACAs is situated in the equatorial region (Fig. 1–13).

The watershed zone is the border between the territories of distribution of two end arteries. Consequently, if the perfusion pressure in the vascular bed supplied by the end arteries falls, the watershed zone, which is an area of comparatively poor vascularity, is most vulnerable to ischemic

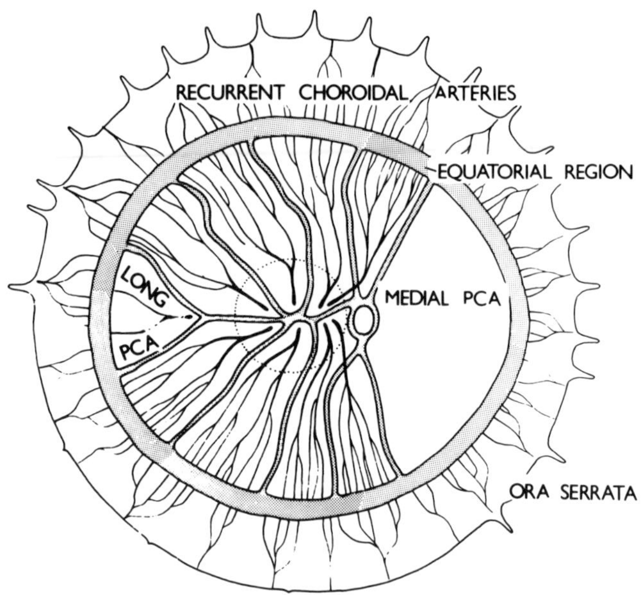

FIGURE 1–13. Diagrammatic representation of the distribution by the various ciliary arteries in the choroid and their watershed zones. The choroid posterior to the equator is supplied by the medial and lateral PCAs. In the area supplied by the lateral PCA are shown the segments supplied by the various short PCAs and the one by the long PCA, with the watershed zones between them (dotted circle in this area indicates the macular region). Recurrent choroidal arteries, from the ACA and supposedly the greater arterial circle of the iris, supply in front of the equator. The watershed zone between the anterior and posterior choroidal arteries lies in the equatorial region. Reproduced from Hayreh SS: *Ophthalmologica* 1981;183:11–19.

disorders. This knowledge is essential to understanding the ischemic disorders of the optic nerve head because PCA circulation is the main source of blood supply to that structure.

Anterior Ciliary Arteries

The ACAs arise from the muscular arteries in the four recti, usually two in each of the recti, except the lateral rectus, which is thought to have only one (Fig. 1–13) (33). Each ACA divides into several branches that include episcleral (to form the episcleral limbal plexus), intrascleral (related to the canal of Schlemm), and large perforating branches (to join the major arterial circle of the iris formed by the two long PCAs) (Fig. 1–14) (34). The major circle, which lies in the ciliary body just behind the root of the iris, gives branches to the ciliary muscle, ciliary processes, iris, and an-

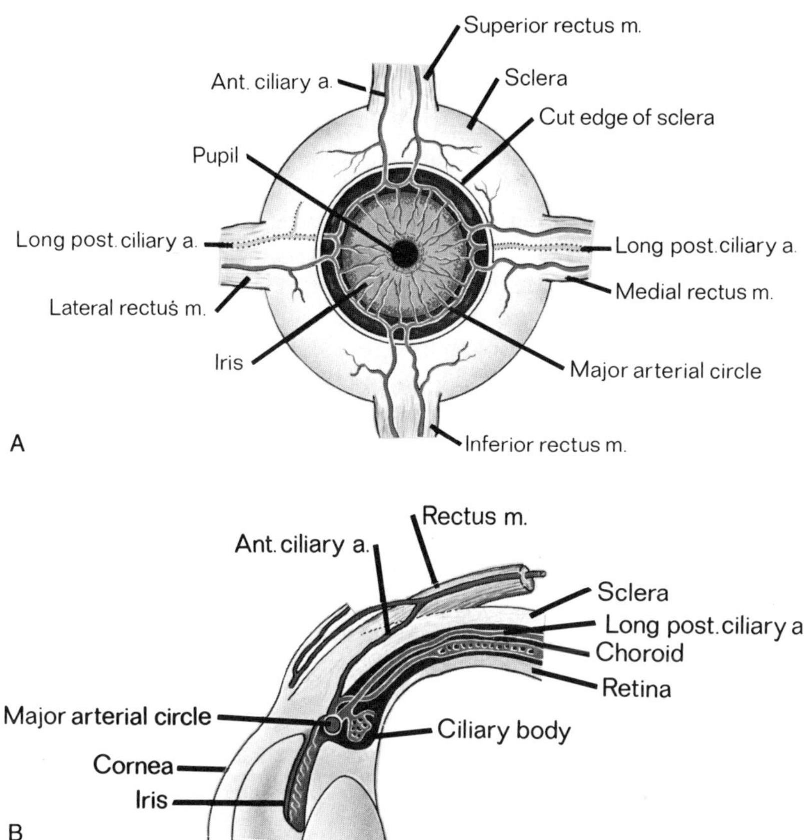

FIGURE 1–14. Schematic representation of the pattern of blood supply of iris and anterior segment, according to textbooks. **A,** As seen from the front. **B,** Schematic longitudinal section of the anterior segment. From Hayreh SS, Scott WE: *Archives of Ophthalmology,* 1978;96:1390–1400. Copyright 1978, American Medical Association. Reprinted with permission. (35)

terior part of the choroid. It has been argued that the so-called major arterial circle of the iris should be able to compensate for the loss of one or more of the ACAs. However, our fluorescein angiographic studies in patients (35) and experimental animals (36) performed after cutting the various vertical recti clearly showed that this is not so. These studies showed that, our knowledge of the anatomy of the greater arterial circle of the iris in man is essentially based on anatomic descriptions dating back more than 125 years (37), with no important new information added since then. In vivo, no appreciable collateral supply is established by the greater arterial circle of the iris. Recent morphologic studies (38), based on examination of morbid casts in monkeys, revealed that the major circle is mostly discontinuous, and its individual centrifugal branches consistently end as arterioles in the iris and ciliary processes. Therefore, this circle is probably less important to collateral flow than previously thought. Moreover, to judge from the recent in vivo fluorescein angiographic studies of the choroid (27,28), the postmortem morphologic vascular pattern does not always correspond with the in vivo circulatory pattern.

Because ACAs are in fact branches of the muscular arteries in the various recti, they arise from the ophthalmic artery as muscular arteries. My studies in humans (2) showed that the muscular arteries to the various recti arose from the ophthalmic artery either as independent branches or, much more frequently, in combination with other orbital arteries (Table 1–6). Each rectus muscle invariably received three branches, either as independent branches from the ophthalmic artery or from other orbital arteries, and the medial rectus in a quarter of the specimens had an additional branch. *The medial muscular artery,* a constant and prominent trunk, usually arose as an independent branch from the ophthalmic artery near the junction of its second and third parts. It soon divided into its various branches, which nearly always supplied the medial and inferior recti and sometimes one of the other recti, usually the lateral rectus. In about 16% of specimens, a *lateral muscular artery,* usually arising from the second part and infrequently from the third part of the ophthalmic artery, supplied lateral and superior recti.

TABLE 1–6. Mode of origin of branches to the various recti from the ophthalmic artery.

	Lateral rectus (%)	Superior rectus (%)	Medial rectus (%)	Inferior rectus (%)
Independent branch	2	29	81	0
With other orbital arteries:				
Lacrimal artery	78	54	3	8
Recurrent meningeal artery	5	2	0	0
Medial muscular artery	45	2	100	98
Lateral muscular artery	14	12	0	5
Supraorbital artery	0	15	0	0
Posterior ethmoid artery	0	7	5	0
Lateral PCA	0	3	0	2
Medial PCA	0	2	0	0
Superior PCA	0	2	0	0
Central retinal artery	0	0	2	0
With other muscular arteries:				
Superior rectus	5	0	2	0
Lateral rectus	0	5	0	0
Medial rectus	0	2	0	0
Total No. of Specimens Examined	58	59	58	59

PCA = posterior ciliary artery.

Collateral Arterial Branches to the Optic Nerve

The collateral arterial branches to the optic nerve arise either directly from the ophthalmic artery (during its intracanalicular and intraorbital parts) or from its various orbital branches (2). One to three minute branches from the intracanalicular part of the ophthalmic artery supply the optic nerve in that region. In the orbit, one to three collateral branches to the optic nerve arise either from the first, second, and/or proximal part of the third part of the ophthalmic artery in about two thirds of the cases, or from other orbital arteries (eg, from medial muscular, medial PCA, and CRA in about 20% to 25% of specimens in each, respectively) and rarely from lacrimal, posterior ethmoid, supraorbital, and muscular arteries to medial rectus, superior rectus, or superior oblique. The collateral branches pierce the dural sheath of the optic nerve to ramify on the pia before supplying the optic nerve.

Acknowledgments. I am grateful to my wife, Shelagh, for her help in the preparation of this manuscript, to Mrs. Ellen Ballas and Mrs. Georgiane Parkes-Perret for their secretarial help, and to the ophthalmic photography department for the illustrations. This paper was supported by an unrestricted grant from the Research to Prevent Blindness, Inc.

Key to abbreviations used in Figures 1–1 to 1–8.

A	Upper margin of the cranial opening of the optic canal.
AE	Anterior ethmoid artery
Ant. Clin. Proc.	Anterior clinoid process
CAR	Central artery of retina
D	Free margin of the crescentic falciform fold of dura.
DIAP. SEL.	Diaphragma sellae
DN	Dorsal nasal artery
DS	Dural sheath of the optic nerve
Dup. OC	Duplicate optic canal
ICA	Internal carotid artery
Lac. A	Lacrimal artery
LPCA	Lateral posterior ciliary artery
LPS	Muscular artery to levator palpebrae superioris
LR	Muscular artery to lateral rectus
MM	Medial muscular artery
MMA	Middle meningeal artery
MP	Medial palpebral artery
MPCA	Medial posterior ciliary artery
MR	Muscular artery to medial rectus
MSO	Muscular artery to superior oblique

Key to abbreviations *(continued)*

OA	Ophthalmic artery
OC	Optic canal
ON	Optic nerve
Orb. Per.	Orbital periosteum
P	Lower margin of the cranial opening of the optic canal.
PCA	Posterior ciliary artery
PE	Posterior ethmoid artery
PPS	Point of penetration of dural sheath
SEL. TUR.	Sella turcica
SO	Supraorbital artery
SOF	Superior orbital fissure
SR	Muscular artery to superior rectus
ST	Supratrochlear artery

References

1. Hayreh SS: *A Study of the Central Artery of the Retina in Human Beings in its Intra-orbital and Intra-neural Course,* thesis, Master of Surgery. Panjab University, India, 1958.
2. Hayreh SS: The ophthalmic artery: III. Branches. *Br J Ophthalmol* 1962;46:212–247.
3. Hayreh SS: Arteries of the orbit in the human being. *Br J Surg* 1963;50:938–953.
4. Hayreh SS: The ophthalmic artery, in Newton TH, Potts DG (eds): *Radiology of the Skull and Brain.* Angiography, vol. 2, book 2. St Louis, The CV Mosby Co, 1974 Chap 61, pp 1333–1350.
5. Hayreh SS, Dass R: The ophthalmic artery: I. Origin and intra-cranial and intra-canalicular course. *Br J Ophthalmol* 1962;46:65–98.
6. Hayreh SS, Dass R: The ophthalmic artery: II. Intra-orbital course. *Br J Ophthalmol* 1962;46:165–185.
7. Singh S, Dass R: The central artery of the retina: I. Origin and Course. *Br J Ophthalmol* 1960;44:193–212.
8. Singh S, Dass R: The central artery of the retina: II. Distribution and anastomoses. *Br J Ophthalmol* 1960;44:280–299.
9. Chanmugam PK: Note on an unusual ophthalmic artery associated with other abnormalities. *J Anat* 1936;70:580–582.
10. Flemming EE: Absence of the left internal carotid. *J Anat Physiol* 1895;29:13–14.
11. Lowery LG: Anomaly in the circle of Willis, due to absence of the right internal carotid artery. *Anat Rec* 1916;10:221–222.
12. Fisher AGT: A case of complete absence of both internal carotid arteries, with a preliminary note on the developmental history of the stapedial artery. *J Anat Physiol* 1914;48:37–46.
13. Quain J: *The Anatomy of the Arteries of the Human Body.* London, Taylor & Walton, 1844.
14. Hayreh SS, Edwards J: Ophthalmic arterial and venous pressures: Effects of acute intracranial hypertension. *Br J Ophthalmol* 1971;55:649–663.

15. Hayreh SS: Blood supply of the optic nerve head and its role in optic atrophy, glaucoma, and oedema of the optic disc. *Br J Ophthalmol* 1969;53:721–748.
16. Hayreh SS: *Anterior Ischemic Optic Neuropathy*. New York, Springer-Verlag, 1975.
17. Hayreh SS: Structure and blood supply of the optic nerve, in Heilmann K, Richardson K, (eds): *Glaucoma*. Stuttgart, Thieme, 1978, pp 78–96.
18. Hayreh SS: The long posterior ciliary arteries: An experimental study. *Albrecht Von Gracfe's Arch Clin Exp Ophthalmol* 1974;192:197–213.
19. Weiter JJ, Ernest JT: Anatomy of the choroidal vasculature. *Am J Ophthalmol* 1974;78:583–590.
20. Ashton N: Observations on the choroidal circulation. *Br J Ophthalmol* 1952;36:465–481.
21. Ring HG, Fujino T: Observations on the anatomy and pathology of the choroidal vasculature. *Arch Ophthalmol* 1967;78:431–444.
22. Ruskell GL: Choroidal vascularization in the rabbit. *Am J Ophthalmol* 1961;52:807–815.
23. Shimizu K, Ujiie K: *Structure of Ocular Vessels*. Tokyo, Igaku-Shoin, 1978.
24. Vilstrup G: *Studies on the Choroid Circulation*. Munksgaard E (ed). Copenhagen, 1952.
25. Wybar KC: A study of the choroidal circulation of the eye in man. *J Anat* 1954;88:94–98.
26. Wybar KC: Vascular anatomy of the choroid in relation to selective localization of ocular disease. *Br J Ophthalmol* 1954;38:513–527.
27. Hayreh SS: Segmental nature of the choroidal vasculature. *Br J Ophthalmol* 1975;59:631–648.
28. Hayreh SS: Physiological anatomy of the choroidal vascular bed. *Int Ophthalmol* 1983;6:85–93.
29. Hayreh SS: Acute choroidal ischaemia. *Trans Ophthalmol Soc UK* 1980;100:400–407.
30. Hayreh SS: Anterior ischemic optic neuropathy. *Arch Neurol* 1981;38:675–678.
31. Hayreh SS: Submacular choroidal vascular pattern: Experimental fluorescein fundus angiographic studies. *Albrecht Von Graefe's Arch Clin Exp Ophthalmol* 1974;192:181–196.
32. Hayreh SS: The choriocapillaris. *Albrecht Von Graefe's Arch Clin Exp Ophthalmol* 1974;192:165–179.
33. Leber T: *Graefe-Saemisch Handbuch der Gesamten Augenheilkunde*, ed 2. Leipzig, Engelmann, 1903, vol 2, part 2, pp 43–50.
34. Ashton N, Smith R: Anatomical study of Schlemm's canal and aqueous veins by means of neoprene casts: III. Arterial relations of Schlemm's canal. *Br J Ophthalmol* 1953;37:577–586.
35. Hayreh SS, Scott WE: Fluorescein iris angiography: II. Disturbances in iris circulation following strabismus operation on the various recti. *Arch Ophthalmol* 1978;96:1390–1400.
36. Virdi PS, Hayreh SS: Anterior segment ischemia after recession of various recti—An experimental study. *Ophthalmology* 1987;94:1258–1271.
37. Mackenzie W: *A Practical Treatise on the Diseases of the Eye*, ed 4. London, Longman, Brown, Green, and Longmans, 1854, p xxiii.
38. Morrison JC, Van Buskirk EM: Anterior collateral circulation in the primate eye. *Ophthalmology* 1983;90:707–715.

CHAPTER 2

Clinical Presentation and Differential Diagnosis of Amaurosis Fugax

Jean-Claude Gautier

Simultaneous permanent loss of vision in one eye with contralateral hemiplegia is diagnostic of internal carotid artery (ICA) occlusive disease, but it is rare (1) and a feature of completed stroke. The concept of an ischemic disorder common to the cerebral and ophthalmic branches of the ICA was put in an entirely new perspective when Fisher (2) reported in 1952 that *transient* monocular blindness (TMB) could *precede* contralateral hemiplegia. This finding provided clinicians with a new major symptom and a new major syndrome, one that could lead to stroke prevention. Fisher stressed that in his cases ICA occlusion ipsilateral to TMB was a prominent finding but gave a long list of various other causes of TMB.

The clinical characteristics of TMBs were well described in the early papers (2–5), but they still deserve attention for many reasons: episodes of TMB are a common issue in clinical practice. The diagnosis of the cause and the differential diagnosis may be difficult. Atherosclerosis is the cause in approximately half the cases but should not be overdiagnosed as overdiagnosis could lead to unnecessary noninvasive or invasive studies and unnecessary surgery. In half the cases a wide range of pathology must be scanned. The prognosis involves sight, brain, and life and varies widely according to the cause. The mechanisms of retinal ischemia vary and are debated or obscure in a number of patients. Understanding of TMBs could shed light on the mechanisms of cerebral ischemia. Many cases remain idiopathic.

The term *amaurosis fugax* is said (6) to have been coined in 1922 by Moore (7). In ophthalmology its meaning was broader than it is now (8,9). In recent times it has come to mean TMB, and it is used in that similar sense in this chapter. The main causes and mechanisms of amaurosis fugax are listed in Table 2–1 (10,11).

Clinical Features

Table 2–2 lists the main studies (12–19) on which most clinical descriptions are based and the number of patients who underwent angiography. The main clinical features were mentioned in the first neurologic account (2):

TABLE 2–1. Causes and mechanisms of amaurosis fugax.

Occlusive retinal arterial disease
- Arterial disease (atherosclerosis)
- Cardiac disease
- Arteritides

Low retinal perfusion pressure
- Multiple occlusions of extracranial cerebral arteries
- Arteriovenous fistulas
- Intracranial hypertension
- Glaucoma

High resistance to retinal perfusion
- Migraine
- Malignant arterial hypertension
- Increased blood viscosity

Miscellaneous causes

No obvious cause

Modified from Ross Russell RW, 1973, 1985 (10, 11).

This type of blindness has many constant features, as well as many that seem to be highly variable. Characteristically, the blindness lasts from a few seconds to a few minutes. Blindness is usually complete in the affected eye, although at times the defect is limited to one sector. The frequency of attacks varies from several a day to a few each year. Symptoms last for years or may disappear completely after a few months. In some cases the course of the complaint is benign, whereas in others a few attacks may result in a severe visual deficit . . . The attacks of blindness seem not to occur at the same time as the other neurological symptoms . . . Usually the attacks of blindness cease with the onset of the stroke . . . The blindness most commonly comes on as through a blind was lowered or raised, and vision returns from the opposite direction . . . The attacks last from a minute or so up to seven minutes or more. The onset as well as the recovery may be sudden or gradual.

Subsequent studies (14–16, 18) have corroborated these features and added some details. In the common TMBs no prodromata occur. There

TABLE 2–2. Main studies with clinical descriptions of amaurosis fugax.

Study	No. of patients	No. with angiography
Cogan, 1961 (12)	25	2
Eadie et al, 1968 (13)	12	8
Marshall, Meadows, 1968 (14)	80	27
Morax et al, 1970 (15)	66	60
Pessin et al, 1977 (16)	43	43
Wilson, Ross Russell, 1977 (17)	80	67
Parkin et al, 1982 (18)	51	38
Nelleman-Sorensen, 1983 (19)	44	7

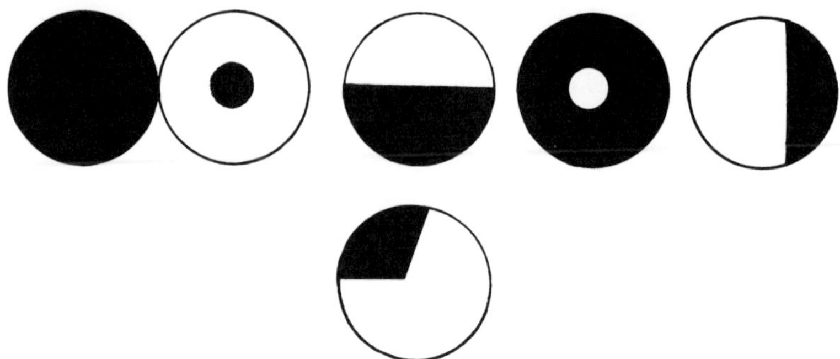

FIGURE 2–1. Types of visual defect. Courtesy Ross Russell RW, 1973 (10).

is no particular frequency at any time of the day. No noticeable postures or types of exertion can be incriminated. The onset is sudden, and the time from the beginning to the full extent of field defect is a matter of seconds. Patients usually state that they see black or gray, like a gray fog. Some frequent types of field involvement are shown in Fig. 2–1. Altitudinal ischemia is suggestive of retinal ischemia (20,21). A nasal defect is suggestive of embolic ischemia because emboli show a marked preference for the temporal circulation (22,23). A vertical defect usually suggests choroidal ischemia, rarely an anomalous branching of the retinal artery (24).

In many cases, from 15%–25% (25) to 65% (17), obscuration of the field develops as if a curtain or shade were coming from above downwards or from below upwards. Less often the shade progresses across the field in a vertical plane. Again, the first type suggests a disorder in the central retinal, the second, in the choroïdal circulation. Presence of a curtain is said to be no more predictive of carotid artery disease than other variants of monocular visual loss (25), and it has been reported in heart disease, migraine (26), and low-pressure retinopathy (11). It is tempting to see curtains as a model that could help in understanding some of the patterns of clinical deficit in transient hemispheric attacks (THAs). Most attacks of amaurosis fugax last less than 10 minutes, and many last less than five minutes. However, longer attacks up to 48 hours are known; some of them have allowed a detailed examination of the fundus (7,18,27,28). Recovery may be as quick or somewhat longer than the onset. Some patients mention having a bluish or white tinge of sight when vision returns. A slight blurring may last minutes or hours. In many patients vision returns in a manner inverse to the onset. In patients with multiple TMBs, the subsequent episodes frequently assume the same pattern of onset and recovery. The total number of attacks is quite variable. Most recorded patients have experienced one episode, and many such cases are likely to go unrecorded. Patients with five to 10 TMBs are frequent. Rare cases with up to 700 or 2,000 episodes are known (15,29). In patients with more than one attack of amaurosis fugax the episodes may occur many times a day for a few days or weeks or at intervals of months or years.

During the episode it is logical that the pupil should be dilated. Fisher (2) mentioned that "usually blindness is total at the height of the attack and the pupil no doubt dilates" but added that he had not seen that personally. An analysis of reports of fundoscopic examinations performed on patients who were having an attack indicated that dilatation of the pupil certainly has been observed (eg, Zentmayer, 1907; Ormond, 1918; Davenport, 1931) (2). In a few detailed cases the pupil reacted sluggisly (5), was completely unreactive to light (30), or was probably normal (31). In other cases the pupil was unremarkable perhaps because of an incomplete involvement of the visual field or an incomplete loss of vision or both. In many cases the characteristics of the pupil have not been recorded.

Some features are significant by their absence. Conversely, their presence should suggest the possibility of an uncommon cause or mechanism. Pain in the eye and head is distinctly rare. This and the brevity of most attacks of amaurosis fugax explain why many patients do not volunteer information about their trouble. Simultaneous THAs are possible (32), but strikingly rare. One case has been reported, but no details were given (18). Transient ipsilateral facial paresthesias may occur concomitantly with TMBs (33). They are poorly explained but obviously raise different kinds of problems. In an individual patient with both TMBs and THAs, either may come first.

Scintillations and diplopia typically are absent. The vast majority of incidents of amaurosis fugax happen in no special circumstances (ie, they happen at rest or during everyday normal activities). Particular circumstances, such as sitting, assuming an upright position, moving the head and neck (15), coming from dim to bright light (34,35) or to sunlight, having a hot bath, entering a hot room (36), or being in a postprandial period (37) have been recorded. Amaurosis fugax is usually unilateral, but bilateral episodes have been recorded (15,18).

In a few cases the fundus has been examined during TMB. The retina and arteries may be normal (12,13,38), suggesting that the occlusive material already has disappeared or that it or the circulatory disturbance is retrolaminal (ie, affects mainly the choroïdal circulation). In addition, retinal vessels may look normal while the CRA is occluded (25).

In other cases no embolic material has been seen, but the retinal arteries and veins were narrowed and the retina became pale (15,30,31). Segmentation of the blood column in arteries and veins (boxcar pattern, cattle-trucking) frequently occurs concomitantly. In such a sequence the carotid artery was normal (27).

The most frequent emboli are cholesterol emboli (4,22) broken off from an upstream, usually carotid, atherosclerotic lesion (20,22,39,40), or, very rarely, from the heart (22). Cholesterol crystals are white but appear yellow-orange, probably because the red blood column shows through because of the thinness of the crystals. They vary in size from 250 μm to less than 10 μm in diameter. They are flat small plaques less than 2 to 3 μm thick (23). According to their angle of impaction, the blood flow may not necessarily be blocked (23,28). They usually lodge in the temporal retinal arteries (22,23). When pressure is applied to the eye, cholesterol emboli may move, most often forward, or they may flip over, presenting their edges and thus becoming invisible to the examiner (23). In 70 patients with cholesterol, platelet-fibrin, and calcific emboli, only those with cholesterol emboli complained of amaurosis fugax (22). Cholesterol emboli usually disappear rapidly from the retina. Fluorescein angiography may show linkage at their points of impaction or may reveal the crystal (22,41). Cholesterol emboli provoke a sheathing reaction of the vessel wall (42), which is suggestive of the diagnosis when it is localized and isolated (22).

Platelet or platelet-fibrin emboli are long white-gray bodies that may progress through the retinal arterioles slowly, intermittently, or rapidly (3,5,22,29). Fragments may break off from their distal ends. Their usual source is an upstream atherosclerotic lesion. In a case that included a pathologic study (43), one microembolus consisted primarily of platelets, a few leukocytes, and a small quantity of lipids, but no fibrin or red blood cells. These emboli have been reported after myocardial infarction when they had broken off from a mural thrombus. Pathologically, the embolic material in the CRA was made of fibrin with emmeshed red and white blood cells (44).

Calcific emboli are usually chalky white, single bodies that block blood flow (11,20,22,45). Thus, they cause permanent loss of vision rather than amaurosis fugax. Calcified aortic or mitral valves are their usual sources. Other types of emboli have been recorded, including fat (46), myxoma (47), septic emboli from bacterial endocarditis, talc (in drug abusers), and silicone after injections of cosmetic material into the face or scalp (11).

Diagnosis

Is It a Monocular Blindness?

The answer is straightforward when the patient has alternately covered each eye. In many cases, however, this has not been done, and a number of patients have one eye or one poor eye. Very brief monocular blurrings also create difficulties in being certain that the event occurred on one side only.

These cases emphasize the usual diagnostic problem, which is to rule out an hemianopia, by no means always an easy task. The following clues help: Hemianopia as a brief, isolated transient ischemic attack (TIA) is rare. Hemianopia usually lasts longer than amaurosis fugax. In partial retinal ischemia the usual defect is characteristically a horizontal one, whereas in more central ischemia of the visual pathways it is characteristically a vertical one (21,48). Scintillations suggest primary involvement of the calcarine cortex. This is all the more true when visual phenomena are far lateral in the temporal field; a location in the center of vision suggests a retinal origin (49). Headache, particularly throbbing headache, suggests migraine. By gently displacing the eyeball rhythmically with the finger tip, the patient may observe that the visual display will move with the eyeball if it arises in the retina but not if it originates in the calcarine region (49). Previous ipsilateral THAs point to TMB. A curtain is highly suggestive of retinal ischemia.

What Is the Cause?

See Table 2–1 for a list of the causes of amaurosis fugax.

Occlusive Retinal Arterial Disease

Lesions of the ICA, particularly of the origin of the ICA, by far rank first as a cause of amaurosis fugax. Trauma, endarterectomy, kinks, dissecting extracranial ICA, and aneurysms are rare causes of TMBs (15). The overwhelming cause, at least in men over the age of 50, is atherosclerosis. Its prevalence has been estimated as 50% (14) or even 78% in a study of hemispheric TIAs due to disease of the ICA (15). It has also been estimated to occur in 40% of patients with symptomatic carotid disease (50). In a series of 95 cases of carotid TIAs, 33 (34%) had pure TMBs, and 43 (45%) had TMBs and (nonsimultaneous) THAs (16). This series also verified that amaurosis fugax is one of the commonest issues in clinical neurology.

The vast majority of ICA lesions that have been correlated to TMB were located on the proximal part of the artery. A bruit at the bifurcation of the common carotid artery was found in from 20% to 47.2% of the patients (14,15). The presence of a bruit in a man more than 50 years old is highly suggestive of an atherosclerotic lesion (15,17). However, the presence or absence of a bruit correlated poorly with the presence or absence of occlusion or tight or moderate ICA stenosis (15). Nevertheless, amaurosis fugax per se suggests stenosis more than occlusion and tight stenosis more than moderate to minimal stenosis (15–18) (Table 2–3). The results of a recent clinicopathologic study (51) supported this view (Table 2–4), which is consistent with the fact that TMBs cease after ICA occlusion (2,16,38). However, amaurosis fugax after ICA occlusion, presumably due to embolism via the external carotid artery or hemodynamic mechanisms, has been reported (36,52–57). The clinical features of episodes of TMB do not correlate with tight *v* moderate stenoses, but the presence of both TMB and THAs suggests tight stenosis (16).

Data about atherosclerosis of the carotid siphon and amaurosis fugax are scanty (58) although the embolic potential of the siphon has been estimated to be between one third and one half that of the carotid bifurcation (59). A few instances of TMB have been attributed to lesions of the siphon

TABLE 2–3. Stenosis and occlusion in amaurosis fugax.

Authors	No. of patients	Tight stenoses	Occlusions	Moderate to minimal stenoses	Normal angiogram
Morax et al, 1970 (15), TMB due to atherosclerosis	54	26	22	6	
Pessin et al, 1977 (16), Pure TMBs	33	14	5	6	8
Wilson, Ross Russell, 1977 (17)	67	18 "stenosis"	7	10 + 6 kinks	26
Parkin et al, 1982 (18)	38	21 "suitable for surgery"	4	12	1

(28,31,60,61). Parkin et al (18) reported that one patient had severe focal irregularity and another one had severe stenosis of the siphon. In addition, they mentioned that most of their patients with proximal artery disease also had disease of various severity in the distal ipsilateral carotid circulation. This problem belongs to the yet unsolved and potentially important aspect of tandem disease. In Gerstenfeld's oft quoted case (30), the ophthalmic artery had an anomalous origin, and the patient had a severe frontal headache. Both of these features suggest that this was not a common atherosclerotic kind of TMB.

According to Adams (62), "Atherosclerosis involves arteries of an order of size which varies from about 0.2 mm up to 3 or 4 mm or larger. It is quite exceptional to see an atheromatous change in vessels of smaller size, at least if one takes as the criterion the presence of an identifiable atherosclerotic plaque." The caliber of the ophthalmic artery at its origin

TABLE 2–4. Pathology of surgically removed plaque in 23 cases of transient monocular blindness.

Finding	No. of cases
Diameter of residual lumen (mm)	
1 or less	19 (90%)
1–2	0
2–3	1
3	1
Mural thrombus	22 (96%)
Ulceration	13 (57%)
Internal carotid artery	11
Common carotid artery	3
Intraplaque hemorrhage	15 (65%)
Cul-de-sacs	2

From Fisher CM, Ojemann RG, 1986 (51).

varies from 0.7 to 1:4 mm (63), and, theoretically at least, it could be involved by atherosclerosis. However, because the ophthalmic artery is not well visualized by means of the usual carotid angiographic techniques, it is commonly impossible to assess the artery with reasonable certainty. A case of a patient with two episodes of amaurosis fugax, no carotid lesion, and approximately 50% stenosis of the origin of the ophthalmic artery has been reported (64). In two cases reported by Parkin et al (18), the ophthalmic artery failed to fill at angiography, but this could have been due to the angiographic difficulties just mentioned or to an anomalous origin of the ophthalmic artery (the most commonly reported is from the middle meningeal artery, 3% of 170 specimens (63). Pickering (65) has reported the case of a 63-year-old man who had three transient attacks of loss of vision in the right eye followed by a fourth attack in which vision was permanently lost, all in the space of two days. Angiography showed slight narrowing at the origin of the ICA. Endarterectomy 3 months later did not show fresh thrombus. The patient died 18 months later of gastric hemorrhage. Pathologic examination showed a relatively healthy ophthalmic artery except for a short segment with severe stenosis, suggesting a recanalized embolus.

The CRA is about 280 μm in diameter at its origin. As it pierces the dura, it gives off a few branches and is reduced to about 180 μm in diameter (2). The diameter of the retinal branches is about 90 μm (50), making atherosclerotic thrombotic occlusion in these vessels unlikely. Thus, occlusions of the CRA and its branches mean the clinician must search for an embolic source.

Turning again to the bifurcation of the common carotid artery, it has been mentioned already that atherosclerosis of the external carotid artery rarely might be a source of retinal embolism. Embolism from the stump of an occluded ICA also is possible (66). Atherosclerosis of the common carotid and innominate arteries and of the aortic arch also is a potential source of retinal emboli.

Transient monocular blindness due to atherosclerosis is a common clinical problem that raises three prognostic questions: (1) risk of blindness, (2) risk of stroke, and (3) risk of death. These questions are dealt with specifically in another part of this volume. The following section presents clinical data only that might help in the evaluation of these risks and in the selection of appropriate diagnostic investigations.

The clinical features of amaurosis fugax (ie, duration, number, frequency of attacks, presence of a shade) are not reliable predictors either of blindness or brain infarction, nor of the angiographic characteristics of the carotid lesion (14–16,18,25).

The risk of blindness has been estimated to be from 5.8% to 11.2% (14,15,18). It has been calculated at 6% by Poole and Ross Russell (67), but some of their cases were due to retinal vein occlusion, and as patients were followed up for an average of 8 years, the risk was probably not more than 1% per year (27). Ackerman (68) followed up patients for an average of 2.3 years after amaurosis fugax and found that only two had a permanent loss of vision. In 136 patients with amaurosis fugax without carotid lesions, no subsequent ocular event occurred. These data have led Ellenberger and Epstein (27) to conclude that prevention of blindness is not an adequate justification for carotid endarterectomy. The benefits of carotid artery surgery for patients with retinal stroke also have been challenged by Savino et al (69).

The risk of stroke has been estimated at 40% (38), 39.3% (15), 34% (TIAs and strokes) (18), and as low as 13% (67). In the last series (66), 16 high-risk cases who had endarterectomies and six cases who had retinal cholesterol emboli were excluded. Nevertheless, the prevalence of first stroke was four times greater than expected, and the authors thought their data might be an underestimate. In 86 patients with retinal artery occlusion or retinal cholesterol emboli, Savino et al (69) also found a stroke risk four to five times greater than expected. Patients with amaurosis fugax and an occluded or narrowed artery have a greater risk of subsequent stroke than those whose carotid angiogram are normal (67). In amaurosis fugax patients silent cerebral embolism has been reported on the basis of electroencephalographic (ECG), angiographic, and regional cerebral blood flow evidence (70).

Two distinct risks of stroke exist after an episode of TMB: the risk of ipsilateral stroke, which to a large extent results from the cause of the TMB; and the risk of strokes in all localizations, which results from the usual atherosclerotic involvement of the whole cerebral arterial tree. In a number of studies this distinction was not specified.

What can help in a particular case? It has been stated that in most instances clinically obvious stroke is preceded by one or more THAs and that TMB tends to precede the first THA if a careful history can be documented (25). Such obviously important clinical clues deserve further study. Whatever the quantitative risk of ipsilateral stroke, many of such strokes occur at short notice. Table 2–5 lists the intervals between TMB

TABLE 2–5. Interval between amaurosis fugax and stroke.

Interval	No. of patients	
24 hr	6	41% (24 hr and 1–7 days)
1–7 days	8	
1–12 weeks	3	
12–52 weeks	3	
1 year	2	
Undetermined	2	

Note—Some data are from Morax et al, 1970 (15).

and stroke in 34 cases. For clinicians, problems about the diagnosis and treatment of TMB should be clarified without delay.

The risk of death after TMB due to atherosclerosis is higher than the risk of blindness and the risk of stroke. Survival is decreased significantly (14,71), although only in men in one study (67). The chief cause of death is ischemic cardiac disease. Thus, the impact of TMB on survival is similar to that of THAs, and a similar management (72) is required.

Because angiography, at least conventional angiography, carries a real risk of mortality and morbidity even in large centers (73), and because carotid surgery also carries a rather high risk of morbidity and mortality, identification of patients at special risk is worthwhile. The following may be useful: Hemodynamically significant stenoses carry a higher risk of mortality and morbidity (68). Patients with retinal stroke have had a diminished survival rate from the third year onwards. Patients with visible retinal emboli have had a diminished survival rate. Patients with retinal arterial occlusions without visible emboli have had a survival rate comparable to a matched control population (69).

On the whole, it appears that TMB carries a risk of death similar to that associated with THAs but probably a lower risk of stroke (67,74,75). In therapeutic trials the two conditions should not be equated (76).

Cardiac Disease

Emboli from the heart can block the retinal arterial supply (77). An occlusion of a branch of the CRA is more suggestive of cardiac embolism than CRA occlusion (78). Cardiac sources include ischemic heart disease, atrial fibrillation, congestive heart failure, aortic stenosis with or without incompetence (11,20), chronic rheumatic heart disease (79), verrucous endocarditis (80), subacute bacterial endocarditis, marantic endocarditis, and myxoma (47). In most cases permanent loss of vision has resulted, and transient blindness is apparently rare in cardiac disease (81). However, it has been mentioned in verrucous endocarditis (80) and was a prominent feature in chronic rheumatic heart disease in which two cases with a curtain (one horizontal, one transverse) were noted (79). In mitral valve prolapse, amaurosis fugax has been reported in 4 (one with a curtain) of 10 cases (82) and in 1 of 18 cases (83). In the study of Lesser et al (84), 13 (22%) of 57 patients with mitral valve prolapse had eye symptoms. Among those 13, 12 had binocular grayouts or blackouts. One only had monocular visual loss lasting 5 to 30 seconds, and another one had both binocular and monocular grayouts lasting 10 to 20 seconds. This suggests that amaurosis fugax may be rare in mitral valve prolapse and that factors other than embolism may play a role.

An important clinical point has been made by Bogousslavsky et al (85). By detailed cardiac examination (electrocardiography [ECG], 2-dimensional echocardiography, and Holter monitoring), every fourth or fifth patient with TMB was shown to have a potential cardiac source of emboli. Most of these patients also have an appropriate potential carotid source. Therefore, finding a carotid lesion does not clinch the diagnosis, and cardiac investigations are warranted.

Low-Pressure Retinopathy

In his 1952 paper, Fisher (2) mentioned that in cases of bilateral ICA occlusion, exertion is prone to bring on transient amaurosis. Subsequently, Kearns and Hollenhorst (57) recognized "venous stasis retinopathy" in about 5% of patients with carotid disease, and they thought that it was usually associated with amaurosis fugax. The condition is known now to result from low retinal perfusion pressure due to multiple occlusions of the extracranial cerebral arteries whichever their cause: atherosclerosis, Takayasu's disease, giant-cell arteritis (86). Ross Russell and Page (36) have reported four cases and reviewed the clinical features and pathogenetic mechanisms. Amaurosis fugax in this setting may have particular characteristics: it may be provoked by exertion, changes in posture, bright light, or heat. In one case the patient experienced simultaneous visual and speech difficulties, a rare and perhaps significant feature, and in another case gray mist passed across the patient's left eye from the temporal to the nasal field and was quite suggestive of a curtain (36). Moderate to severe pain may be present in the affected eye (57). Characteristic changes of the fundus oculi must be distinguished from those of diabetic retinopathy, retinal vein occlusion, and caroticocavernous fistulas (36). Secondary glaucoma may develop because of anterior segment ischemia (57). In one case, low-pressure retinopathy developed in one eye in which abnormal IOP had been recorded previously (33). In addition, in this case an episode of TMB lasted 1 week.

Arteriovenous Fistulas

Diversion of arterial blood and elevated venous and intraocular pressure may result in low retinal perfusion (36). Episodes of TMB were the presenting symptom in a patient with a dural arteriovenous fistula fed partly by a branch of the ipsilateral ophthalmic artery (87).

Intracranial Hypertension

Amaurosis fugax has been reported in patients who have tumors, most often with papilledema. It is then likely to be related to posture and may be accompanied by headache and pain in the eye (12). In one case with pseudotumor cerebri and papilledema, a painless monocular loss was due to a subretinal neovascular membrane (88).

Glaucoma

Elevated intraocular pressure reduces the perfusion pressure of the eye and may reduce blood flow to the choroid, retina, and disk (89). In addition, more spontaneous central vein occlusions are observed when the IOP is elevated (33). Amaurosis fugax tends to occur in poor light when the pupil is dilated (76). Transient monocular blindness may happen in transient ocular hypertension and glaucomatous iritis (19). Postprandial, painful amaurosis fugax may occur with narrow-angle glaucoma (37). A case with increased visual disorders after pupillary dilatation has been recorded (90). Therefore, the ocular pressure should be checked in patients who present with TMB.

Migraine

Monocular transient or permanent loss of vision is well recognized in migraine in adults (4) and children (91) and is a source of diagnostic difficulty. The subject has been reviewed recently (92). It has been stated that the characteristics of TMB in migraine and in atherosclerotic and cardiac disease preclude a definitive distinction (93). Presence of scintillations, headache, and a previous personal or family history of migraine are considered elements for the diagnosis, but all may be absent or uncertain. The pathogenesis of retinal migraine is poorly understood; both venous and arterial abnormalities have been reported (94). An underlying pathology may be present; 15 of 33 patients with migrainous amaurosis fugax had immediate or remote evidence of vascular disease, and 45% of the 33 had complications of that disease as compared to only 13% of the patients with homonymous attacks (4).

Fisher proposed late-life migrainous accompaniments as a large diagnostic category for cases that may closely mimic TIAs. As far as TMBs are concerned, in 1979 Fisher (49) reported only one TMB (with paresthesias) among 120 patients. In 1986, in a report of further cases (95), "Cases of benign transient monocular blindness occurring in the absence of detectable cerebrovascular disease, although widely accepted as 'migrainous' were not included in the present series."

Other Causes of High Resistance to Retinal Perfusion

Malignant hypertension, increased blood viscosity (polycythemia rubra vera, thrombocytemia, sickle cell disease, macroglobulinemia, coagulopathies), and, very rarely, Raynaud's phenomenon (when spasm is a possible mechanism) may be associated with TMB (2,76,96). Arteritis, particularly giant-cell arteritis, deserves special mention because in the arteritic form of ischemic optic neuropathy, TMB occurs premonitory to definitive loss of vision (96–100). In the idiopathic ("arteriosclerotic")

TABLE 2–6. Transient monocular blindness in patients less than 40 years of age.

				Cause						
Reference	No. of cases	Males	Females	Atherosclerosis	Migraine	Raynaud's Phenomenon	Pregnancy or menses	Other	Psychologic problems	Unknown
Fisher, 1952 (2)	57	25	32	5	15	1	1	5	0	30
Cogan, 1961 (12)	12	6	6	0	0	0	1	5	5	1
Poole et al, 1987 (100)	16	5	11	0	1	2	1	0	0	12
Total	85	36	49	5	16	3	3	10	0	43

form, TMB is usually absent. However, Boghen and Glaser (97) reported it in 2 of 37 cases.

Miscellaneous Causes

Fisher (2) has recorded and reviewed acute sharp pain, irrigation of the antrum, blowing the nose, epilepsy, jaundice, cold sensitivity, menstruation (one case during pregnancy (12), malaria, and retinal tuberculosis associated with TMB. Both Fisher (2) and Cogan (12) mentioned that some of these patients had been relieved by amyl nitrite.

No Obvious Cause

There is an additional group of patients (Table 2–6) in which women less than 40 years of age predominate (12,14,18,19,100) and in which young subjects, less than 21 years of age may be present (46). This group is probably quantitatively important; it accounted for 50% in a series of 44 unselected patients (19). A cause cannot be firmly identified. Some cases are perhaps of a migrainous nature. Some patients incriminate an "emotional stress," and Nelleman-Sorensen (19) suggested that one third of his young patients might come into this category. The diagnosis of "hysteria" sometimes is offered. Studies on visual symptoms of hysteria mention blindness, amblyopia, and field defects that can affect only one eye (101–103), but precise descriptions appear to be lacking. The diagnosis of hysteria should not be a loose one but should be based on positive symptoms and signs (103); the clinician always should be on the lookout for organic disease. Ophthalmologic anomalies, such as hyaline bodies of the optic nerve, refractive errors (myopia), and congenital dysplasias of optic disc also have been mentioned as possible causes of transient visual loss (96). Noninvasive studies are warranted, but, as the prognosis of TMBs in this group of patients is generally benign, invasive investigations should be considered only with great care.

References

1. Castaigne P, Lhermitte F, Gautier JC, et al: Corrélations cliniques et artériographiques dans 250 cas d'accidents ischémiques du cerveau d'origine athérosclèreuse. *Rev Neurol* 1962;106:497–501.
2. Fisher CM: Transient monocular blindness associated with hemiplegia. *Am Arch Ophthalmol* 1952;47:167–203.
3. Ashby M, Oakley N, Lorentz I, et al: Recurrent transient monocular blindness. *Br Med J* 1963;2:894–897.
4. Hedges TR, Lackman RD: Isolated ophthalmic migraine in the differential diagnosis of cerebro-ocular ischemia. *Stroke* 1976;7:379–381.
5. Ross Russell RW: Observations on the retinal blood vessels in monocular blindness. *Lancet* 1961;2:1422–1428.

6. Walt AJ: The carotid and the eye: Their historical connection, in Berguer R, Weiss H (eds): *The Carotid and the Eye*. New York, Praeger Scientific, 1985.
7. Moore RF: *Medical Ophthalmology* Philadelphia, P Blakiston Son and Co, 1922.
8. Duke-Elder WS: *Text Book of Ophthalmology*. London, Henry Kimgton, 1940, vol. 3.
9. Wagener HP: Amaurosis fugax. *Am J Med Sci* 1952;224:229–236.
10. Ross Russell RW: Histoire naturelle des cécités monoculaires transitoires, *in* Géraud J, Lazorthes G, Bès A (eds): *Ischémie cérébrale dans le territoire carotidien. Rev Med Toulouse,* 1973; suppl.
11. Ross Russell RW The clinical significance of retinal emboli, in Berguer T, Weiss H (eds): *The Carotid and the Eye*. New York, Praeger Scientific, 1985.
12. Cogan DG: Blackouts not obviously due to carotid occlusion. *Arch. Ophthalmol* 1961;66:180–187.
13. Eadie MJ, Sutherland JM, Tyrer JH: Recurrent monocular blindness of uncertain cause. *Lancet* 1968;1:319–321.
14. Marshall J, Meadows S: The natural history of amaurosis fugax. *Brain* 1968;91:419–434.
15. Morax PV, Aron-Rosa D, Gautier JC: Symptômes et signes ophtalmologiques des sténoses et occlusions carotidiennes. *Bull Soc Ophtalmol France* 1970; suppl.
16. Pessin MD, Duncan GW, Mohr JP, et al: Clinical and angiographic features of carotid transient ischemic attacks. *N Engl J Med* 1977;296:358–362.
17. Wilson LA, Ross Russell RW: Amaurosis fugax and carotid artery disease: Indications for angiography. *Br Med J* 1977;2:435–437.
18. Parkin PJ, Kendall BE, Marshall J, et al: Amaurosis fugax: Some aspects of management. *J Neurol Neurosurg Psychiatry* 1982;45:1–6.
19. Nelleman-Sorensen P: Amaurosis fugax: A. Unselected material. *Acta Ophthalmol* 1983;61:583–588.
20. Ross Russell RW: The source of retinal emboli. *Lancet* 1968;2:789–792.
21. Smith P: Reflex amblyopia and thrombosis of the retinal artery. *Ophthalmol Rev* 1884;2:1.
22. Arruga J, Sanders MD: Ophthalmologic findings in 70 patients with evidence of retinal embolism. *Ophthalmology* 1982;89:1336–1347.
23. Hollenhorst RW: Vascular status of patients who have cholesterol emboli in the retina. *Am J Ophthalmol* 1966;61:1159–1165.
24. Wolpow ER, Lupton RG: Transient vertical monocular hemianopia with anomalous retinal artery branching. *Stroke* 1981;12:691–692.
25. Mohr JP, Pessin MS: Extracranial carotid artery disease, in Barnett HJM, Stein BM, Mohr JP, et al (eds): *Stroke*. New York, Churchill Livingstone, 1986.
26. Ewing CC: Recurrent monocular blindness. *Lancet* 1968;1:1035–1036.
27. Ellenberger C Jr, Epstein AD: Ocular complications of atherosclerosis: What do they mean? *Semin Neurol* 1986;6:185–193.
28. Hooshmand H, Vines FS, Lee HM, et al: Amaurosis fugax: Diagnostic and therapeutic aspects. *Stroke* 1974;5:643–647.
29. Fisher CM: Observations of the fundus oculi in transient monocular blindness. *Neurology* 1959;9:333–347.

30. Gerstenfeld J: The fundus oculi in amaurosis fugax. *Am J Ophthalmol* 1964;58:198–205.
31. Dyll LM, Margolis M, David NJ: Amaurosis fugax: Fundoscopic and photographic observations during an attack. *Neurology* 1966;16:135–138.
32. Fisher CM (1976). *Tenth Princeton Conference on Cerebrovascular Diseases*, Scheinberg P (ed). New York, Raven Press pp 50–52.
33. Neupert JR, Brubaker RF, Kearns TP, et al: Rapid resolution of venous stasis retinopathy after carotid endarterectomy. *Am J Ophthalmol* 1976;81:600–602.
34. Brigham RA, Youkey JR, Clagett GP, et al: Bright-light amaurosis fugax: An unusual symptom of retinal hypoperfusion corrected by external carotid revascularization. *Surgery* 1985;97:363.
35. Furlan AJ, Whisnant JP, Kearns TP: Unilateral visual loss in bright light: An unusual symptom of carotid artery occlusive disease. *Arch Neurol* 1979;36:675–676.
36. Ross Russell RW, Page NGR: Critical perfusion of brain and retina. *Brain* 1983;106:419–434.
37. Eisenberg E, Bental E: Postprandial transient painful amaurosis fugax. *J Neurol* 1986;233:209–211.
38. Hollenhorst RW: The neuro-ophthalmology of strokes, in Lawton-Smith J (ed): *Neuro-ophthalmology*. St Louis, The CV Mosby Co, 1965.
39. Ehrenfeld WK, Hoyt WF, Wylie EJ: Embolization and transient blindness from carotid atheroma. *Arch Surg* 1966;93:787–794.
40. Ross Russell RW: Atheromatous retinal embolism. *Lancet* 1963;2:1354–1356.
41. Muci-Mendoza R, Arruga J, Edward WO, et al: Retinal fluorescein angiographic evidence for atheromatous microembolism. *Stroke* 1980;11:154–158.
42. Dark AJ, Rizk SN: Progressive focal stenosis of retinal arteries: A sequel to impaction of cholesterol emboli. *Br Med J* 1967;1:270–271.
43. McBrien DJ, Bradley RD, Ashton N: The nature of retinal emboli in stenosis of the internal carotid artery. *Lancet* 1963;1:697–699.
44. Zimmerman LE: Embolism of central retinal artery secondary to myocardial infarction with mural thrombus. *Arch Ophthalmol* 1965;73:822–826.
45. Brockmeier LB, Adolph RJ, Gustin BW, et al: Calcium emboli to the retinal artery in calcific aortic stenosis. *Am Heart J* 1981;101:32–37.
46. Cogan DG, Kuwabara T, Moser H: Fat emboli in the retina following angiography. *Arch Ophthalmol* 1964;71:308–313.
47. Jampol LM, Wong AS, Albert DM: Atrial myxoma and central retinal artery occlusion. *Am J Ophthalmol* 1973;75:242–249.
48. Uhtoff W: Periodische Verdunkelunger der Augen. *Klin Monatsbl Augenh* 1925;75:469.
49. Fisher CM: Late-Life transient cerebral ischemia of obscure nature: Migrainous accompaniments? in *Deuxièmes Conférences de la Salpêtrière*. Paris JB Baillère Publishers, 1979.
50. Fisher CM: Concerning recurrent transient cerebral ischemic attacks. *Can Med Assoc J* 1962;86:1091–1099.
51. Fisher CM, Ojemann RG: A clinico-pathologic study of carotid endarteriectomy plaques. *Rev Neurol* 1986;142:573–589.

52. Bogousslavsky J, Regli F, Hungerbühler JP, et al: Transient ischemic attacks and external carotid artery: A retrospective study of 23 patients with an occlusion of the internal carotid artery. *Stroke* 1981;12:627–630.
53. Bogousslavsky J, Regli F: Accidents ischémiques transitoires avant et après occlusion de l'artère carotide interne. *Rev Neurol* 1983;139:625–634.
54. Bogousslavsky J, Regli F: Delayed TIAs distal to bilateral occlusion of carotid arteries: Evidence for embolic and hemodynamic mechanisms. *Stroke* 1983;14:58–61.
55. Burnbaum MD, Delhorst JB, Harbison JW, et al: Amaurosis fugax from disease of the external carotid artery. *Arch Neurol* 1977;34:532–535.
56. Ehrenfeld WK, Lord RA: Transient monocular blindness through collateral pathways. *Surgery* 1969;63:911–915.
57. Kearns TP, Hollenhorst RW: Venous stasis retinopathy of occlusive disease of the carotid artery. *Mayo Clin Proc* 1963;38:304–312.
58. Gautier JC, Mohr JP: Intracranial internal carotid artery disease, in Barnett HJM, Stein BM, Mohr JP, et al (eds): *Stroke*. New York, Churchill-Livingstone 1986.
59. Saunders FW, Shedden P: The carotid siphon: A scanning electron microscope assessment of its embolic potential. *Can J Neurol Sci* 1985;12:263–266.
60. David NJ: Amaurosis fugax and after, in Glaser JS (ed): *Neuro-Ophthalmology*. St Louis, The CV Mosby Co, 1979, vol 9. Chapter 2, pp 22–24.
61. Wechsler LR, Kistler JP, Davis KR, et al: The prognosis of carotid siphon stenosis. *Stroke* 1986;17:714–718.
62. Adams RD: Pathology of cerebral vascular disease, in Wright IS, Millikan CH, eds: *Cerebral vascular disease. Second Princeton Conference*. New York, Grune and Stratton, 1958.
63. Hayreh SS: Arteries of the orbit in the human being. *Br J Surg* 1963;50:938–953.
64. Weinberger J, Bender AN, Yang WC: Amaurosis fugax associated with ophthalmic artery stenosis: Clinical simulation of carotid artery disease. *Stroke* 1980;11:290–292.
65. Pickering G: Arterial occlusion, especially of the coronary arteries and of the subclavian and carotid arteries. *Bull John Hopkins* 1963;113:105–157.
66. Barnett HJM, Peerless SJ, Kaufman JCE: "Stump" of the internal carotid artery: A source for further cerebral embolic ischemia. *Stroke* 1978;9:448–456.
67. Poole CJM, Ross Russell RW: Mortality and stroke after amaurosis fugax. *J Neurol Neurosurg Psychiatry* 1985;48:902–905.
68. Ackerman RH: Visual disturbances and carotid disease. Presented at the 10th International Joint Conference on Stroke and the Cerebral Circulations, New Orleans, February 1985.
69. Savino PJ, Glaser JS, Cassady J: Retinal stroke: Is the patient at risk? *Arch Ophthalmol* 1977;95:1185–1189.
70. Harrison MJG, Marshall J: Evidence of silent cerebral embolism in patients with amaurosis fugax. *J Neurol Neurosurg Psychiatry* 1977;40:651–654.
71. Pfaffenbach DD, Hollenhorst RW: Morbidity and survivorship of patients with embolic cholesterol crystals in the ocular fundus. *Am J Ophthalmol* 1973;75:66–72.

72. Adams HP Jr, Kassell NF, Mazuz H: The patient with transient ischemic attacks: Is this the time for a new therapeutic approach? *Stroke* 1984;15:371–375.
73. Toole JF, Yuson CP, Janeway R, et al: Transient ischemic attacks: A prospective study of 225 patients. *Neurology* 1978;28:746–753.
74. Harrison MJG: Foster Elting Bennet Memorial Lecture: United Kingdom Trials of Medical and Surgical Management of TIA. Presented at the annual meeting of the American Neurological Association, Chicago, October 3, 1985.
75. Hurwitz BJ, Heyman A, Wilkinson WE, et al: Comparison of amaurosis fugax and transient cerebral ischemia: A prospective clinical and arteriographic study. *Ann Neurol* 1985;18:698–704.
76. Ross Russell RW: Transient cerebral ischemia, in Ross Russell RW (ed): *Vascular Disease of the Central Nervous System*. Edinburgh, Churchill Livingstone, 1983.
77. Gowers WR: On a case of simultaneous embolism of central retinal and middle cerebral arteries. *Lancet* 1875;2:794–796.
78. Wilson LA, Warlow CP, Ross Russell RW: Cardiovascular disease in patients with retinal arterial occlusion. *Lancet* 1979;1:292–294.
79. Swash M, Earl CJ: Transient visual obscurations in chronic rheumatic heart disease. *Lancet* 1970;2:323–326.
80. D'Alton JG, Preston DN, Bormanis J, et al: Multiple transient ischemic attacks, lupus anticoagulant and verrucous endocarditis. *Stroke* 1985;16:512–514.
81. Slepyan DH, Rankin RM, Stahler C Jr, et al: Amaurosis fugax: A clinical comparison. *Stroke* 1975;6:493–496.
82. Wilson LA, Keeling PWN, Malcolm AD, et al: Visual complications of mitral leaflet prolapse. *Br Med J* 1977;2:86–88.
83. Barnett HJM, Boughner DR, Cooper PF, et al: Further evidence relating mitral valve prolapse to cerebral ischemic events. *N Engl J Med* 1980;312:139–144.
84. Lesser RL, Heineman MH, Borkowski H, et al: Mitral valve prolapse and amaurosis fugax. *J Clin Neuro-Ophthalmol* 1981;1:153–160.
85. Bogousslavsky J, Hachinski VC, Barnett HJM: Causes cardiaques et artérielles de cécité monoculaire transitoire. *Rev Neurol* 1985;141:774–779.
86. Hollenhorst RW: Effect of posture on retinal ischemia from temporal arteritis. *Trans Am Ophthalmol Soc* 1967;65:94–105.
87. Bogousslavsky J, Vinuela F, Barnett HJM, et al: Amaurosis fugax as the presenting manifestation of dural arteriovenous malformation. *Stroke* 1985;16:891–893.
88. Todd Troost B, Safit RL, Grand G: Sudden monocular visual loss in pseudotumor cerebri. *Arch Neurol* 1979;36:440–442.
89. Best M, Blumenthal M, Futterman HA, et al: Critical closure of intraocular blood vessels. *Arch Ophthalmol* 1969;82:385.
90. Fisher CM: Some neuro-ophthalmological observations. *J Neurol Neurosurg Psychiatry* 1967;30:383–392.
91. Hachinski VC, Porchawka J, Steele JC: Visual symptoms in the migraine syndrome. *Neurology* 1973;23:570–579.

92. Tatemichi TK, Mohr JP: Migraine and stroke, in Barnett HJM, Stein BM, Mohr JP, et al (eds): *Stroke*. New York, Churchill Livingstone, 1986.
93. Goodwin JA, Gorelick P, Helgason C: Transient monocular visual loss: Amaurosis fugax versus migraine, abstracted. *Neurology* 1984;34(suppl 1):246.
94. Coppeto JR, Lessell S, Sciarra R, et al: Vascular retinopathy in migraine. *Neurology* 1986;36:267–270.
95. Fisher CM (1986). Late-life migraine accompaniments: Further experience. 1986;17:1033–1042.
96. Glaser JS: *Neuro-Ophthalmology*. Hagerstown, Md, Harper & Row Publishers Inc, 1978.
97. Boghen DR, Glaser JS: Ischaemic optic neuropathy: The clinical profile and natural history. *Brain* 1975;98:689–708.
98. Eagling EM, Sauders MD, Miller SJM: Ischaemic papillopathy: Clinical and fluorescein angiographic review of forty cases. *Br J Ophthalmol* 1974;58:990–1008.
99. Wagener HP, Hollenhorst RW: The ocular lesions of temporal arteritis. *Am J Ophthalmol* 1958;45:617–630.
100. Poole CJM, Ross Russell RW, Harrison P, et al: Amaurosis fugax under the age of 40 years. *J Neurol Neurosurg Psychiatry* 1987;50:81–84.
101. Spaeth EB: The differentiations of the ocular manifestations of hysteria and of ocular malingering. *Arch Ophthalmol* 1930;4:911–938.
102. Svynos AN: Des amblyopies et des amauroses transitoires. Thèse Med. Paris. 1873
103. Turner RG: Hysterical blindness, in Rose FC (ed): *Medical Ophthalmology*. London, Chapman and Hall, 1976.

CHAPTER 3

Neurologic Mechanisms of Visual Loss

Louis R. Caplan

Fleeting loss of vision can result from any process that temporarily interrupts the normal functioning of the human visual system. The transient nature of the symptoms usually indicates that the cause has been temporary and corrected. Less often, the visual defect remains, but (1) the defect has become less severe and so less noticeable to the patient; (2) the visual functions have been assumed, at least partially, by other undamaged structures; or (3) other factors, such as spatial neglect or impaired cognitive function, limit the patient's recognition and description of the persistent visual deficit.

Almost always loss of vision is caused by a lesion of the afferent visual perceptual pathway that transmits light and visual stimulus information to the retina and, subsequently, through the optic nerve, optic chiasm, and optic tracts to the lateral geniculate body and then to the calcarine visual cortex. This system allows a person to "see" a visual stimulus in contrast to the occulomotor apparatus that subserves exploration of visual space, allowing a person to "look" for or at a stimulus (1). Patients with oculomotor abnormalities occasionally do report blurred or unclear vision. "Looking" abnormalities can be separated from "seeing" abnormalities by careful questioning and examination.

Oculomotor (Looking) Abnormalities

Vestibular Dysfunction

Dysfunction of the vestibular system alters patients' normal perceptions of where they are in space. The vestibular nuclei are intimately connected to the eye movement system (vestibulo-ocular reflex) to allow vision during movement (2). Peripheral and central vestibular lesions cause nystagmus, often with the perception that things are moving, turning, spinning, or teetering. Oscillopsia, the sensation of objects moving, jiggling, or oscillating, may be described as blurred vision. Brightness is not altered, and the patient, when questioned, will describe oscillation of objects similar to that seen on a malfunctioning television set in which the picture is moving slightly but quickly and rhythmically up and down or sideways. Loss of the normal vestibulo-ocular reflex can cause momentary difficulty in fixation when the patient moves the head, as when fixating on an object to the side or when trying to read in a moving vehicle. Clues to a vestibular dysfunction include symptoms of motion or rotation, accompanying nausea, nystagmus, and occurrence after or during head or body motion.

Dysconjugate Gaze

When the two normally seeing eyes do not work conjugately in a field of gaze, the visual stimulus does not fall simultaneously on the macula of each eye. This asymmetry in perception usually is recognized as diplopia by most intelligent observers, especially if the objects obviously are separated by a distance. When the objects merely overlap, the patient may describe "blurred vision," not recognizing the disorder as double vision. Some patients recognize that the visual blurring occurs in only one field of gaze and identify the abnormal eye; thus, a patient with a palsy of the sixth left cranial nerve may tell the physician that the left eye was "temporarily blurred." Diplopia can be due to weakness of individual oculomotor nuclei or their nerves (III, IV, VI) or to weakness of the extraocular muscles themselves. Myasthenia gravis and transient brainstem ischemia produce temporary dysfunction of these structures. Ocular skew and intranuclear opthalmoplegia also cause diplopia and are due to lesions in the central brain stem. Patients should be questioned carefully as to whether they closed one eye at a time to see if that maneuver helped the visual dysfunction, and they should be examined carefully for abnormalities of eye movement.

Lid and Pupillary Abnormalities

Iridoplegia affects the amount of light input to the retina. Blurred vision is almost universal after instillation of eye drops that dilate the pupil and is caused by an inability to shade the retina from overexposure. Dilatation of the pupil can be caused by local or systemic administration of pupillary-dilating drugs, iris ischemia or inflammation, dysautonomia, or dysfunction of the third cranial nerve. Unilateral pupillary abnormalities can occur during migraine and are especially frequent during an attack of cluster headache or Raeder's syndrome (3). The physician should look for coexisting headache or pain in the forehead or around the eye, dilatation and abnormal pupillary reactivity, and eye muscle weakness that indicate dysfunction of the third cranial nerve.

Rarely, patients with ptosis do not realize that their visual dysfunction, monocular or binocular, is due to the fact that the eyelid obscures their vision. I vividly recall a patient who called her daughter because the patient suddenly could not see, and the room had "gone black." The patient first thought that the electric company had shut off the lights. By touch, she was able to call her daughter for help. When the daughter arrived, she told her mother, "Of course, you can't see, your eyes are shut." The patient had developed a midbrain infarction (4) with bilateral third nerve palsies and complete ptosis. Because she had not willed her eyes shut, she was unaware that bilateral lid closure had occurred.

Afferent (Seeing) Abnormalities

Abnormalities of the Anterior Visual Media and Retina

Lesions that affect the anterior media that block transmission of visual input to the retina seldom are transient. Hyperglycemia, usually caused by uncontrolled diabetes, alters the viscosity of the visual media and leads to blurred vision, usually in both eyes. Abnormalities of the cornea (eg, keratitis, ulcers), anterior chamber (eg, inflammation, glaucoma), iris (eg, iritis), lens (eg, cataract), and vitreous humor (eg, tumors, bleeding, neovascularization, inflammation) nearly always cause lasting symptoms. Moreover, if the patient cannot see out, the physician should have difficulty seeing "in" through the opthalmoscope. Occasionally, a "floater" precipitate in the aqueous or vitreous humor can block vision temporarily, but the blockage is corrected by head or eye movement.

Transient retinal ischemia is due to abnormal delivery of oxygen and metabolites to the retina through the ICA, ophthalmic artery, CRA pathway. Clues to a retinal localization include dimming, darkening, or blackness of vision. Sometimes sparks of light or colors (eg, a red and gray grating) are described. A drop in systemic perfusion pressure (such as occurs in syncope or cardiac dysfunction) causes dim vision in both eyes, usually along with sweating, pallor, muffled hearing, and feelings of faintness. Hypoglycemia or hypovolemia (as might occur with gastrointestinal hemorrhage or brisk diuresis) also limit delivery of high-energy blood to the retina and cause blurred vision. In patients with postural hypotension due to hypovolemia or to dysfunction of the autonomic nervous system, visual blurring occurs only when the patient is standing or sitting upright and is alleviated when the patient lies down. Increase in intraocular pressure (as in glaucoma) also can reduce effective retinal perfusion pressure and promote ischemia.

Temporary unilateral ischemia (TMB) can be caused by low flow to the retina when there is obstruction of the common carotid artery, ICA, ophthalamic artery, or CRA. When the patient stands up, a decrease in blood pressure (especially after treatment with new hypertensive medicines), or hypovolemia, can accentuate the visual symptoms. When the occlusive lesion causes low flow, TMB often is repeated, brief, and positional. Exposure to bright light also can cause transient monocular dimming, presumably by increasing retinal metabolism in the presence of fixed, limited retinal blood flow (5). Signs of chronic retinal ischemia (eg, venous stasis retinopathy) are often demonstrable by fundoscopy (6).

Probably more often TMB is due to an embolus transiently blocking the CRA or its branches. At times, cholesterol crystals, red clotlike material, or fibrin-platelet plugs (7) can be seen in the retinal arteries. Attacks probably are longer and less frequent in these cases than in patients with hemodynamic insufficiency, and examination may show an embolic source in the heart or carotid arteries. Polycythemia, thrombocytosis, and hyperviscosity states (eg, Waldenstrom's macroglobulemia) can cause temporary sludging of blood in the retinal arteries and symptomatic ischemia.

Functional constriction of retinal arteries ("spasm") is probably the underlying mechanism in retinal migraine (8,9). Attacks usually last 15 to 30 minutes but may persist for hours. The visual loss is monocular and usually is described as blindness or blackness, sometimes with sparks of light or colors. Formed images or shapes are not noticed. Some patients with migraine describe spotty darkening in the periphery of vision in one eye that is followed by gradual constriction of the field until only small clear spots remain in the center (10). Monocular blindness remains for one to two minutes and clears from the periphery toward the center. Transient constriction of the retinal artery, loss of the pupillary light reflex, and regions of retinal edema have been seen when the patient could be examined during an attack (10). A past history of migrainous headache, family history of migraine, concurrent headache or headache after the visual loss clears, and previous symptoms compatible with classic migraine are helpful in diagnosis. Patients with ophthalamic migraine are usually younger and more often female than patients with arteriosclerotic disease, and risk factors for atherosclerosis are present less often. Evaluation does not show an occlusive lesion or an embolic source.

Abnormalities of the Optic Nerve

The blood supply to the optic nerve is different from that of the retina. The most superficial part of the prelaminar optic nerve head is supplied by CRA branches, but the nerve just anterior to the lamina cribrosa and the laminar parts of the optic nerve are supplied by direct branches of the PCAs or their peripapillary choroidal artery branches (11,12). These are small penetrating arteries that are damaged by hypertension, diabetes, and "arteritis" more often than by classical atherosclerosis.

Ischemia of the optic nerve usually is called anterior ischemic optic neuropathy (AION). This syndrome occurs in elderly patients with hypertension and/or diabetes and also in patients with giant-cell arteritis. Usually, visual loss is sudden and permanent and affects one eye or both sequentially. The visual loss in patients with AION can range from only a slight reduction in visual acuity to complete loss of light perception. Typically, an altitudinal loss of vision occurs, most often in the inferior part of the field, but the defect also can include a sectorial scotoma (13). In patients with arteritis, systemic symptoms usually precede the visual loss. Headache, scalp tenderness, limb and joint pain, malaise, anorexia, and jaw claudication are common, and usually the patient just has not felt well for a while. Some patients describe having a shadow, spots, veil, or curtain in the visual field before the more permanent visual loss develops. Transient visual loss with recovery during minutes or hours also has been reported (12). Sometimes visual loss progresses during a week or more (13,14). Swelling of the optic nerve, local or diffuse nerve head pallor, and flame-shaped hemorrhages at or near the disc margins are present sometimes.

Lesions that increase ICP also can cause papilledema, especially in the young. The optic nerve is enclosed by a nonyielding dural envelope. Swelling of the optic nerve due to ICP, inflammation (optic neuritis) or infiltration by tumor (especially optic glioma or meningioma) compresses the nutrient arteries and veins within the optic nerve, causing secondary ischemia. Patients with papilledema (eg, pseudotumor cerebri) often report transient visual obscurations that may be binocular or monocular. Headache is present almost invariably. Maneuvers that increase ICP (eg, coughing or straining) or that decrease perfusion pressures (eg, bending or stooping) may provoke the attacks of transient visual obscuration, which are invariably very brief (less than 1 to 2 seconds) and repeated. The optic disc looks swollen when viewed through the ophthalmoscope, and spontaneous venous pulsations are not visible. Testing of the visual field may show concentric constriction of the periphery of the visual field and enlargement of the blind spot.

Abnormalities of the Optic Chasm

The afferent visual fibers in the optic chiasm and the entering fibers in the optic nerves and exiting fibers in the proximal optic tracts are supplied by small penetrating branches of the major arteries of the circle of Willis. A superior group of arteries branch from the internal carotid, anterior cerebral, and anterior communicating arteries, and inferiorly, branches arise from the basilar, posterior cerebral, and posterior communicating arteries. Ischemia to these visual fibers has not been reported after intracranial occlusive lesions, probably because of the multiplity of feeding vessels and the potential for collateral circulation. However, as in the optic nerve, the axons with their myelin sheaths and blood supply are enclosed in a relatively tight perineural envelope of connective tissue. Swelling, such as might occur in demyelinating disease, and extrinsic compression of the chiasm can compromise the nutrient blood supply and lead to temporary or permanent visual loss. The nature of the visual defect depends on the location of the compression. Compression of the optic nerve would cause a monocular visual loss, usually with reduced acuity, abnormal light reflex, and a central scotoma. Chiasmatic pressure causes a bitemporal field defect, often with associated monocular visual loss if the compression is from one side. More posteriorly placed lesions that affect the optic tract cause a congruous contralateral hemianopia. Pituitary adenomas, especially those that undergo rapid enlargement due to hemorrhage or ischemia (so-called pituitary apoplexy), frequently compress the chiasm or extend laterally to affect the optic nerve and the structures within the cavernous sinus. Large aneurysms of the intracranial ICA or the anterior cerebral anterior communicating artery complex also can compress the optic nerves or chiasm. Usually, the visual loss is not transient, and headache and extraocular muscle weakness also are present. Clinical signs of pituitary insufficiency and radiologic signs of enlargement of the sella turcica with suprasellar extension usually are present when sudden visual loss is caused by pituitary adenomas. Contrast-enhanced CT may show a large aneurysm near the chiasm. Inflammatory lesions near the chiasm and optic nerves (eg, luetic or tuberculosis meningitis, Wegner's granulomatosis, or arachnoiditis) can compromise the blood vessels supplying the chiasmatic region and cause visual loss, usually with coexistent headache, pleocytosis, and other cranial neuropathies.

Abnormalities of the Optic Tract, Lateral Geniculate Body, Geniculocalcarine Tract, and Striate Visual Cortex

The optic tracts are supplied mostly by branches of the anterior choroidal arteries (15), with some contribution by direct branches from the ICA. The lateral geniculate body is supplied primarily by the anterior choroidal arteries and lateral posterior choroidal branches of the posterior cerebral arteries. The geniculocalcarine tracts anteriorly near the atria of the lateral ventricles are supplied by branches from the inferior trunk of the middle cerebral arteries (16); the more posterior portions of the visual radiations and the striate cortex are supplied by the posterior cerebral arteries. Occlusive lesions or emboli within these arteries usually produce a hemianopia. When the ischemia is limited to the superior part of the visual radiation or the upper bank of the calcarine fissure (cuneus), the visual deficit is an inferior quadrantanopia, and when the lesion affects the inferior visual radiation fibers or the lower bank of the calcarine cortex (lingual gyri), the deficit is a superior quadrantanopia. Usually, patients with posteriorly placed lesions are aware of their visual defects and speak of a void, darkness, or limitation of vision to their right or left. Many patients, naive about the distinction between their eyes and visual fields, speak of loss of vision in their right or left eyes. Occasionally, the hemianopia can be transient. When the ischemia affects the parietal lobe (either affecting the territory of the middle cerebral artery or the parietal and tempero-parietal branches of the posterior cerebral artery), an accompanying visual neglect may occur so that the patient is unaware of the hemianopia and may report blurred vision, temporary visual loss to one side, or bumping into objects on that side. Inexplicably, some patients with unilateral lesions of the posterior cerebral hemisphere, who show a hemianopia when examined, complain of temporary blindness at the onset of their strokes. Perhaps the combination of forced eye deviation and hemianopia make it difficult to see well anywhere within the visual fields.

In lesions of the calcarine cortex (area 17) or associative visual cortex (areas 18 and 19), patients may report visual allusions, formed visual objects, visual perservations, or altered size and shape of objects (17). When the lesion within the posterior cerebral territories affects the fusiform and lingual gyri and the hippocampi, agitated delirium (18,19) and memory loss (20) may impair the patient's ability to recognize and accurately report the nature of the visual loss. Cognitive dysfunction probably best explains Anton's syndrome (ie, lack of awareness of blindness). More subtle visual defects (eg, Balint's syndrome (21) also can be caused by infarction in the posterior cerebral artery territory or by hypotension with bilateral border zone infarctions between the posterior cerebral and middle cerebral artery territories. Occlusive lesions within the basilar artery or bilateral vertebral arteries do cause episodic blindness or dim vision, usually described by the patient as bilateral. Most often the patient has accompanying signs and symptoms (eg, dizziness, diplopia, bilateral weakness or numbness, and ataxia of vertebrobasilar occlusive disease (22,23).

Seizures arising in the posterior hemispheres usually cause positive visual symptoms (eg, lights, colors, and formed visual objects), but, after the seizure, temporary postictal visual loss may occur. Visual accompaniments in classical migraine usually are related to dysfunction of the occipital lobe and are characterized by moving, flickering, scintillating objects described as balls, lines, zig-zags, heat waves, angles, or fortifications. These move within the visual fields, leaving in their wake a region of darkness or scotoma. The visual dysfunction typically lasts 15 minutes to an hour and often is followed or accompanied by a headache.

References

1. Tyler HR: Looking and seeing and their relation to visual cognition, in Smith, JL (ed): *Neuro-Ophthalmology*. St Louis, The CV Mosby Co, 1968, vol 4, pp 249–265.
2. Leigh RJ, Zee D: *The Neurology of Eye Movements*. Philadelphia, FA Davis Co, 1983, pp 11–38.
3. Toussaint D: Raeder's syndrome, in Vinken PJ, Bruyn GW (eds): *Handbook of Clinical Neurology*. Amsterdam, North-Holland, 1968, vol 5: *Headaches and Cranial Neuralgias*, pp 333–336.
4. Growden J, Winkler G, Wray S: Midbrain ptosis. *Arch Neurol* 1974;30:179–181.
5. Furlan A, Whisnant J, Kearns T: Unilateral visual loss in bright light. *Arch Neurol* 1979;36:675–676.

6. Carter JE: Chronic ocular ischemia and carotid vascular disease. *Stroke* 1985;16:721–728.
7. Fisher CM: Observations of the fundus occuli in transient monocular blindness. *Neurology* 1959;9:333–347.
8. Carroll D: Retinal migraine. *Headache* 1970;10:9–13.
9. Copetto JR, Lessell S, Sciarra R, et al: Vascular retinopathy in migraine. *Neurology* 1986;36:267–270.
10. Corbett JJ: Neuro-Ophthalmic complications of migraine and cluster headaches, in Smith CH, Beck. RW: *Neurologic Clinics*. Philadelphia, WB Saunders Co, 1983, vol 1, pp 973–995.
11. Miller NR: Anterior ischemic optic neuropathy, in *Walsh and Hoyt's Clinical Neuro-Ophthalmology,* ed 4. Baltimore, The Williams & Wilkins Co, 1982, pp 212–226.
12. Lieberman MF, Maumenee AE, Green WR: Histologic studies of the vasculature of the anterior optic nerve. *Am J Ophthalmol* 1976;83:405–423.
13. Boghen DR, Glaser JS: Ischemic optic neuropathy. *Brain* 1975;98:689–708.
14. Knox DL, Duke JR: Slowly progressive ischemic optic neuropathy. *Trans Am Acad Ophthalmol Otolaryngol* 1971;73:1065–1068.
15. Helgason C, Caplan LR, Goodwin J, et al: Anterior choroidal artery territory infarction: Case report and review. *Arch Neurol* 1986;43:681–686.
16. Caplan LR, Kelly M, Kase CS, et al: Infarcts of the inferior division of the right middle cerebral artery: Mirror image of Wernicke's aphasia. *Neurology* 1986;36:1015–1020.
17. Caplan LR: "Top of the basilar" syndrome. *Neurology* 1980;30:72–79.
18. Horenstein S, Chamberlain W, Conomy J: Infarction of the fusiform and calcarine regions: Agitated delirium and hemianopia. *Trans Am Neurol Assoc* 1967;92:85–89.
19. Medina J, Rubino F, Ross E: Agitated delirium caused by infarction of the hippocampal formation and fusiform and lingual gyri. *Neurology* 1974;24:1181–1183.
20. Caplan LR, Hedley-White T: Cuing and memory dysfunction in alexia without agraphia. *Brain* 1974;97:251–262.
21. Hecaen H, DeAjuriaguerra J: Balint's syndrome (psychic paralysis of visual fixation) and its minor forms. *Brain* 1954;77:373–400.
22. Caplan LR: Vertebrobasilar occlusive disease, in Barnett HJ, Mohr JP, Stein BM, et al (eds): *Stroke: Pathophysiology, Diagnosis and Management*. New York, Churchill-Livingstone, 1985, pp 549–619.
23. Caplan LR, Stein RW: *Stroke: A Clinical Approach*. Boston, Butterworths (Publishers) Inc, 1986 pp 139–166.

CHAPTER 4

Angiography of Retinal and Choroidal Vascular Disease

Joseph B. Michelson and Mitchell H. Friedlaender

Amaurosis fugax, or "fleeting loss of vision", presents as a painless, sudden monoculor loss of vision. The patient describes an acute total loss of vision, often beginning as an abrupt dimming or darkening of the visual field, proceeding to total darkness. The return of vision is characteristic. The patient likens this to a "curtain rising up again" after two to ten minutes in a sectional or piecemeal return. Generally, vision returns to absolutely normal immediately after initial episodes of amaurosis. The frequency of these episodes may vary to an isolated event to multiple "attacks" each day. Amaurosis fugax is reported to be the most common symptom of carotid artery disease (1).

Not all episodes of fleeting visual loss and other forms of visual TIAs are caused by thrombotic microembolization from carotid artery disease. Other causes of amaurosis fugax include temporal arteritis, pseudotumor cerebri, migraine attacks with cerebrovascular spasm, structural cardiac defects, atrial myxoma, stenosis or aneurysm of the ophthalmic artery, hematologic causes (eg, leukemia), ocular hypertension, arterial hypertension, and intra-arterial embolization of drugs associated with intravenous (IV) drug abuse in an ever-growing population of young and middle-aged persons who have a history of bizarre complaints and symptoms, often with amaurosis fugax as a prominent feature (2,3).

During an amaurosis fugax attack the retina may show hemiocclusion or total occlusion of the central retinal artery, occlusion of its branches, partial or complete retinal infarction or a whitening, with isolated emboli or "showers" of emboli, either migrating through the arteriolar tree, or lodged at bifurcations. The retina may even appear normal (4).

The importance of recognizing the TIA of amaurosis fugax as a transient phenomenon is that it is frequently associated with atheromatous ulcerative disease of the ipsilateral extracranial carotid artery (Figs. 4–2, 4–3). Microembolization of this ulcertive lesion is the mechanism responsible for the amaurosis fugax. One third of all patients with an untreated attack of amaurosis fugax can be expected to have a stroke in the future. This rate is approximately four times the incidence in an age-matched population.

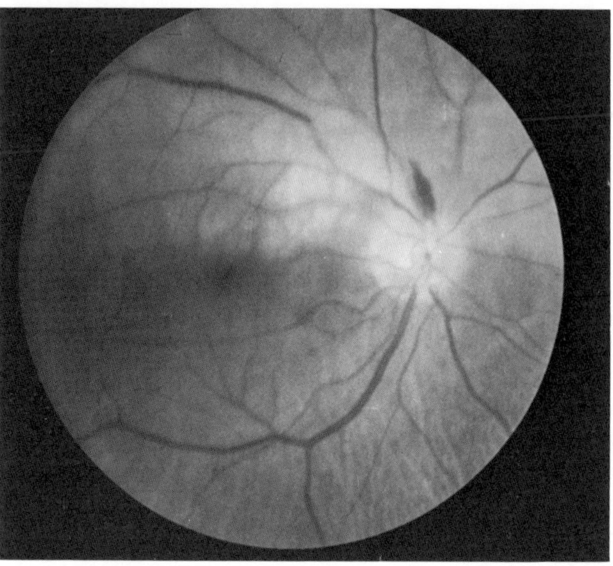

FIGURE 4–1. Clinical photograph of the retina shows hemiretinal scotoma secondary to embolism from ulcerative atheromatous disease of the ipsilateral extracranial carotid artery. Note the flame-shaped hemorrhage just above the area of a Hollenhorst plaque in the CRA on the optic nerve head. Note how this hemiretinal infarction obeys the horizontal median raphé.

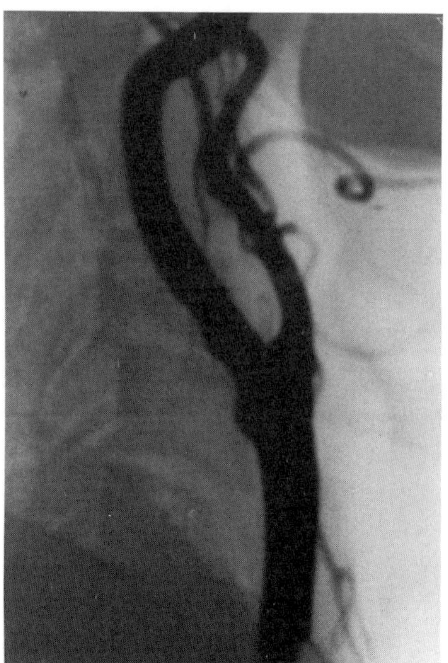

FIGURE 4–2. Angiogram of atheromatous ulcerative disease of the extracranial carotid artery shows a small plaque on the vessel wall, which is capable of causing profound damage to the retina as an embolic phenomenon (see Fig 4–1).

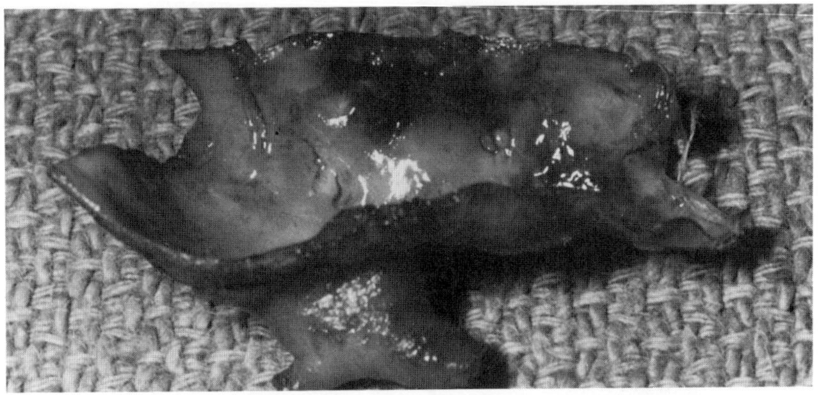

FIGURE 4–3. Diseased ulcerated atheromatous carotid artery section removed from patient shown in Figs 4–1 and 4–2 shows the small, but potentially lethal or blinding, atheromatous disease process.

Types of Emboli

Cholesterol Emboli

(Acute arterial occlusions are due to emboli that are sometimes visible ophthalmoscopically.) Experiments have shown that the retina can withstand about 100 minutes of total CRA occlusion (7). While some few patients can recover vision even hours after a subtotal CRA occlusion, most do not. Most patients will demonstrate some lasting loss of visual field. Acute occlusions may involve either a branch artery, a cilioretinal artery (Fig. 4–4), the CRA (Fig. 4–5, with sparing of the cilioretinal artery), or the ophthalmic artery.

Cholesterol emboli, or "Hollenhorst Plaque" (Fig. 4–6) are glistening, bright yellow or orange, irregular shapes and appear to be larger than the blood vessel in which they are lodged. They flow into the circulation, moving more and more distal until they lodge at the smallest bifurcation from which they can no longer pass. (Fig. 4–6). When a more central occlusion is observed in the eye, the ophthalmologist may attempt to lower the pressure in the eye by using medicines, digital means, or paracentesis to try to force the obstructive plaque downstream so that less of the retina will be affected when the embolus migrates to a smaller, more distal bifurcation. Such emboli generally do not produce complete obstruction of the CRA but can produce localized partial obstruction of the arteriole, which may be accompanied by retinal infarction and dilatation of the vein. (8).

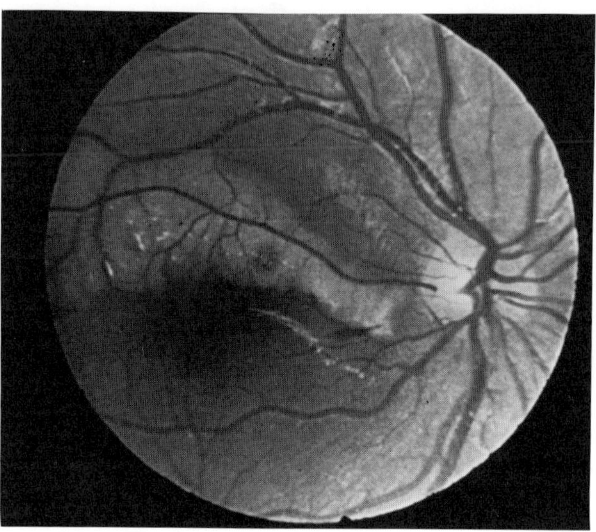

FIGURE 4–4. Clinical photograph of the retina shows occlusion of the cilioretinal artery in a patient in whom the CRA was spared.

Transient obstructions producing amaurosis fugax are common. Some of these emboli remain unchanged ophthalmoscopically for long periods of time in the retina. Others disappear completely and are transient in nature, seen passing into the more distal retinal circulation. In some patients an inflammatory segmental perivascular cuff will appear gradually at the site of cholesterol lipid embolization.

This focal inflammatory reaction may obscure the embolus completely (9,10). This obscurative sheathing most probably is due to damage to the endothelial cells. It may disappear completely in time, leaving a narrow blood column behind as a consequence (9). Digital pressure on the globe occasionally may cause the embolus to "flash" and become more apparent to the observer; it may enable the embolus to pass into the more distal circulation as well, where its occlusive capacity will cause little or no compromise to the retina. However, further pressure sometimes may cause the embolus to move retrograde toward the optic disk as the CRA partially collapses and be responsible for a more profound infarction (9). In some cases the embolization has disappeared ophthalmoscopically by the time the patient seeks ophthalmologic attention. The retina may only manifest ischemic or infarction changes. Fluorescein angiography then provides evidence of microembolization in the form of distinctive focal arteriolar changes suggestive of embolic phenomena (11). These cholesterol emboli are the direct result of ulceration of an atheromatous plaque in the ipsilateral extracranial carotid artery.

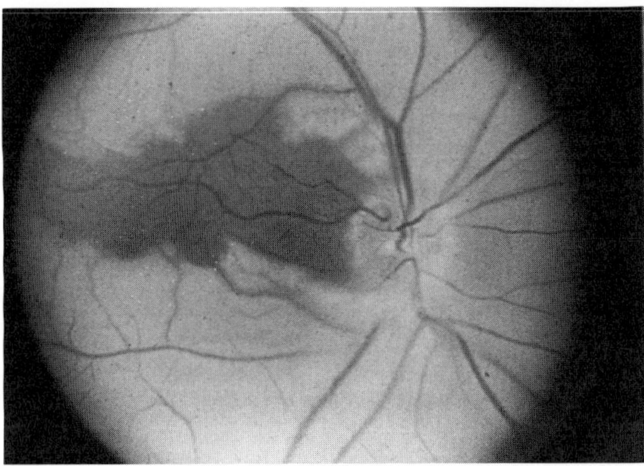

FIGURE 4–5. Clinical photograph of the retina shows occlusion of the CRA in a patient who has a patent cilioretinal artery and sparing of the macula and central acuity, although all the peripheral vision was lost.

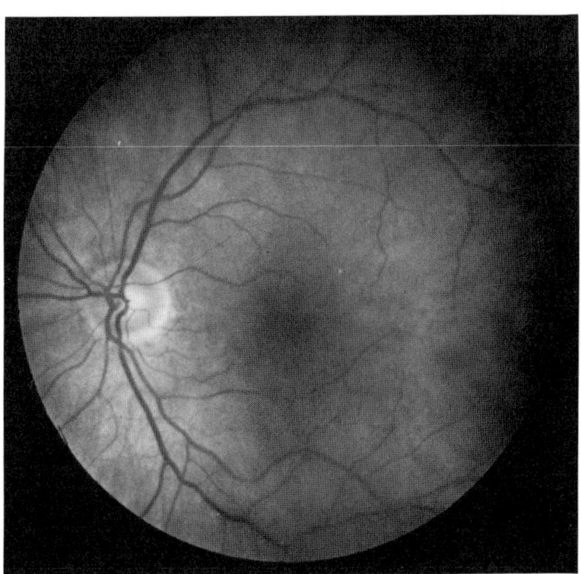

FIGURE 4–6. Retinal photograph shows a Hollenhorst plaque, which is seen as a highly refractile body at the end of the superotemporal arteriole just above the macular area.

Platelet-Fibrin Clots

A second type of endogenous emboli are platelet fibrin clots. These gray or white amorphous particles that are approximately the same size as the blood column, occur with less frequency than cholesterol emboli. They may be seen as a shower of emboli in the eye that changes position from one examination to the next due to the fact that they fragment more easily and in so doing, move more quickly through the circulatory tree, passing into the distal circulation where they "disappear" more rapidly and easily than the "harder" cholesterol plaques. They may be totally asymptomatic but also can produce an amaurosis fugax attack or an occlusion of a branch retinal artery (9). Because of the fleeting nature of platelet-fibrin emboli as compared with cholesterol emboli, the former are seen less often when patients present for ophthalmoscopy (9). These emboli are composed primarily of platelet aggregates, having been shunted off the surface of a thrombus in the ipsilateral extracranial carotid artery (12,13).

Calcific Vegetations

A third type of microemboli noted in the retinal circulation, and responsible for occlusion of the retinal vessels and retinal infarction, is due to valvular heart disease, and not associated with extracranial carotid artery disease at all. Calcific or vegetative emboli, which are sharp gray or white, the same size or larger than the arterial lumen, in which they are lodged are the "hardest" of the emboli, and fragment the least. These may also be infectious in nature but are usually responsible only for occlusive phenomena. They lodge at bifurcations closer to the optic disk, and may produce a more central, and hence, more profound retinal occlusion and infarction. These are fragments of calcifications or vegetation on the heart valves which are spun off into the circulation and ultimately lodge in the retinal circulation, as well as elsewhere such as the brain, liver, spleen, etc.

The importance of cholesterol emboli or platelet-fibrin emboli as a sign of carotid disease has been well established. 69% of patients in the study with cholesterol emboli experienced either a TIA or a full-blown stroke within 10 days of being examined (14). Patients with cholesterol or platelet-lipid emboli have increased death rates when compared with age-matched subjects (15). Interestingly, the most frequent cause of death in these patients, however, is not cerebrovascular accident but uncontrollable cardiovascular disease (16).

Microembolisms from Drug Abuse

Yet a fourth type of retinal microembolization is being noted with increased frequency: showers of emboli associated with IV drug abuse. Patients inject themselves with contaminated materials that are, at first, well filtered by the lung but then, with subsequent reinjections and the development of pulmonary hypertension, become less well filtered and are shunted into the arterial system where they shower the eye, central nervous system (CNS), liver, spleen, and so forth. The disregard for aseptic technique, the use of contaminated illicit drugs and diluting substances, the sharing of injection paraphernalia by several persons, and the direct infusion of organisms into the bloodstream or subcutaneous tissue are all responsible for these infectious and embolic complications. Atlee (17), in 1972, first described talc retinopathy in 17 drug addicts who had injected methylphenidate hydrochloride (Ritalin) IV. Since that time, talc retinopathy has been reported in association with IV abuse of methylphenidate hydrochloride, heroin, methadone, codeine, meperidine hydrochloride (Demerol), and pentazocine. Methylphenidate tablets contain talc (magnesium silicate) and cornstarch as fillers and binders and are designed for oral use. However, the abuser prepares a suspension for injection by dissolving the crushed tablets in boiling water. The turbid solution may be passed through cotton or other homemade filters to remove the larger impurities. The solution is then injected IV, subcutaneously (SQ), or intramuscularly (IM). The particles embolize to the lungs, causing pulmonary hypertension and cor pulmonale. After some time, collateral vessels develop around the normal circulation with pulmonary hypertension and hence, embolize to the eye and set up a focus of inflammation and embolization. As this pattern of embolization has become more apparent, numerous case studies (6,17) have described intraretinal emboli of talc, cornstarch, cotton, and other particles that embolized through the lungs as a result of IV substance

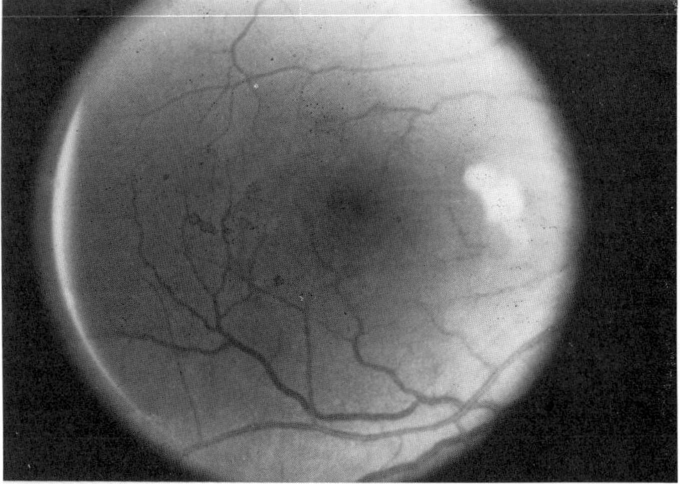

FIGURE 4–7. Clinical photograph of the retina of a 28-year-old white man who had a sudden loss of vision due to a cascade of colored lights secondary to a talc embolism to the eye from intravenous (IV) drug abuse (6).

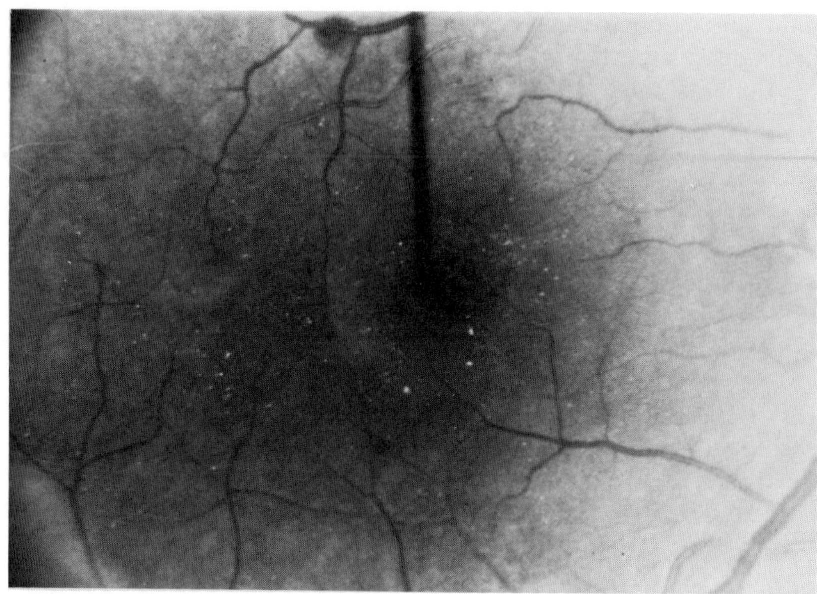

FIGURE 4–8. Clinical photograph of the retina shows multiple talc emboli to the retina scattered around the macular region in a young patient who was an IV abuser of methylphenidate.

abuse (Figs. 4–7 to 4–9). It is now generally regarded that if a young person who has not undergone ocular surgery has what appears to be intraretinal microembolization in a shower pattern or has metastatic endophthalmitis or panuveitis as a consequence of this, IV drug abuse should be suspected until proven otherwise. Drug abuse is a growing worldwide problem, and its ocular manifestations are so well recognized now that it ushers in a host of wholly new considerations in the medical management of young patients with mysterious ocular complaints and illnesses (Figs. 4–7 to 4–9).

Retinal Physiology

The retinal inner layers receive nutrition from the intraretinal circulation. The outer retinal layers receive nutrition by diffusion from the underlying choroidal circulation. Blood traverses a microcirculatory bed composed of vascular end units of the CRA; the central retinal vein; and the inner postterminal arterioles, venules, and capillaries. With the exception of a cilioretinal artery, (which is present in 15% to 30% of subjects) (Fig. 4–5), the CRA is the sole afferent retinal vessel and any compromise of flow will result in immediate ischemia. There are inter-connections of the cap-

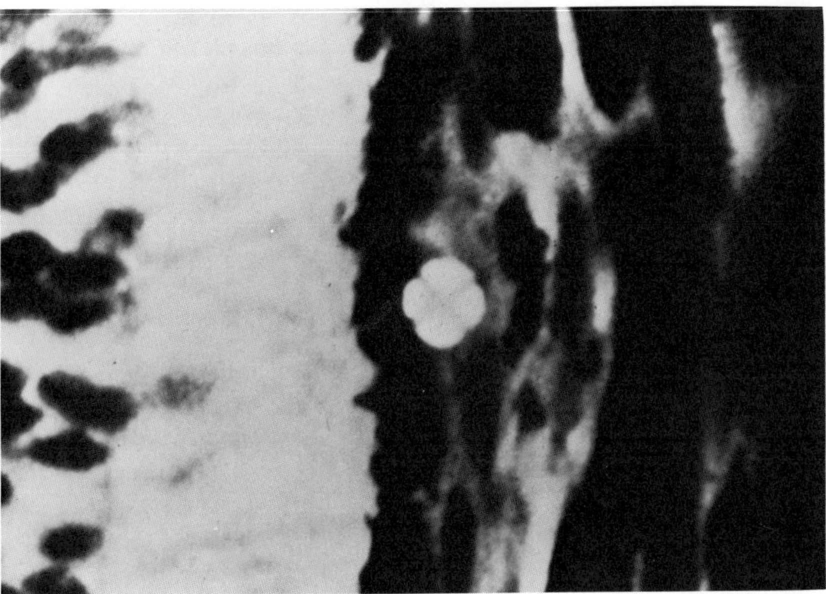

FIGURE 4–9. Intraretinal cotton embolism in the retina in an IV drug abuser who died from an overdose. These cotton strands are the source of embolization and were the consequence of inadequate and inappropriate "filtering" of the abused substance and the homemade paraphernalia.

illaries of the optic nerve head (derived from the choroidal circulation) with the adjacent intraretinal capillaries but this is insufficient to present ischemia and infarction of the retina in central and branch retinal artery occlusion.

Venous Stasis Retinopathy

Another clinical situation of carotid artery flow occlusion which results in chronic obstruction is the Venous Stasis Retinopathy syndrome. This is produced by stenosis of the ipsilated extracranial carotid artery, and not due to the acute changes of micro-embolization. It was reported first by Hedges (18) and was termed venous stasis retinopathy by Kearns and Hollenhorst (19). Although this term is not descriptive, it refers to a basic mechanism of hypoperfusion of the arterial inflow, not a reduction of the venous outflow. The condition is characterized by dot-and-blot hemorrhages in the mid-peripheral to peripheral retina, venous tortuosity and engorgement, microaneurysms, and occasional sludging and box-carring (of the blood within the vein). Fluorescein angiography generally shows areas of capillary nonperfusion and microaneurysms in the midperiphery.

The condition usually does not affect the posterior pole of the eye and patients usually have normal visual acuity. For this reason, this condition may only be observed on routine ophthalmologic examination. The entire periphery of the eye usually is involved, although one quadrant often has more hemorrhages than another. Although patients occasionally have some ocular discomfort or eye pain, they have a normal IOP. Reduction of OAP is a pathognomonic feature of this disorder. Usually, disk edema and optic disk collateral vessels are not present. This disease is associated with a chronic stenosis of the ophthalmic artery and a hyperlipoproteinemia as a concommitant with hypertension. These patients may have much more profound cardiovascular disease than their "benign" fundus presentation of peripheral dot and blot hemorrhage would lead one to expect.

Fluorescein Angiography

Fluorescein angiography can be effective in the study of these embolic and ischemic vascular disorders. For some conditions not mentioned here (eg, branch vein occlusion and diabetic retinopathy), the fluorescein angiogram is the most useful guide for determining appropriate therapy. For the disorders mentioned here (eg, occlusion of branch arteries or the CRA), angiograms may be an effective means for estimating a patient's visual prognosis.

With the exception of those who have a cilioretinal artery, most patients rely on a CRA to supply the entire nutrition to the inner layers of the retina. Because there is no anastomotic circulation in the retina as there is in the choroid, any obstruction of blood flow leads to severe ischemia and loss of function in the affected area. Fluorescein angiograms clearly show the affected vessel branches and thus play a meaningful role in demonstrating recovery and possible return of blood flow to ischemic areas.

As illustrated in the figures in this chapter, occlusion of branch arteries is associated with a lack of perfusion of fluorescein-containing blood into a branch of the artery. The involved sector of the retina has a ground-glass appearance due to retinal edema secondary to ischemia. The point of occlusion usually can be pinpointed with great accuracy on the angiogram. The veins in the area of the retina fed by the blocked portion of the artery do not contain fluorescein. Laminar flow occurs in the veins adjacent to the area of nonperfused retina. The blood column in the veins does not mix. Sometimes a retrograde flow of fluorescein-containing blood into the branches of the artery or veins in the area of the occlusion is seen. When a branch artery is occluded only partially, filling will be delayed in the affected area, staining and possible leakage of the artery will occur in areas that are damaged by hypoxia or emboli, and if a trypsin digest study of such an area is done, marked loss of endothelial cells can be expected.

Fig. 4–10 shows occlusion of the CRA. The artery is dark and the part

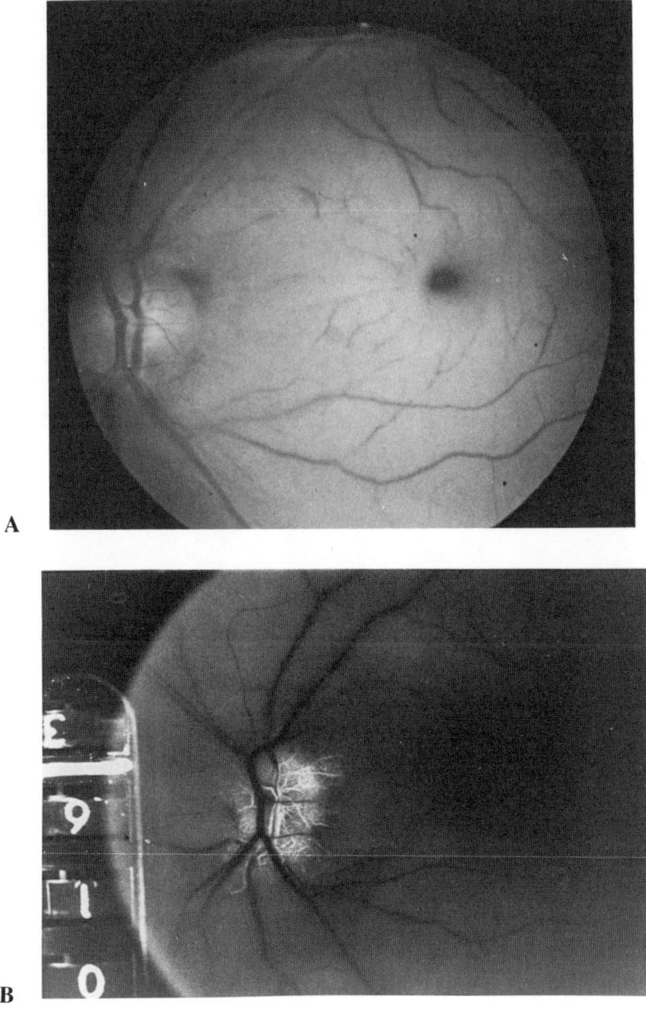

FIGURE 4–10. CRA occlusion. **A,** Clinical photograph shows a ground-glass appearance of the macula. The cherry-red spot of the fovea is due to the thinness of that area of the retina and allows the underlying choroidal circulation to show through as a red spot while the rest of the edematous retina appears yellowish as in ground glass. **B,** Fluorescein angiogram shows absence of fluorescein filling of the retina and presence of filling in the capillary network of the optic nerve head.

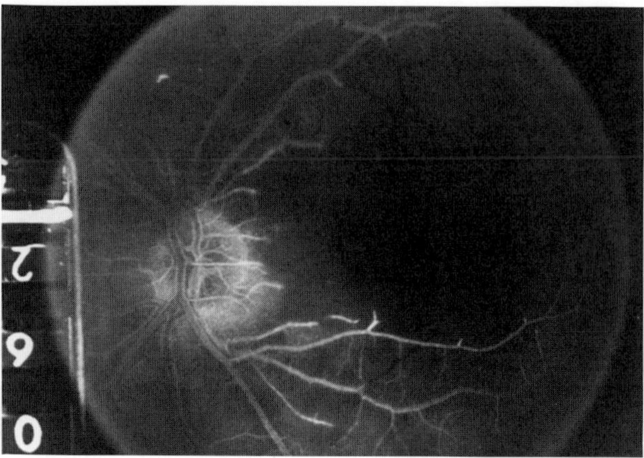

FIGURE 4–11. Late phase of fluorescein angiogram at 62 seconds shows continued absence of arterial filling with some retinal venous drainage of fluorescein and very tortuous retinal veins.

that is on the optic nerve cannot be discerned. The retina is not perfused and appears edematous because of tissue swelling. Early laminar flow will occur in some branches of the veins. Blood in the upper branch of the inferior vein contains fluorescein on the side of the vein that has a normally perfused retina (Fig. 4–11). Fig. 4–12 is a fluorescein angiogram that shows how a previously blocked vessel can be seen in a subsequent examination to be open and carrying blood. The background fluorescence can be discerned then as normal, and edema will have subsided.

In an occlusion of the CRA, vision is affected severely unless a cilioretinal artery (Fig. 4–5) is present to supply circulation to the macula itself. However, obstruction of the cilioretinal artery also can occur (Fig. 4–4). In the acute phase of CRA occlusion circulation in the retina is decreased markedly, especially compared with flow in the opposite eye. In some instances retinal circulation may be reestablished, but the filling time is long, and the circulation is sluggish. In these cases the retinal arteries characteristically remain narrow. In addition to an abnormally long circulation time, the retinal vessels begin to fill long after the choroidal vessels have filled and have emptied already. The retinal arteries may fill to variable degrees, ranging from none to complete but delayed filling. Optic atrophy is common, and the optic nerve head shows less fluorescence than usual because of its decreased capillary network, although some of its circulation will be supplied by collateral vessels from the choroid. The discontinuity of fluorescein dye in the vessels shows the lack of blood flow in the vessels themselves. In some situations, circulation in the retina is virtually absent, even after prolonged waiting. In other cases, with an older, more chronic CRA occlusion, some perfusion of the retinal circulation is present. However, the circulation time is long and the vessels

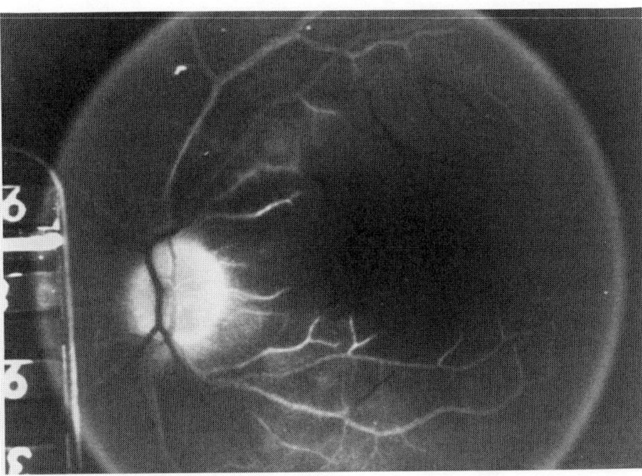

FIGURE 4–12. Angiogram of CRA occlusion in very late phases shows atrophy of the optic nerve head secondary to the artery occlusion. (Compare Figs 4–10 and 4–11, which showed a profuse capillary network in the optic nerve head itself.) This frame shows the atrophy and pallor of the optic nerve head with an absence of its own papillary circulation.

are narrowed extraordinarily. This usually is associated with atrophy of the optic nerve head, which is accompanied by an absence of the capillary network on the nerve and the absence of fluorescein dye in the nerve head itself (Fig. 4–12).

Occlusion of Branches of the Retinal Vein

Although occlusion of branches of the retinal vein is not usually discussed in association with amaurosis fugax, it does occur, usually in advanced arteriosclerotic disease in the elderly. Some authorities (19,20) also ascribe this type of occlusion to giant-cell arteritis, which has its primary pathology on the arterial side of the circulation. These authorities state that the venule may be obstructed by pressure as a result of arteriolar thickening and narrowing due to inflammation in the arteriole itself. The arteriole closes off at the retinal venule crossing, where the arteriole and venule share a common syncytium. This presumably results in occlusion of the branch vein. The superior temporal branch vein is affected most commonly by occlusion. The inferior temporal branch is affected less commonly, and the nasal branches are affected rarely. Occlusion of a branch vein is almost always seen at the site of the arteriovenous crossing and may occur frequently in patients with chronic hypertension. Visual acuity is affected only if the retinal involvement is contiguous with the macula and results in macular edema.

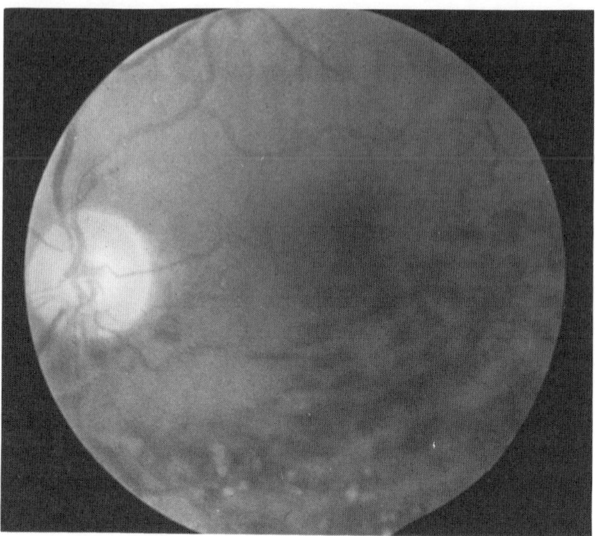

FIGURE 4–13. Angiogram of a retina with branch vein occlusion shows the triangular area of retinal edema with adjacent flame-shaped hemorrhages and some macular edema collecting inferior to it. The flame-shaped hemorrhages in this triangle point to the area of obstruction.

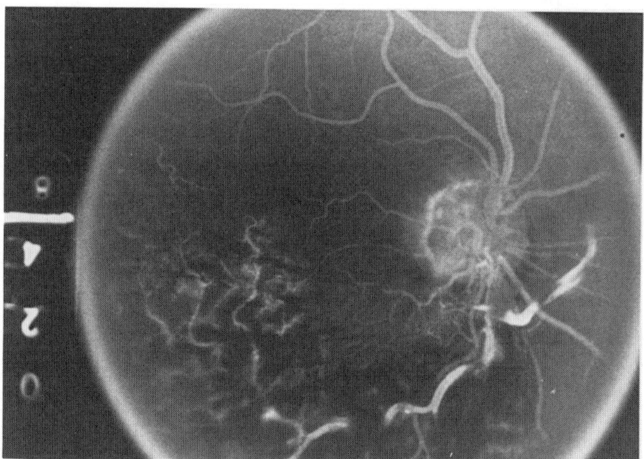

FIGURE 4–14. Fluorescein angiogram of this occlusion of the retinal branch vein shows partial obstruction of the retina superiorly, fluorescein staining with leakage, development of tortuous vessels with collaterals distal to the ischemic area, and an area without capillary perfusion superiorly. This is not to be confused with those areas that show the choroidal fluorescence blocked by the intraretinal hemorrhage.

Giant-Cell Arteritis

Giant-cell arteritis is a disease of large and medium-sized arteries and may not involve the arterioles. According to Hayreh (20), the most common ocular artery to be involved is one of the main posterior ciliary arteries. The CRA or the ophthalmic artery is involved less frequently. Hayreh himself (20) has found no evidence of intraocular arteries being affected by giant-cell arteritis.

The appearance of the retina is diagnostic in occlusion of a branch vein. Retinal edema occurs with adjacent numerous flame-shaped hemorrhages which point to the area of obstruction (Figs, 4–13, 4–14). On fluorescein angiograms, the involved vein usually is obstructed only partially, is engorged, and shows fluorescein staining with leakage. The capillary bed may be dilated in the involved area, and variable amounts of leakage from the capillary bed may occur (Fig. 4–14). Capillary leakage may be seen in the early stages of occlusion, or it may become evident later when some healing has occurred. The degree of leakage from the capillary bed can help determine whether laser treatment to diminish macular edema will be effective in a particular patient. Thus, the fluorescein angiogram provides a useful guide to therapy in such patients. In older occlusions of branch veins, evidence of repair and reestablishment of circulation with collateral vessels may be present. Neovascularization may be seen at the

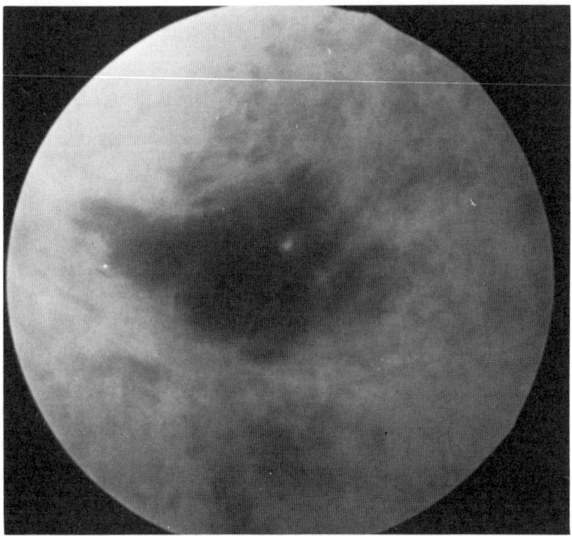

FIGURE 4–15. Clinical photograph of the retina shows an apparent example of a vein occlusion, with an area of intraretinal hemorrhage that does not observe the horizontal raphé.

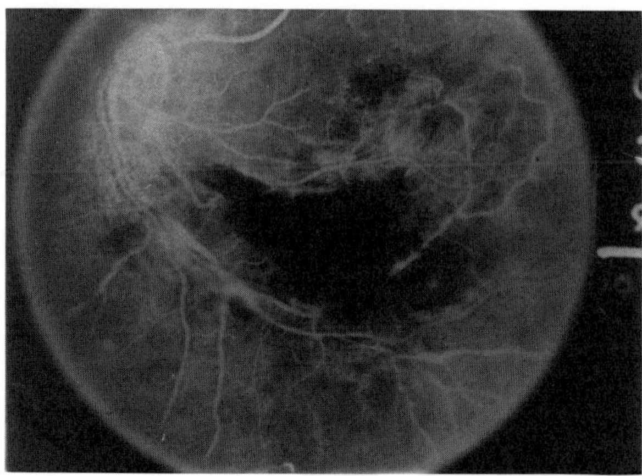

FIGURE 4–16. Fluorescein angiogram of the eye in Fig 4–15 shows retinal edema extending beyond the horizontal raphé and areas of nonperfusion, which should not be confused with hemorrhage both superior and inferior to the vein occlusion itself.

site of the occlusion or from the optic nerve head itself as a consequence of ischemia and infarction of the retina.

Usually the site of occlusion, which may be partial or complete, can be seen on the fluorescein angiogram. Staining of the wall of the affected branch vein occurs in the occluded area. Sometimes a bright stain is seen at the site of occlusion. Ischemia of the capillary bed occurs in the retinal area drained by the vein itself, and leakage from the remaining unobstructed capillaries occurs in the affected retinal area. In older occlusions persistent retinal edema may be present in the occluded area, and the capillary network in the macular area may be involved as well, with loss of central visual acuity. Formation of collateral vessels with neovascularization may take place as the healing occurs. The presence of neovascularization in the retina, and more importantly on the disk, mitigates the usefulness of laser treatment to the eye. Blockage of fluorescence may occur as a result of residual hemorrhage in the nerve fiber layer of the retina.

In Fig. 4–14, the branch vein is occluded at the point of intersection with the adjacent branch of the artery. In Figs. 4–15 and 4–16, the area of nonperfusion of the retinal capillary network extends beyond the horizontal raphé to involve some of the adjacent retina. The area of nonperfusion extends into the macula, almost reaching the foveolar pit. The retinal capillary bed is abnormal in the area of involvement and shows vessel staining and fluorescein leakage into the retina. Dilatation and staining of the vessel walls also are evident. Collateral vessels cross in irregular patterns, and extensive areas of nonperfusion are present in the area affected by the occlusion, as seen by the totally dark areas with no gray fluorescein diffusion. It is this ischemia, with its demonstrable areas of nonperfusion, that results in neovascularization. Although neovascularization seemingly is a protective mechanism in theory, it causes great harm to the eye, producing fragile, unstable blood vessels that will bleed later. This ultimately may lead to total retinal detachment if unchecked. It is for these reasons that laser treatment is advocated to diminish and ablate retinal neovascularization, as in a diabetic patient.

Hypertensive Retinopathy

Hypertension also may be a cause of TIAs in the retinal and cerebral circulation. In benign hypertension, some narrowing of the retinal arterioles and capillaries occurs. With more severe hypertension, areas without capillary perfusion also may be present, as is seen with branch vein occlusion and arteriolar occlusion with staining and leakage of fluorescein dye from adjacent capillaries. In addition, the capillaries may be dilated and tortuous, with possible formation of microaneurysms. The classic ''cotton-wool'' spots represent areas of ischemic infarction within the retina. Patients with malignant hypertension show retinal changes in addition to possible papilledema and more profound narrowing changes in the retinal vessels. Diffuse retinal edema may result from leakage of the retinal vessels. Other findings may include staining of retinal vessels, extensive nonperfusion due to areas of capillary bed closure, and leakage from the swollen optic disk. In malignant hypertension, choroidal vessels also are

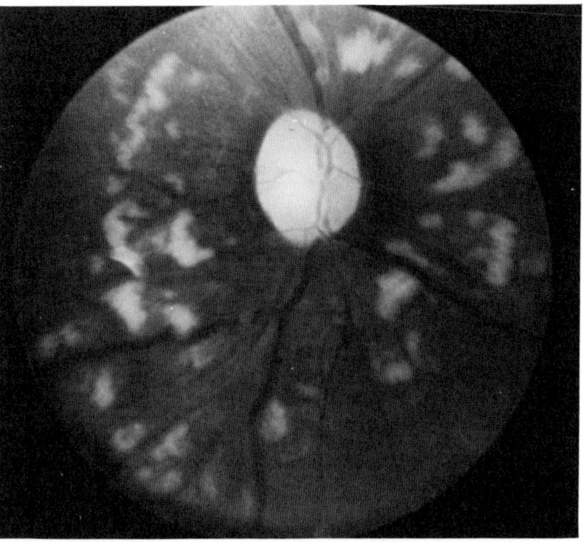

FIGURE 4–17. Clinical photograph of the retina shows the optic nerve pallor and profuse cotton-wool exudates in a patient with advanced hypertensive retinopathy.

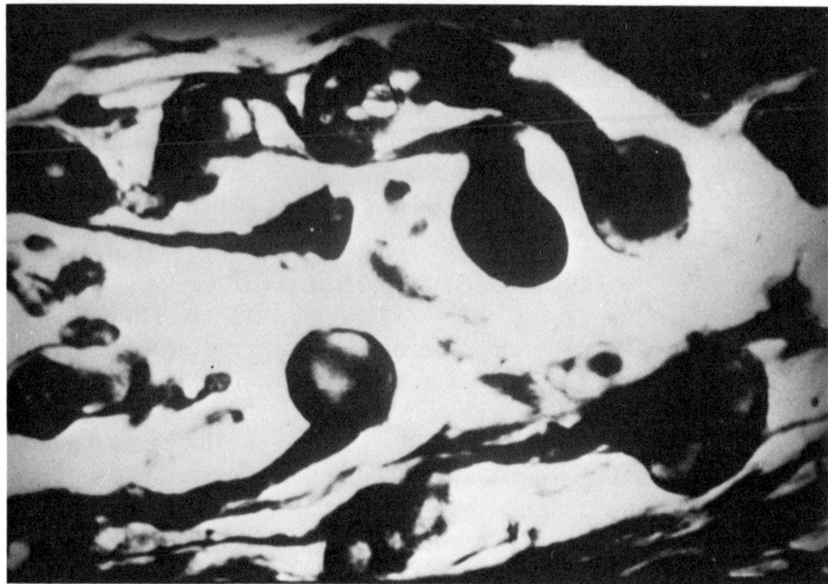

FIGURE 4–18. Histologic specimen shows cytoid bodies, which represent Wallerian degeneration of the nerve fiber layer of the retina.

affected, and these can be seen angiographically as areas of chorioretinal atrophy and pigment disturbance. Abnormalities in vessel caliber are apparent, especially in the retinal arterioles. Staining of the vessel walls occurs in areas of vascular damage, and leakage from damaged vessels can be seen accompanied by retinal edema. If hemorrhage is present, the underlying fluorescence of the choroid and the outer layer of the retina will be blocked by the hemorrhage and may simulate areas of nonperfusion. Careful attention to detail will separate areas of intraretinal hemorrhage and surrounding areas of nonperfusion (Fig. 4–16). Cotton-wool spots, which are areas of ischemic infarction, produce a ground-glass or edematous appearance in the involved retinal area. (A red-free photograph would better delineate the occluded vessel with exudate around the vessel and a large cotton-wool spot.) So-called cytoid bodies, although not a clinical ophthalmoscopic sign as such, do represent infarction of the nerve fiber layer of the retina (Figs. 4–17, 4–18) and Wallerian degeneration of the nerve fiber layer caused by a direct ischemia. Cytoid bodies should not be cited as a clinical finding. Rather, they should be called cotton-wool spots or infarctions of the nerve fiber layer of the retina. The term cytoid body should be reserved for the histologic feature of Wallerian degeneration of the nerve fiber layer as seen microscopically in Fig. 4–18.

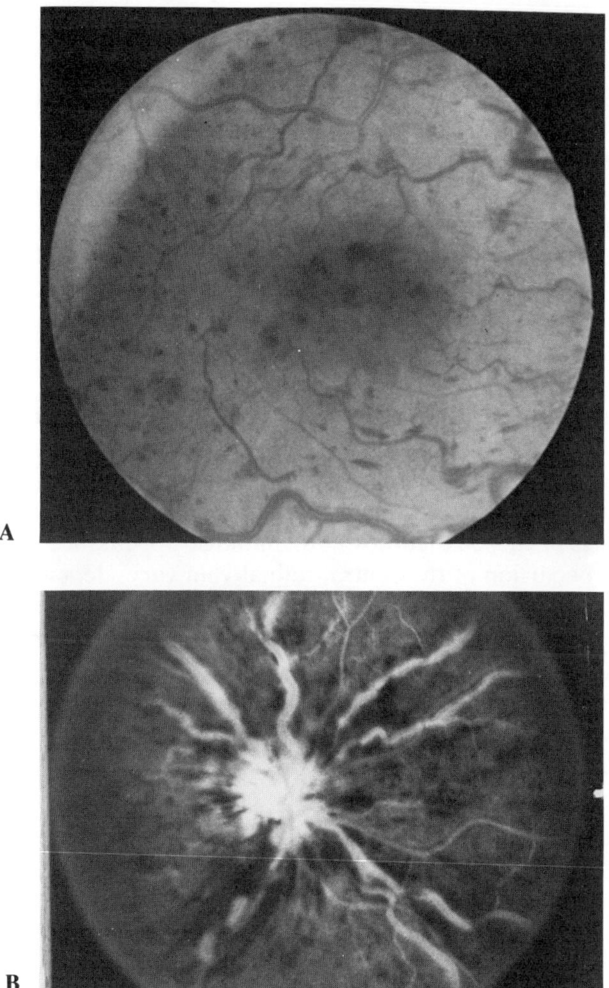

FIGURE 4–19. **A,** Clinical photograph of the retina shows blood-and-thunder appearance of marked hemorrhage and some exudate in the macula of a patient who sustained an occlusion of the central retinal vein. **B,** Fluorescein angiogram shows the optic nerve head, dilated tortuous vessels, and the numerous flame-shaped hemorrhages in the retina that block the underlying choroidal fluorescence in this case of occlusion of the central retinal vein.

Occlusion of the Central Retinal Vein

Occlusion of the central retinal vein usually is due to hypertensive disease or arteriosclerotic disease and has clinical features very different from those outlined for arteriolar obstruction. Occasionally, the onset of occlusion of the central retinal vein may be slow, incipient, and mild. More often a patient reports a sudden, acute, severe loss of vision in the affected eye. The ophthalmic signs also vary from the "blood-and-thunder" fundus of a swollen optic nerve head, dilated and tortuous veins, retinal edema with poor capillary perfusion, and a profound number of flame-shaped hemorrhages at the posterior pole of the eye that may be likened to a child throwing ketchup over the retinal fundus. Dilatation of the retinal veins often is present, minimal edema occurs sometimes, and retinal capillary perfusion may be preserved. If the perifoveal capillary network is preserved and perfused, the retinal edema is minimal to absent, and vision actually can be quite good, although the patient may say it is diminished. Hayreh (20) has proposed that the ophthalmologic appearance and clinical symptoms of occlusion of the central retinal vein vary, depending on the degree of retinal hypoxia associated with the occlusion.

The milder form of occlusion is associated with vision, particularly with preservation of the central acuity; occasional or no cotton-wool exudates; complete perfusion of the capillary bed; and a low prevalence of neovascular glaucoma. This condition, referred to as "incomplete occlusion," may be manifested as venous stasis retinopathy, but it may develop into the more severe form of occlusion of the central retinal vein over time. In this type of occlusion, aside from the profound blood-and-thunder appearance of the retinal fundus (Fig. 4–19), filling of the retinal vessels is delayed markedly, with relatively normal filling of the choroid underneath. Abnormalities occur in the caliber of the arterioles and venules, some leakage from the optic nerve head occurs because of secondary optic disk edema, and staining of the retinal vessel wall occurs because of ischemic injury and damage. The degree of ischemia depends on the perfusion of the retinal capillary network, which may vary from quite poor and almost absent to quite good and almost complete. In the early stage of the angiographic examination, late background fluorescence from filling of the choriocapillaries is visible, and filling of the retinal arteries will be just beginning. Retinal circulation time is delayed, and the variation in caliber of the retinal veins is evident. The late-phase fluorescein angiogram shows leakage from the optic nerve disk and staining of the walls of the veins due to damage. This staining is nonspecific and indicates damage to the vessel wall itself because of endothelial cell loss.

Acknowledgment. We acknowledge Sohan Singh Hayreh for reviewing the manuscript and suggesting important revisions.

References

1. Hollenhorst RW: Ocular manifestations of insufficiency or thrombosis of the internal carotid artery. *Trans Am Ophthalmol Soc* 1958;56:474–479.
2. Michelson JB, Friedlaender MH: Endophthalmitis of drug abuse. *Int Ophthalmol Clin* 1987; (in press).
3. Michelson JB, Whitcher JP, Wilson S, et al: Foreign body granuloma of the retina associated with intravenous cocaine addiction. *Am J Ophthalmol* 1979;87:278–282.
4. Hollenhorst RW: The neuro-ophthalmology of stroke. *Neuro-ophthalmology* 1965;2:109–115.
5. Goldner JC, Wisnant JP, Taylor WF: Long-term prognosis of transient cerebral ischemic attacks. *Stroke* 1971;2:160–167.
6. Fisher CM: Observation of the fundus oculi in transient monocular blindness. *Neurology* 1959;9:333–347.
7. Hayreh SS, Kolder HE, Weingeist TA: Central retinal artery occlusion and retinal tolerance time. *Ophthalmology* 1980;87:75–79.
8. Hoyt WF: Ocular symptoms and signs, in Wylie EJ, Ehrenfeld WK (eds): *Extracranial Cerebrovascular Disease: Diagnosis and Management.* Philadelphia, WB Saunders Co, 1970, pp. 64–95.
9. Arruga J, Sanders MD: Ophthalmologic findings in 70 patients with evidence of retinal embolism. *Ophthalmology* 1982;89:1336–1338.
10. Dark AJ, Rizk SN: Progressive focal sclerosis of retinal arteries: A sequel to impaction of cholesterol emboli. *Br Med J* 1967;1:1270–1274.
11. Muci-Mendoza R, Arruga J, Edwards WO, et al: Retinal fluorescein angiographic evidence for atheromatous microembolism. *Stroke* 1980;11:154–158.
12. McBrien DJ, Bradley RD, Ashton N: The nature of retinal emboli in stenosis of the internal carotid artery. *Lancet* 1963;1:697–699.
13. Ross Russell RW: Observations on the retinal blood vessels in monocular blindness. *Lancet* 1961;2:1422–1428.
14. Hollenhorst RW: Vascular status of patients who have cholesterol emboli in the retina. *Am J Ophthalmol* 1966;61:1159–1165.
15. Pfaffenbach DD, Hollenhorst RW: Morbidity and survivorship of patients with embolic cholesterol crystals in the ocular fundus. *Am J Ophthalmol* 1973;75:66–72.
16. Savino PJ, Glaser JS, Cassady J: Retinal stroke: Is the patient at risk? *Arch Ophthalmol* 1977;95:1185–1189.
17. Atlee WE Jr: Talc and corn starch emboli in the eyes of drug abusers. *JAMA* 1972;219:49–51.
18. Hedges TR: Ophthalmoscopic findings in internal carotid artery occlusion. *Bull Johns Hopkins Hosp* 1962;3:89–93.
19. Kearns TP, Hollenhorst RW: Venous stasis retinopathy of occlusive disease of the carotid artery. *Mayo Clin Proc* 1963;38:304–312.
20. Hayreh SS: Central retinal vein occlusion: differential diagnosis and management. *Trans Am Arch Ophthalmol Otolaryngol* 1977;83:OP379–OP391.

CHAPTER 5

Visual Aspects of Extracranial Internal Carotid Artery Disease

Shirley H. Wray

The visual symptoms of ipsilateral internal extracranial carotid disease are sudden transient monocular visual loss (amaurosis fugax); sudden persistent visual loss and ischemic eye pain.

The funduscopic signs include a normal fundus, a visible retinal embolus, occlusion of the central retinal artery (CRA) or branch retinal artery, venous stasis low-pressure retinopathy, anterior ischemic optic neuropathy (AION) and hypertensive retinal signs and arcus senilis restricted to the nonoccluded side.

Monocular Amaurosis Fugax

Amaurosis fugax is a major visual symptom that may herald stroke. The four types of monocular amaurosis fugax are 1, due to transient retinal ischemia; 2, due to retinal vascular insufficiency; 3, due to angiospasm; and 4, idiopathic.

Amaurosis Fugax Type 1

The visual disturbance in amaurosis fugax type 1 is a sudden attack of partial or complete transient monocular blindness (TMB), lasting seconds to minutes, with total recovery. Partial visual impairment may be described by the patient as a grayout, as an ascending or descending curtain (altitudinal hemianopia, 20/35 cases), or as a blind moving sideways across the eye (hemianopia, 6/35 cases). Occasionally, the patient will describe moving tracks of light. Ipsilateral headache is rare (2/35 cases) (1).

In 1952, Fisher (2) drew attention to the association of amaurosis fugax of this brevity, with contralateral hemiplegia. Since then, amaurosis fugax has come to be regarded as one variety of carotid artery distribution transient ischemic attack (TIA). Like other TIAs, this symptom means the patient has an above average risk of stroke. By extrapolation from data for TIAs in general, the risk of stroke and/or death is probably about 10%

per annum (3), but death more often is due to ischemic heart disease than to stroke (4). In a recent study (5), cerebral vascular symptoms (TIA or stroke) occurred in 22 patients (43%) either before or after amaurosis fugax. Of 44 patients with no cerebral ischemic symptoms before the onset of amaurosis fugax, 15 (34%) subsequently had TIAs or strokes. Yet, the neurologic prognosis for the patient who has isolated amaurosis fugax still remains difficult to determine on the basis of clinical findings.

The majority of attacks of amaurosis fugax type 1 are due to embolism of fresh thrombus into the ophthalmic circulation from a source in the carotid artery, notably, the bifurcation of the common carotid artery in the neck or from the aorta or heart. Careful funduscopy looking for retinal emboli or other vascular changes (eg, central retinal or branch artery occlusion), ischemic optic neuropathy, or asymmetric hypertensive retinopathy is the most important examination to perform next to auscultation of the neck for a carotid artery bruit. The retinal microcirculation is visualized best if the pupil is dilated with 10% phenylephrine (Neosynephrine) eye drops after the visual acuity is measured and the pupillary response recorded. The ophthalmoscopic appearance of a retinal embolus can provide specific information about the embolic material and its possible source.

Bright, yellowish, glinting lipid emboli (Hollenhorst plaques) are the most common emboli seen in the eye. They are associated mostly with atheromatous changes of the ipsilateral carotid artery or aortic arch disease (6,7). The embolic material has been confirmed to be cholesterol.

Calcific emboli are characteristically matte-white, nonscintillating and somewhat wider than the blood column. Calcific emboli may be dislodged by the surgical manipulation of calcified heart valves at the time of valvulotomy or may occur spontaneously from rheumatic valvular vegetation.

Some of the circulating microemboli that pass through the retina, so-called migrant, pale emboli, are believed to be composed of platelets. Their occurrence is associated with thrombocytosis. The emboli that occur after myocardial infarction fall into the category of fibrin plugs. They are especially frequent in patients who have neurologic complications after open heart surgery. The heart lesions traditionally associated with thromboembolism have been myocardial infarction producing mural thrombus; mitral stenosis, with or without atrial fibrillation; and vegetative valvular lesions, bacterial or nonbacterial. Previously unrecognized potential sources of emboli have come to light: mitral-annulus calcification may be the origin of cerebral and retinal emboli in the elderly (8–10), and the prolapsing mitral valve may be the source in younger patients (11–13). In the case of embolic seeding from a myxoma of the heart, the histopathology of the embolus is like that of the original tumor (14).

Clinical experience has shown that the risk of permanent visual loss in patients with amaurosis fugax type 1 is relatively low, perhaps 3% per annum. In one series only 11% of patients with CRA occlusion and 18%

with occlusion of the branch retinal artery could remember a previous episode of amaurosis fugax (1). Complete monocular blindness, when it occurs, is due to a CRA occlusion. Partial blindness may be the sequelae to an occlusion of the retinal artery or to ischemia of the optic nerve. There is no correlation between multiple attacks of amaurosis fugax, defined as more than 20 before presentation, and subsequent permanent visual loss (5).

The results of carotid angiography in patients with amaurosis fugax type 1 has confirmed the high prevalence of ipsilateral carotid disease. A carotid bruit, a history of cerebral TIA, and hypertension all increase the yield of abnormal findings (5). For patients with carotid stenosis or ulceration localized to the origin of the vessel, endarterectomy is still the treatment of choice.

A clear association also is known between symptoms of recurrent retinal ischemia, amaurosis fugax, and reversed ophthalmic artery flow ipsilateral to a complete internal carotid artery (ICA) occlusion (15–19). The proposed pathogenic mechanisms responsible for recurrent amaurosis fugax and cerebral TIAs in such a case have differed. On the one hand, it has been suggested that prominent retrograde ophthalmic artery flow seen in these circumstances may reflect a steal phenomenon from the ophthalmic artery-retinal circulation, and that in this situation, the orbital collateral channels are conscripted by the ipsilateral cerebral hemisphere at the expense of ocular perfusion needs. Consequently, surgical augmentation of intracranial blood flow by means of an ipsilateral external carotid-internal carotid bypass has been suggested as a beneficial procedure. On the other hand, others (15) have suggested that episodic ophthalmic artery hypotension and an ocular steal phenomenon are inadequate explanations for the recurrent intermittent attacks of acute transient ischemia of the retina or brain when robust orbital collaterals are evident angiographically. Their opinion is that microembolism from the stump of the occluded ICA to the symptomatic retina and hemisphere is the pathogenic mechanism, and ipsilateral external carotid endarterectomy with excision of the adjacent ICA stump is the procedure of choice.

Separate considerations arise when the ophthalmic artery has an anomalous origin. In a patient with stenosis of the external carotid artery, ipsilateral amaurosis fugax occurred. Angiography in this case showed that the ophthalmic artery originated from the middle meningeal artery and the retinal ischemic attacks ceased after the patient had an external carotid endarterectomy (19).

The importance of amaurosis fugax as a marker for generalized arteriosclerotic vascular disease should be noted. A recent study (5) reported a correlation with hypertension (18%), hyperlipidemia (61%), and ischemic heart disease or peripheral vascular disease at presentation (25%) and at follow-up in an additional number of patients (18%). A family history of ischemic heart disease, peripheral vascular disease or stroke before the age of 60 years was present in 37% of the cases.

Amaurosis fugax type 1 also may occur in patients with nonarteriosclerotic vasculopathies: fibromuscular hyperplasia, granulomatous angiitis (as opposed to giant-cell or temporal arteritis), congophilic angiopathy, systemic lupus erythematosus, Behçet's syndrome, and moyamoya disease. These rare angiopathies affect small-caliber arteries and, collectively, must be considered in any TIA.

Additionally, states of altered coagulability and thrombocytosis (eg, the altered viscosity of the red cells in sickle cell disease and the altered blood viscosity in polycythemia) are associated with TIA.

Amaurosis Fugax Type 2

Amaurosis fugax of a different type may occur in patients with extensive, extracranial arterial occlusive disease. Amaurosis fugax type 2 is due to retinal vascular insufficiency. Temporary attacks of visual or cerebral disturbance that are hemodynamic occur before permanent structural changes develop in the eye and brain. The temporary episodes of monocular visual loss, characteristic of amaurosis fugax type 2, in comparison with the brief transient attacks of amaurosis fugax type 1, are less rapid in onset and longer in duration (the visual loss develops over minutes rather than seconds and lasts minutes up to two hours). Recovery also takes place gradually. Visual acuity may not be altered significantly during the attacks, but contrast acuity is. Bright objects appear brighter, whereas dark objects may become difficult to see. The edges of bright objects can appear to flicker. When the bright, dazzling sensation is marked, the overall effect is one of overexposure, and the patient may experience difficulty reading because of the dazzle of white paper. Yet, although patients may not see to read, they can discern shapes and identify colors. When sight becomes fragmented and patchy, patients describe the appearance as a photographic negative. Occasionally, they note a transient closing in of the peripheral vision. Sometimes the attacks are accompanied by dull pain over the eye. Symptoms of generalized cerebral ischemia (faintness, fatigue, impaired concentration) often coexist but are mild compared with the visual symptoms.

Factors that provoke attacks of amaurosis fugax type 2 are systemic hypotension, venous hypertension, and extracerebral steal. They occur on stooping or straining when venous pressure rises, on standing or during exercise, on exposure to bright lights or warm surroundings (20,21). This pattern to the attacks suggests a temporary failure of retinal homeostasis. In the unique case of a man with amaurosis fugax type 2 provoked by facial heating with a hair dryer, the mechanism of the visual loss was postulated to be diversion of blood to a dilated external carotid facial vascular bed, resulting in temporary ocular oligemia on the affected side (21).

These unusual visual symptoms are of retinal origin. Investigations (21), including retinal photo-stress tests, have shown no indication of delayed retinal metabolism. Ophthalmodynamometry shows a low resting retinal perfusion pressure and further reduction during an attack of amaurosis. The retina thus appears to be a more sensitive indicator of vascular insufficiency than the brain.

Important compensatory mechanisms in the retinal circulation accompany a progressive reduction in retinal perfusion pressure. A low-pressure retinopathy is characteristic (22). The earliest change is venous distension, irregularity of the vein wall, and leakage of fluorescein from the venules. Blot hemorrhages and microaneurysms develop in the retinal periphery. Low-pressure retinopathy has been detected in 20% of patients with ICA occlusion (16,23). Reconstructive surgery is sometimes possible in the proximal neck arteries, and external carotid–internal carotid bypass may be helpful if the external carotid is spared.

Compensation becomes inadequate when both the external and internal carotid arteries are stenotic or occluded. Florid microaneurysms develop, and arteriovenous shunts form. Recurrent vitreous hemorrhage may lead to retinal detachment and blindness. Signs of anterior segment ischemia usually coexist: rubeosis of the iris, neovascular changes in the anterior chamber, secondary glaucoma, and cataract formation. At this stage, transcranial bypass is no longer practical.

In the majority of patients suffering from extensive occlusion of the major arteries arising from the aortic arch, the cause is severe atherosclerosis. In young women, the cause may be inflammatory arteritis of a type similar to that reported in Takayasu's arteritis. Such cases also may have ischemic exercise pain in jaw muscles from chewing. Amaurosis fugax type 2 also has been noted in giant-cell arteritis when a similar state of critical retinal perfusion exists (24).

Amaurosis fugax type 1 or type 2 may be the herald symptom of three common ocular strokes: CRA occlusion, occlusion of a branch retinal artery, and AION.

Amaurosis Fugax Type 3

The visual disturbance in amaurosis fugax type 3 is similar to that described for amaurosis fugax type 2, but the eye involved usually shows no persistent or progressive signs of impaired retinal perfusion. The mechanism suggested for amaurosis fugax type 3 is that of simple angiospasm of the ophthalmic, retinal, or choriodociliary circulation. This mechanism may explain the transient monocular visual aura and visual loss in cases of ocular migraine. Ocular migraine is rare, however, and the diagnosis should be made only after all other causes are excluded.

The following is a description of an episode of migrainous amaurosis fugax from a personal case:

> At the onset, floating bright, white lines were present, descending slowly from the top of the visual field over several seconds to involve the entire field. The lines slightly shimmered but neither pulsed nor flashed on and off. When the lines

reached the bottom of the field, the pattern changed to a persistent gray-white, speckled pattern that impaired vision. The patient said this pattern resembled the background design of the Ishihara plates after being shown the test plate 12 and also mentioned that it resembled the interference pattern on a television screen. At the time, however, believing that her vision was impaired because the eye lid was shut, the patient inspected her eyes in the mirror. No accompanying symptoms occurred, in particular, no eye or head pain. The episode cleared abruptly, over seconds, within 15 minutes of the onset and was described as being like "a lid being lifted off my vision." Sight returned to normal. Repeated stereotypic attacks occurred twice a day for nine days in spite of treatment with IV heparin. A carotid angiogram, erythrocyte sedimentation rate (ESR), and other investigations showed no abnormality. The patient had a positive family history for migraine but was not known to experience migraines herself.

In patients in whom the fundus has been observed during an amaurotic attack of migraine, retinal arteriolar and venous narrowing, retinal edema, venous dilatation, and delayed fluorescein filling of retinal vessels have been noted (25,26). Infarction results if retinal ischemia is severe. Rarely, migrainous patients may suffer a CRA occlusion (27) or anterior ischemic optic neuropathy.

Treatment of ocular migraine poses a problem, even though propranolol has been used successfully in both the acute and prophylactic treatment of classic migraine. Caution is warranted; a single case of migrainous CRA occlusion coincident with the initiation of propranolol therapy has been reported (27). Experimental evidence suggests that adrenergic mechanisms are involved in the pathophysiology of migraine (28) and that alpha-adrenergic receptors mediate vasoconstriction and beta-adrenergic receptors mediate vasodilatation. The pharmacologic effect of beta-blockers in peripheral vascular beds is to allow alpha-adrenergic action to be unopposed and thereby cause vasoconstriction. This pharmacologic effect may be potentiated, however, in the microcirculation to the eye because the CRA has a network of adrenergic nerve fibers superimposed on its muscular coats (29–31). Also, beta-blockade in treatment of amaurosis fugax type 3 may change the autonomic tone of the vessels and thereby exacerbate the vasoconstrictive phase of migrainous angiospasm and thus increase the risk of CRA occlusion.

Amaurosis Fugax Type 4

The classification of amaurosis fugax into types 1, 2, and 3 is based on my analysis of over 850 cases of amaurosis fugax. However, in this large population, another group of patients was identified who did not fit into any one of the defined types. Many of these cases were young adults under the age of 30 years who had no detectable abnormalities on comprehensive examinations. For example, in 1982, in a review of 209 of 850 unselected cases of amaurosis fugax, 23 (about 11%) of the 209 patients were 30 years or younger at the onset of their symptoms. Of those, 10 (about 43%) gave a history of more than 10 attacks when first seen. As might be expected, this percentage increased during the follow-up period because of recurrent transient monocular attacks. The type of visual disturbance in this young idiopathic group resembled most closely type 1, except in the duration of the attack, which frequently was too long (30 to 60 minutes) or too short (for seconds only). Rarely did the episodes resemble the temporary loss of contrast vision typical of amaurosis fugax type 2.

For practical purposes, this group of patients with idiopathic amaurosis fugax has been separated out and categorized as amaurosis fugax type 4. Such cases are thought to have a benign prognosis. A prospective study of this small group is underway. Follow-up of all idiopathic cases is essential, and the physician should keep an open mind as to the ultimate pathophysiology.

Sudden Permanent Visual Loss

Sudden permanent visual loss is the presenting complaint of a patient who has suffered an occlusion of the CRA.

Anterior ischemic optic neuropathy also may cause sudden visual loss and a persistent defect in the visual field (see chapter by Savino, *this volume*). Anterior ischemic optic neuropathy may occur in the eye ipsilateral to disease of the ICA.

Ischemic Eye Pain

Ischemic eye pain is relatively rare. It may occur in association with disease of the ophthalmic artery. The pain is experienced as a deep ache over the orbit, worse when the patient is in the upright position and relieved by recumbency. In severe occlusive disease of the ipsilateral internal and external carotid artery, ischemia of the eye may be profound, and eye pain may become constant.

References

1. Wilson IA, Warlow CP, Ross Russell RW: Cardiovascular disease in patients with retinal arterial occlusion. *Lancet* 1979;1:292–294.
2. Fisher CM: Transient monocular blindness associated with hemiplegia. *Am Arch Ophthalmol* 1952;47:167–203.
3. Warlow CP: Transient ischemic attacks, in Matthes WB, Glaser GH (eds): *Recent Advances in Clinical Neurology*. Edinburgh. Churchill-Livingstone, 1982, pp 191–214.
4. Cartlidge, NEF, Whisnant JP, Elveback LR, et al: Carotid and vertebral-basilar transient cerebral ischemic attacks: A community study, Rochester, MN. *Mayo Clin Proc* 1977;52:117–120.

5. Parkin PJ, Kendall BE, Marshall J, et al: Amaurosis fugax: Some aspects of management. *J Neurol Neurosurg Psychiatry* 1982;45:1–6.
6. Hollenhorst RW: The ocular manifestations of internal carotid arterial thrombosis. *Med Clin North Am* 1960;44:897–908.
7. Hollenhorst RW: Significance of bright plaques in the retinal arterioles *JAMA* 1961;178:123–129.
8. D'Cruz IA, Cohen HC, Prabhu R, et al: Clinical manifestations of mitral-annulus calcification, with emphasis on its echocardiographic features. *Am Heart J* 1977;94:367–377.
9. Guthrie J, Fairgrieve J: Aortic embolism due to myxoid tumor associated with myocardial calcification. *Br Heart J* 1963;25:137–140.
10. diBono DP, Warlow CP: Mitral-annulus calcification and cerebral or retinal ischemia. *Lancet* 1979;2:383–385.
11. Barnett HJM: Transient cerebral ischemia pathogenesis, prognosis and management. *AnnR Coll Physicians Surg* Canada 1974;7:153–173.
12. Barnett HJM: Delayed cerebral ischemic episodes distal to occlusion of major cerebral arteries. *Neurology* 1978;28:769–774.
13. Barnett HJM, Boughner DR, Cooper PF, et al: Further evidence relating mitral valve prolapse to cerebral ischemic events. *N Engl J Med* 1980;302:139–144.
14. Cogan DG, Wray SH: Vascular occlusions in the eye from cardiac myxomas. *Am J Ophthalmol* 1975;80:396–403.
15. Countee RW, Vijayanathan T, Chavis P: Recurrent retinal ischemia beyond cervical carotid occlusions. *J Neurosurg* 1981;55:532–542.
16. Kearns TP, Siekert RG, Sundt TM Jr: The ocular aspects of bypass surgery of the carotid artery. *Mayo Clin Proc* 1979;54:3–11.
17. Sundt TM Jr, Siekert RG, Piepgras DG, et al: Bypass surgery for vascular disease of the carotid system. *Mayo Clin Proc* 1976;51:677–692.
18. Whisnant JP: Extracranial-intracranial arterial bypass. *Neurology* 1978;28:209–210.
19. Weinberg PE, Patronas NJ, Kim KS, et al: Anomalous origin of the ophthalmic artery in a patient with amaurosis fugax. *Arch Neurol* 1981;38:315–317.
20. Furlan AJ, Whisnant JP, Kearns TP: Unilateral visual loss in bright light: An unusual symptom of carotid artery occlusive disease. *Arch Neurol* 1979;36:675–676.
21. Ross Russell RW, Page NGR: Critical perfusion of brain and retina. *Brain* 1983;106:419–434.
22. Kearns TP, Hollenhorst RW: Venous stasis retinopathy of occlusive disease of the carotid artery. *Mayo Clin Proc* 1963;38:304–312.
23. Edwards MS, Chater NL, Stanley JA: Reversal of chronic ocular ischemia by extracranial-intracranial arterial bypass: A case report. *Neurosurgery* 1980;7:480–483.
24. Hollenhorst RW: Effects of posture on retinal ischemia from temporal arteritis. *Trans Am Ophthalmol Soc* 1967;65:94–105.
25. Kline LB, Kelly CL: Ocular migraine in a patient with cluster headaches. *Headache* 1980;20:253–257.
26. Wolter JR, Burchfield WJ: Ocular migraine in a young man resulting in unilateral transient blindness and retinal edema. *J Pediatr Ophthalmol* 1971;8:173–176.
27. Katz B: Migrainous central retinal artery occlusion. *J Clin Neuro-ophthalmol* 1986;6:69–75.

28. Tokola R, Hokkanen E: Propranolol for acute migraine. *Br Med J* 1978;2:1089.
29. Ehinger B: Adrenergic nerves to the eye and to related structures in man and in the cynomolgus monkey. *Invest Ophthalmol Vis Sci* 1966;5:42–52.
30. Laties AM: Central retinal artery innervation. *Arch Ophthalmol* 1967;77:405–409.
31. Laties AM, Jacobowitz D: A comparative study of the autonomic innervation of the eye in monkey, cat, and rabbit. *Anat Rec* 1966;156:383–395.

CHAPTER 6

Occlusion of the Central Retinal Artery

Shirley H. Wray

The central retinal artery (CRA) is the feeder artery to the inner retinal layers of the eye and the only directly visible artery in the human body. Familiarity with the anatomic features of this artery is vital to an overall understanding of transient monocular visual loss, or amaurosis fugax. It is equally important to the understanding of sudden monocular blindness and ocular stroke.

The CRA usually arises as the first and smallest branch of the ophthalmic artery but the site, order, and mode of origin of this artery from the ophthalmic trunk may vary. (see chapter by Hayreh, *this volume*). To reach the optic nerve the CRA must penetrate the dural sheath, the vaginal space, and the optic nerve. Branches from the intravaginal and intraneural segment of the vessel provide an important nutrient circulation to the optic nerve anterior to the point of entry of the artery into the nerve.

To reach the fundus the CRA must penetrate the lamina cribrosa, an inelastic lattice of glial-lined collagen fibers at the level of the sclera. At this point the trunk of the CRA is probably at its narrowest, and the periarterial fibrous tissue presents a mechanical barrier to expansion of the artery. Most of the pathology responsible for disease of the CRA probably occurs at this location. This may well be the site of vulnerability for occlusion of the CRA by sclerotic, inflammatory, or embolic lesions. Unfortunately, the area cannot be visualized with the ophthalmoscope, and the retrobulbar central retinal artery cannot be imaged by carotid angiography. Therefore, symptoms must be interpreted with an anatomist's understanding of their place in the scheme of things.

Pathogenesis

There are five principle causes of occlusion of the CRA:

1. An embolic obstruction
2. Occlusion in situ in association with atheromatous disease when the narrowed arterial lumen becomes obliterated by superimposed thrombosis or hemorrhage (1)

3. A sequela of inflammatory endarteritis, such as temporal arteritis (2) thromboangiitis obliterans (3), polyarteritis nodosa with involvement of the choroidal and retinal arteries (4)
4. As the result of simple angiospasm, a rare cause that may be the mechanism of CRA occlusion associated with Raynaud's disease (5) or with migraine (6,7)
5. Arterial occlusion that occurs hydrostatically with either the high intraocular pressure (IOP) of glaucoma or with the low retinal blood pressure of carotid stenosis or the aortic arch syndrome or severe hypotension

Amaurosis fugax as a premonitory symptom of CRA occlusion suggests an embolic cause. In patients under the age of 40, the heart is the leading source of emboli (8) in association with rheumatic valvular disease or cardiac myxomata (9). In older patients, the source of the embolus may be cardiac (10), or it may be atheromatous ulceration of the aorta or the ipsilateral internal carotid artery (ICA).

What might be happening at the level of the CRA can be inferred if the following also are found on examination: (1) a retinal embolus with or without cardiac disease, (2) hypertension, and/or (3) disease of other arteries, notably the ophthalmic or temporal artery or the ICA in the neck. However, even in cases of embolic genesis, an embolus may not be seen because emboli frequently impact behind the lamina cribrosa.

Trauma is also an important cause of CRA occlusion. Compression of the globe may be self-inflicted in the setting of heavy alcohol and drug consumption followed by stupor (8,11). The spontaneous occurrence of this syndrome outside a hospital setting is unusual. Iatrogenic CRA occlusion has been reported of patients undergoing surgery where prolonged pressure to the orbit has occurred inadvertently in association with a period of hypotension during anesthesia (12,13).

Clinical Presentation

Occlusion of the CRA causes an infarction in the glioneuronal layer of the retina down to and including part of the bipolar cell layer. Such an ocular stroke is a medical emergency. Sudden blindness with persistent visual loss is the major symptom, but, occasionally, amaurosis fugax is the herald symptom. Pain in the eye rarely occurs. If present and severe, it suggests involvement of the ophthalmic artery.

Blindness is confirmed by failure of the pupil to react to light. If, however, a portion of the retina is supplied by a cilioretinal artery fed from the choroidal circulation, perception of light or hand movement may be preserved in a small central segment of the visual field.

Diagnosis

The diagnosis of CRA occlusion is usually straightforward. Arrest of the retinal arterial circulation, partial or complete, produces unmistakable ophthalmoscopic signs. What is seen depends on how soon after the occlusion the examiner has the opportunity to look. If the fundus is examined within the first few minutes while the occlusion persists, the most striking finding is the presence of discontinuity in the circulation of the retina. Segmentation of the blood column (box-car segmentation) with slow streaming of the flow is present in the veins. The blood in the arteries is dark, and a few areas may show segmentation (clear areas alternating with areas where the cells appear clumped together), but this is nowhere so obvious as in the veins. Frequently, ophthalmoscopy is not performed within the first hour or so, by which time the circulation may be restored. Inspection of the fundus then shows surprisingly little. Typically, the disk shows no more than mild pallor, and the arteries are only slightly attenuated. Gentle digital pressure on the globe (digital ophthalmodynamometry) during ophthalmoscopy nevertheless may elicit segmentation of the blood column, indicating the presence of a slow, but not completely arrested, circulation.

Another subtle sign of diminished flow in the CRA is the type of collapse induced in the artery by gentle pressure on the globe. Instead of demonstrating the crisp pulsation that occurs normally when the IOP exceeds the retinal diastolic pressure, the obstructed artery may merely collapse and show a comparatively slow refill as the pressure is removed (14). Total obstruction posterior to the lamina cribrosa is present if no pulsation is observed in the retinal arteries upon increasing globe pressure. Restoration of normal pulsation indicates removal of the obstruction, a useful sign in evaluating therapy.

In the normal eye, the systolic and diastolic opthalmic artery pressure (OAPs) are 80/40 to 90/50 mm Hg (Bailliart ophthalmodynamometer) in a normotensive patient with normal IOP. Reproducible differences of 15% or more between the two eyes is quite significant, but a difference of 20% to 25% is diagnostic of ipsilateral carotid insufficiency on the side of the lower pressure.

Measuring systemic blood pressure and IOP is important. When obstruction of the CRA is secondary to occlusion of the ophthalmic artery, the IOP will be pathologically low, in the range of 4 to 6 mm Hg instead of 20 mm Hg.

Complete occlusion of the CRA that lasts one hour or more, causes an infarction in the retina. Cloudy swelling of the ganglion cells causes loss of transparency, and the retina appears milky-white, especially in the thickest region around the macula. The opalescent halo accentuates the normal fovea, an area devoid of ganglion cells, through which the red choroidal color is transmitted. This gives the appearance of a central cherry-red spot (Fig. 6–1; see color plate).

Within several days the retinal opacification disappears. The ischemic ganglion cells disintegrate and death of the cell, as evidenced by loss of the pattern electroretinogram, occurs (Wray, unpublished data). Optic atrophy of the primary type develops with loss of the retinal nerve fiber layer.

Differential Diagnosis

The differential diagnosis of sudden persistent monocular visual loss includes AION, acute occlusion of the central retinal vein, detachment of the retina, acute closed-angle glaucoma, sudden vitreous or macular hemorrhage, and factitious visual loss.

Diagnostic Approach

The approach to the patient with sudden persistent loss of vision and a suspected occlusion of the CRA follows the classic format of the complete elucidation of a history followed by physical examination. Each question or step in the ordered examination is structured to provide information on which subsequent steps are based. The initial question, "Is the occlusion acute (less than 24 hours) or chronic?" is critically important because immediate ophthalmic treatment and/or steroid therapy must be undertaken in selected cases in an effort to restore vision.

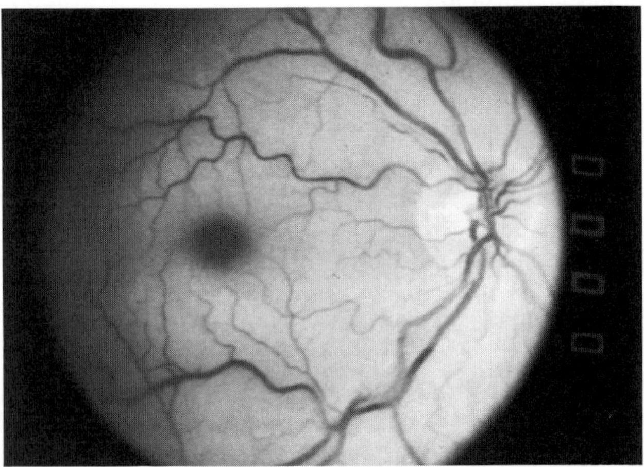

FIGURE 6–1. Opacification of the retina and macula cherry red spot following occlusion of the central retinal artery. For color reproduction of this figure, see frontispiece.

Treatment

The appropriate treatment for CRA occlusion is controversial, no doubt because only anecdotal evidence points to the efficacy of the maneuvers currently used (15,16). Some ophthalmologists never attempt treatment even when the case is diagnosed within the first few minutes to hours after the acute event—clearly the ideal time for emergency intervention.

However, a CRA occlusion or ocular stroke must be equated with a major cerebral stroke, and therapy should begin immediately in most patients. Heroic measures should be taken urgently, even if 24 hours have elapsed. Gratifying recovery of vision has been reported in eyes treated 6, 8, and 12 hours after the event (15,17).

The therapeutic regimen used is designed to increase retinal blood flow by the reduction of pressure intracular and by dilatation of the retinal vasculature. Intraocular pressure is lowered by means of digital massage of the globe, anterior chamber paracentesis, and administration of agents that block aqueous secretion. Vasodilatation is produced by inducing a buildup of carbon dioxide by means of rebreathing into a paper bag or inhaling a carbogen mixture (95% oxygen and 5% carbon dioxide) and by injecting vasodilator agents retrobulbarly. Anterior chamber paracentesis appears to be the most efficacious. The sudden drop in ocular pressure may dislodge an impacted embolus from behind the lamina cribrosa, promote distal migration of visible retinal emboli, and restore some vision within minutes of the procedure.

Heparin anticoagulation is useful in the treatment of impending CRA occlusion, and systemic steroids are essential in the therapy of suspected inflammatory arteritis. There is no rationale for using these drugs or systemic vasodilators in patients with a completed nonarteritic CRA occlusion.

Prognosis for Vision

The prognosis for vision in untreated cases of occlusion of the CRA is extremely poor. After the acute event the affected eye is usually blind and only a few eyes retain vision.

The prognosis for visual recovery is also bad. The ultimate level of visual function can be predicted fairly accurately because it correlates closely with the severity of the acute visual loss and the extent of the visual field deficit. Data suggest that more than 50% of eyes have no useful visual acuity left, and 30% lack light perception. In most cases, the visual field loss is profound, and the field unchartable even to a large isopter. In less than one third of affected eyes, a very small remnant of field remains, usually in the temporal periphery.

A central scotoma with an intact peripheral field in an eye lacking a cilioretinal artery is a rare residual defect after CRA occlusion (Wray, unpublished data). Such central scotomata may be the result simply of a temporal factor.

Associated Cardiovascular Disease

Heart disease is frequently present in patients with CRA occlusion. In a retrospective study of patients with CRA occlusion Appen et al (8) found that 30% of younger and 23% of older patients had associated cardiac valvular disease. In a prospective study (18), 56% of patients under the age of 50 had a potential cardiac source of embolism, compared with 24% in the older age group. Aortic stenosis was the most frequent lesion, but mitral leaflet prolapse was an isolated finding in 10 patients. The data emphasize the vital importance of careful cardiac assessment, especially in young patients.

Occlusion of the CRA also may be a consequence of disease in situ. Potentiation of atheroma in the ophthalmic or central retinal artery by hypertension accounts for some cases, and a significantly greater prevalence of hypertension in patients with CRA occlusion has been noted in comparison with patients with an occlusion of a retinal branch artery (18). The data suggest a different pathogenic mechanism in the two ocular stroke groups (Tables 6–1 and 6–2).

Associated Major Artery Disease

Ophthalmic Artery

The prevalence of disease of the ophthalmic artery in CRA occlusion is, regrettably, unknown, even though this vessel is readily visualized angiographically.

Obstruction of the ophthalmic artery produces the classic signs of a CRA occlusion, accompanied acutely by a marked reduction in the IOP. To confirm the site of the arterial block (ie, occlusion of the ophthalmic artery trunk *v* an isolated distal occlusion of the CRA), a noninvasive test can be used, the flash electroretinogram (FERG). In blockage of the ophthalmic artery with associated CRA occlusion, the FERG is severely reduced or absent because of infarction of the outer retinal layers supplied by the short ciliary branches of the ophthalmic artery in addition to infarction of the inner glioneuronal layer. With a patent ophthalmic artery and occlusion confined to the distal CRA, only the inner retinal layers are infarcted, and the outer retinal layers are preserved. In this situation the FERG is affected only minimally (19).

TABLE 6–1. Preceding vascular events in occlusion of branch and central retinal artery arteries.

	Retinal artery occlusion	
Preceding event	Branch*	Central†
Amaurosis fugax	12 (18)	4 (11)
Transient cerebral ischemia	8 (12)	1 (3)
Stroke	2 (3)	4 (11)
Ischemic heart disease	15 (22)	2 (6)
Claudication	5 (7)	2 (6)

* 43 male, 25 female patients; mean age 55. Numbers in parentheses are percentages.
† 23 male, 12 female patients; mean age 36.
Based on data in Wilson LA, Warlow CP, Ross Russell RW: Cardiovascular disease in patients with retinal artery occlusion. *Lancet* 1979; 1:292–294.

TABLE 6–2. Clinical findings in occlusion of branch and central retinal arteries

	Retinal artery occlusion	
Clinical finding	Branch (n = 68)	Central (n = 35)
Hypertension	17 (25)*	20 (57)
Carotid bruit	12 (18)	5 (14)
Visible retinal embolus	46 (68)	4 (11)
Cardiac valvular abnormality	23 (34)	6 (17)

* Numbers in parentheses are percentages.
Based on data in Wilson LA, Warlow CP, Ross Russell RW: Cardiovascular disease in patients with retinal artery occlusion. *Lancet* 1979; 1:292–294.

Temporal Artery

Occlusion of the CRA occurs in 5% to 10% of elderly patients with temporal arteritis, even in the absence of classic cranial and systemic symptoms. Risk of blindness in the fellow eye is extremely high, and all cases warrant immediate measurement of the Westergren ESR, which, if elevated, indicates the need for steroid therapy and a temporal artery biopsy. Immediate steroid therapy also is advisable when the clinical index of suspicion is high for temporal arteritis in the presence of a normal ESR, pending estimation of the blood fibrinogen level and the result of the biopsy.

Internal Carotid Artery

The association between CRA occlusion and extracranial ICA disease has not been clearly delineated. In one study (20), significant ICA disease was found by carotid angiography in nine out of nine patients who had CRA occlusion. Three patients had complete occlusion of the ICA on the same side, four had significant stenosis, and three had evidence of an ulcerated plaque.

In a second report (21) of 62 patients with CRA occlusion, 25 of whom underwent carotid angiography, 56% (14/25) had ipsilateral extracranial internal carotid disease. Somewhat surprisingly, these patients generally did not have carotid bruits and had normal findings on noninvasive carotid tests. Ten of these 14 underwent ipsilateral carotid endarterectomy; they had either an embologenic ulcerated plaque or tight ICA stenosis. In this study, 11 patients had normal angiograms and 13 who did not undergo angiography had clinical evidence of other etiologic factors. The remaining 24 patients had no diagnostic workup. Unfortunately, follow-up data (mean 34 months) was reported in only six cases who underwent endarterectomy. No strokes were reported.

Occlusion of the CRA in complete occlusion of the ipsilateral ICA may be due to propagation of thrombus from the carotid syphon into the ophthalmic artery (22). Combined data (7,20,23) suggest that if no cause is apparent clinically for the retinal stroke, and no alternative cause is evident, it is likely that the ipsilateral carotid artery is occluded or stenosed or ulcerated and that one patient in seven will go on to have an ipsilateral stroke.

Prevention

Hypertension is an important factor in the genesis of all strokes. The early detection of hypertension, its vigorous treatment, and close surveillance might be expected to reduce the increasing prevalence of CRA occlusion. Prompt treatment of other associated cardiovascular and systemic diseases also may be beneficial, together with early recognition of operable occlusive ICA disease in the late decades of life.

References

1. Dahrling BE: The histopathology of early central retinal artery occlusion. *Arch Ophthalmol* 1965;73:506–510.
2. Cullen JF: Occult temporal arteritis. *Trans Ophthalmol Soc UK* 1963;83:725–736
3. Gresser EB: Partial occlusion of retinal vessels in a case of thromboangitis obliterans. *Am J Ophthalmol* 1932;15:235–237.
4. Goldsmith J: Periarteritis nodosa with involvement of the choroidal and retinal arteries. *Am J Ophthalmol* 1946;29:435–446.

5. Anderson RG, Gray EB: Spasm of the central retinal artery in Raynaud's disease. *Arch Ophthalmol* 1937;17:662–665.
6. Krapin D: Occlusion of the central retinal artery in migraine. *N Engl J Med* 1964;270:359–360.
7. Katz B: Migrainous central retinal artery occlusion. *J Clin Neuro-ophthalmol* 1986;6:69–75.
8. Appen RE, Wray SH, Cogan DG: Central retinal artery occlusion. *Am J Ophthalmol* 1975;79:374–381.
9. Cogan DG, Wray SH: Vascular occlusions in the eye from cardiac myxomas. *Am J Ophthalmol* 1975;80:396–403.
10. Zimmerman LE: Embolism of central retinal artery secondary to myocardial infarction with mural thrombosis. *Arch Ophthalmol* 1965;73:822–826.
11. Jayam AV, Hass WK, Carr RE, et al: Saturday night retinopathy. *J Neurol Sci* 1974;22:413–418.
12. Givner I, Jaffe N: Occlusion of the central retinal artery following anesthesia. *Arch Ophthalmol* 1950;43:197–201.
13. Hollenhorst RW, Svien HJ, Benoit CF: Unilateral blindness occurring during anesthesia for neurosurgical operation. *Arch Ophthalmol* 1954;52:819–830.
14. Cogan DG: *Ophthalmic Manifestations of Systemic Vascular Disease. Major Problems in Internal Medicine*. Philadelphia, WB Saunders Co, 1974, vol 3, p 102.
15. Stone R, Zink H, Klingele T, et al: Visual recovery after central retinal artery occlusion: Two cases. *Ann Ophthalmol* 1977;9:445–450.
16. Burde RM, Savino PJ, Trobe JD: *Clinical Decisions in Neuro-Ophthalmology*. St Louis, The CV Mosby Co, 1985, p 53.
17. Castracane S, Wray SH: Amaurosis fugax, temporal arteritis and carotid disease. *Neurology* 1987 (in preparation).
18. Wilson LA, Warlow CP, Ross Russell RW: Cardiovascular disease in patients with retinal arterial occlusion. *Lancet* 1979;1:292–294.
19. Henkes HE: Electroretinography in circulatory disturbances of the retina: II. The electroretinogram in cases of occlusion of the central retinal artery or of one of its branches. *Arch Ophthalmol* 1954;51:42–53.
20. Kollarits CR, Lubow M, Hissong SL: Retinal strokes: I. Incidence of carotid atheromata. *JAMA* 1972;222:1273–1275.
21. Sheng FC, Quinones-Baldrich W, Machleder HI, et al: Relationship of extracranial carotid occlusive disease and central retinal artery occlusion. *Am J Surg* 1986;152:175–178.
22. Ross Russell RW: Observations on the retinal blood vessels in monocular blindness. *Lancet* 1961;2:1422–1428.
23. Savino PJ, Glaser JS, Cassady J: Retinal stroke: Is the patient at risk? *Arch Ophthalmol* 1977;95:1185–1189.

CHAPTER 7

Retinal Cholesterol Emboli and Retinal Stroke

Peter J. Savino

Amaurosis fugax is a dramatic occurrence of partial or total monocular visual loss that lasts less than 10 minutes. This transient visual loss may be due to hypoperfusion (eg, arrhythmia or steal syndromes), thrombosis (eg, giant-cell arteritis), or embolus. The source of the embolic material may be the heart (atrial myxoma, intracardiac hematoma), heart valves (rheumatic heart disease, mitral valve prolapse), or carotid atheromas.

Fisher's description (1) of the intra-arterial material observed on funduscopy during an episode of amaurosis fugax lent credence to embolism as the cause of amaurosis fugax. Hollenhorst (2) described bright, orange plaques in retinal arterioles of patients with vascular disease and suggested that these plaques originated at the ulcerated atheroma within the ICA. He described the emboli of this origin as having a characteristic appearance. David et al (3) proved that these bright plaques were composed of cholesterol and that carotid atheromas were the source.

The pendulum now has swung to the point where all patients with amaurosis fugax are suspected of having thromboembolic disease of the ipsilateral ICA, are investigated for this, and often are subjected to carotid endarterectomy as prophylaxis for further retinal or cerebral stroke. Although the efficacy of this surgical procedure in accomplishing these aims never has been established unequivocally, a huge increase has occurred in the number of these procedures performed annually.

Retinal stroke or amaurosis fugax is assumed to have the same prognostic significance with regard to cerebral stroke as cerebral TIAs do. However, the true prevalence may be lower. Recent data have indicated that the risk for stroke after a bonafide episode of amaurosis fugax is 1.8% per year, well below the 5%–10% per year that occurs after cerebral TIAs (4).

When considering the patient with retinal emboli (with or without retinal stroke), the question arises whether the presence (or absence) of visible retinal emboli has prognostic significance with respect to the occurrence of stroke or to life expectancy.

Pfaffenbach and Hollenhorst (5) have discussed the morbidity and survival of patients with cholesterol crystals. They noted that 15% of such patients died within 1 year, 29% within 3 years, and 54% within 7 years; the majority of deaths were due to coronary artery disease. Cerebral ischemic phenomena (completed strokes or TIAs) were present in 131 (63%) of 208 patients before or concurrent with observed cholesterol crystals, and 26 additional patients subsequently developed ischemic conditions. Of 94 patients with completed strokes, the strokes were in the cerebral hemisphere ipsilateral to the retinal emboli in 63%, contralateral in 19%, and in the vertebrobasilar arterial system in 13%.

Savino et al (6) examined patients with retinal arterial occlusive disease and/or the presence of bright plaques in the retinal arterioles. The observation of a bright plaque was associated with decreased survival for the 49 patients studied (Fig. 7–1). Patients with retinal arterial occlusion but no emboli had a likelihood of survival identical to that of the control population (Fig. 7–2). The major finding, however, was that patients died of cardiac causes more frequently than of stroke.

This finding was confirmed in a prospective study that examined the cardiac status of patients with TIAs or mild strokes. Twenty-nine of the 50 patients studied had significant coronary artery disease, compared with a 7% prevalence of the condition in other patients of similar age at the same institution (7). It appears, therefore, that patients with retinal emboli are at greater risk of early death independent of the degree of their retinal arteriolar occlusion. This risk and decreased survival is due to coronary artery disease more often than to stroke.

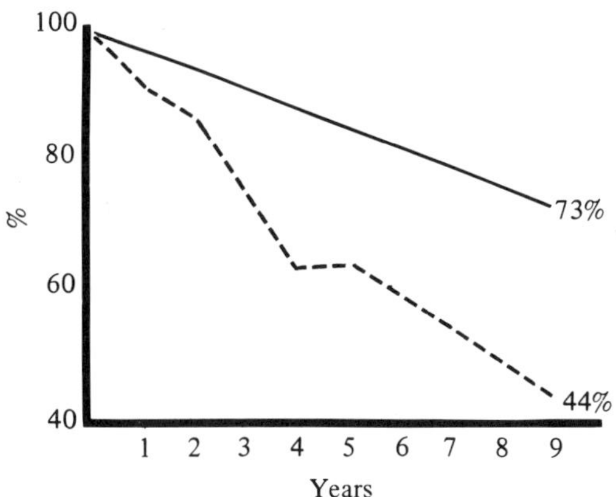

FIGURE 7–1. Survival of 49 patients with visible retinal emboli (dashed line) in retinal arterial occlusive disease compared with an age- and sex-matched control population (solid line).

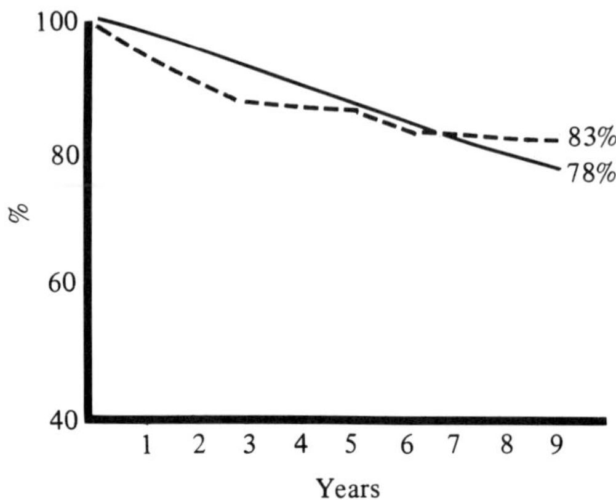

FIGURE 7–2. Survival of 37 patients with retinal arterial occlusions without visible retinal emboli (dashed line) compared with an age- and sex-matched control population (solid line).

References

1. Fisher CM: Observations of the fundus oculi in transient monocular blindness. *Neurology* 1959;9:333–347.
2. Hollenhorst RW: Significance of bright plaques in the retinal arterioles. *JAMA* 1961;178:23–29.
3. David NJ, Klintworth GK, Friedberg SJ, et al: Fatal atheromatous cerebral embolism associated with bright plaques in the retinal arterioles. *Neurology* 1963;13:708–713.
4. Poole CJM, Ross Russell RW: Mortality and stroke after amaurosis fugax. *J Neurol Neurosurg Psychiatry* 1985;48:902–905.
5. Pfaffenbach DD, Hollenhorst RW: Morbidity and survivorship of patients with embolic cholesterol crystalization in the ocular fundus. *Am J Ophthalmol* 1973;75:66–72.
6. Savino PJ, Glaser JS, Cassady J: Retinal stroke: Is the patient at risk? *Arch Ophthalmol* 1977;95:1185–1189.
7. Rokey R, Rolak LA, Harati Y, et al: Coronary artery disease in patients with cerebrovascular disease: A prospective study. *Ann Neurol* 1984;16:50–53.

CHAPTER 8

Acute Ischemia of the Optic Nerve

Sohan Singh Hayreh

Acute ischemia of the anterior part of the optic nerve is one of the most common causes of impaired vision in persons past middle age—a fact not fully appreciated by most physicians. I have called it *anterior ischemic optic neuropathy* (AION) (1). In contrast, I have designated acute ischemic lesions of the posterior part of the optic nerve as *posterior ischemic optic neuropathy* (PION) (2); this is, as far as one can tell, much less common than AION. Acute ischemia of the optic nerve, particularly of the optic nerve head, is an important cause of amaurosis fugax, which commonly is seen with giant-cell or temporal arteritis (3–9) and with marked optic disk edema due to raised intracranial pressure (10–23) or any other etiology. In these cases the development of amaurosis fugax is an ominous sign of impending AION and permanent visual loss in that eye, particularly in patients with giant-cell arteritis in whom blindness may occur within the next few hours or several days. Amaurosis fugax in these cases frequently is precipitated by a change in posture, e.g., suddenly standing up from a prone position (orthostatic hypotension) or stooping. Thus, the onset of amaurosis fugax in these conditions is usually a sign of impending AION and visual disaster.

Clinical Diagnosis

I have published detailed accounts of the clinical findings in AION and PION elsewhere (2, 7, 8, 24–30); briefly these are as follows:

(a) AION: It is easy to diagnose because of the classic symptomatology and clinical findings. Typically a sudden, painless visual loss is usually detected on waking up in the morning, optic disk-related visual field defects occur with normal to markedly defective visual acuity, and optic disk edema is usually seen with splinter hemorrhage(s) at the disc margin during the initial stages (Fig. 8–1); optic atrophy occurs after about 2 months.

(b) PION: A combination of the following findings is highly suggestive of this condition: sudden onset of monocular visual disturbance, with or

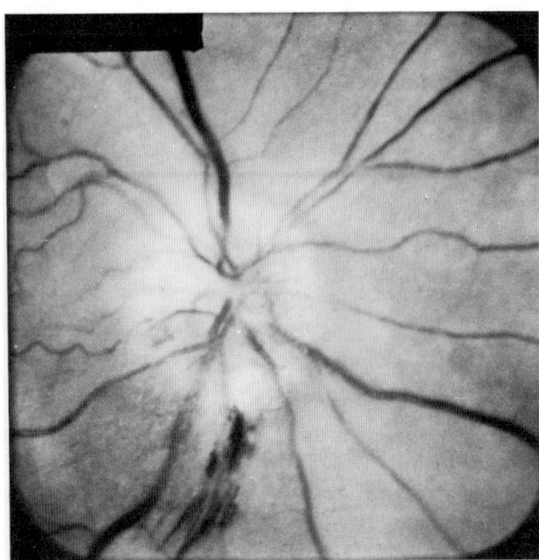

FIGURE 8–1. Right eye of a 61-year-old man with nonarteritic AION, inferior altitudinal hemianopia of sudden onset 10 days previously, visual acuity 6/12, and optic disk edema with a splinter hemorrhage. [Reproduced from Hayreh SS, 1975 (8).]

without deterioration of central visual acuity, optic nerve-related visual field defects in the involved eye, a normal optic disk and no other fundus abnormality at onset, but developing optic atrophy 5 to 6 weeks later. It is difficult to make a firm diagnosis of PION until other possible causes of the visual loss have been ruled out carefully.

For a proper understanding of the acute ischemic disorders of the optic nerve, it is imperative to understand the arterial supply of the optic nerve.

Arterial Supply of the Optic Nerve

I have discussed this in detail elsewhere (8, 31–36). Following is a very brief account. For a discussion of the arterial supply of the optic nerve, the nerve can be divided into anterior and posterior parts. The anterior part of the optic nerve can be subdivided further into (a) the optic nerve head and (b) anterior orbital segment. The posterior part of the optic nerve consists of the rest of the orbital part, and intracanalicular and intracranial parts.

Arterial Supply of the Anterior Part of the Optic Nerve (Figs. 8–2, 8–3)

(a) The optic nerve head: From back to front the optic nerve head consists of (Fig. 8–2):

(i) The region of the lamina cribrosa: This is continuous on the sides with the sclera. It is supplied by centripetal branches from the short posterior ciliary arteries (PCAs) and in a few cases by the so-called arterial circle of Zinn and Haller. Contrary to the prevalent impression, the circle

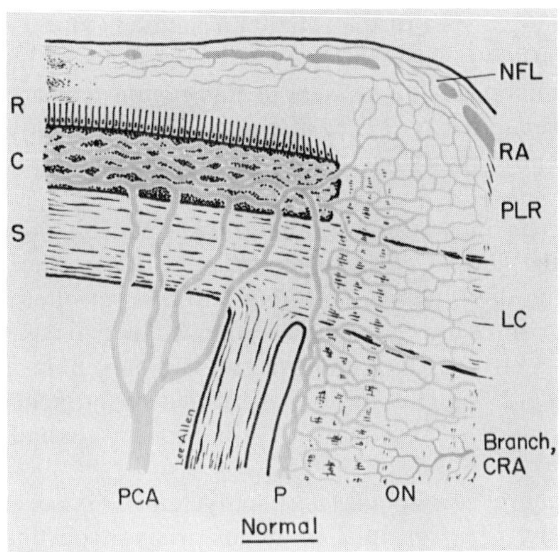

FIGURE 8–2. Schematic representation of blood supply of the optic nerve head and retrolaminar optic nerve. [Reproduced from Hayreh SS, 1978 (35).] For color reproduction of this figure, see frontispiece.

Abbreviations used in Figs. 8–2 to 8–4: A, arachnoid; Ant. Sup. Hyp. Art., anterior superior hypophyseal artery; C, choroid; CAR and CRA, central retinal artery; Col. Br., collateral branches; CRV, central retinal vein; C2, circle of Zinn and Haller; D, dura; ICA, internal carotid artery; LC, lamina cribrosa; LPCA, lateral posterior ciliary artery; Med. Mus., medial muscular artery; MPCA, medial posterior ciliary artery; NFL, surface nerve fiber layer of the disk; OA, ophthalmic artery; OD, optic disk; ON, optic nerve; P, pia; PCA, posterior ciliary artery; PR and PLR, prelaminar region; R, retina; RA, retinal arteriole; Rec. Br. CZ, recurrent pial branches from peripapillary choroid/CZ; S, sclera; SAS, subarachnoid space.

of Zinn and Haller is an uncommon finding in the human eye and, when seen, usually is an incomplete circle. The central retinal artery gives off no branches in this region.

(ii) The prelaminar region: This is situated in front of the lamina cribrosa, at the level of the choroid and outer layers of the retina. Essentially, it is supplied by centripetal branches from the peripapillary choroidal arteries. This region also may receive some contribution from the vessels in the region of the lamina cribrosa. No branches arise from the central retinal artery in this region. Fluorescein angiographic studies strongly suggest that the temporal part of the prelaminar region is much more vascular than the rest and that it receives a maximum contribution from the adjacent peripapillary choroid.

(iii) The surface nerve fiber layer: The nerve fibers from the retina converge to this area to bend posteriorly to form the optic nerve. This layer of nerve fibers contains the main retinal vessels and a large number of capillaries that are a part of the retinal circulation. Thus, this part of the optic nerve head is supplied mainly by branches from the retinal arterioles. It is not uncommon to find vessels in this region that are derived from the adjacent prelaminar part (i.e. of choroidal origin—mostly in the temporal sector); these may arise from the cilioretinal arteries, when those are present.

(b) The anterior intraorbital segment: This part includes the area extending from the lamina cribrosa to the point where the central retinal artery enters the optic nerve, i.e., about 10 mm retrobulbar optic nerve (Fig. 8–3). This part of the optic nerve is supplied by two vascular systems:

(i) The axial centrifugal vascular system: It is present in 75% and absent in the remaining 25%. This system is formed by branches arising from the intraneural part of the central retinal artery (usually one to four branches).

(ii) The peripheral centripetal vascular system: This is seen in all nerves and is formed by recurrent pial branches arising from the peripapillary choroid and the circle of Zinn and Haller (when it is present), and by pial branches from the central retinal artery and from the collateral branches of the ophthalmic artery or of its various intraorbital branches (Figs. 8–3, 8–4). Because the retrolaminar region of the anterior intraorbital part of the optic nerve is supplied mainly by the recurrent pial branches from the peripapillary choroid and/or circle of Zinn and Haller, it forms an integral part of the optic nerve head (Fig. 8–2).

Arterial Supply of the Posterior Part of the Optic Nerve (Figs. 8–3, 8–4)

There is no centrifugal vascular system in this region except very rarely when for 1 to 4 mm adjacent to the anterior orbital segment a small recurrent branch from the central retinal artery may run posteriorly in the center of the optic nerve and give centrifugal branches. The entire posterior part of the optic nerve is supplied by the peripheral centripetal vascular system. This is formed by the pial vessels, which in turn come from the collateral arteries usually arising directly from the ophthalmic artery and less commonly from its intraorbital branches (Figs. 8–3, 8–4). No strict division exists between the pial branches of the anterior and posterior segments of the optic nerve.

Anterior Ischemic Optic Neuropathy

This account is based essentially on my prospective clinical studies on over 500 cases of this disorder, and on experimental studies in primates (1, 2, 8, 14, 26–30, 36–39). It is important to have a complete understanding of the marked inter-individual variation in the blood supply of the anterior

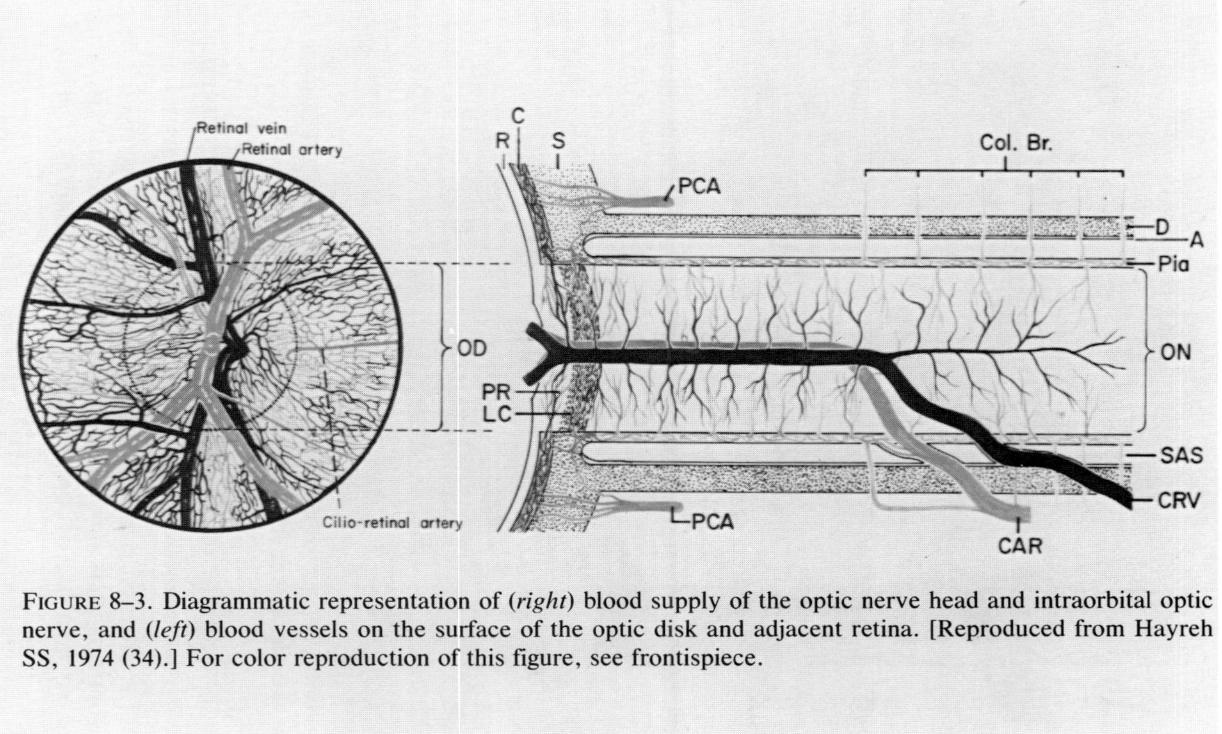

FIGURE 8–3. Diagrammatic representation of (*right*) blood supply of the optic nerve head and intraorbital optic nerve, and (*left*) blood vessels on the surface of the optic disk and adjacent retina. [Reproduced from Hayreh SS, 1974 (34).] For color reproduction of this figure, see frontispiece.

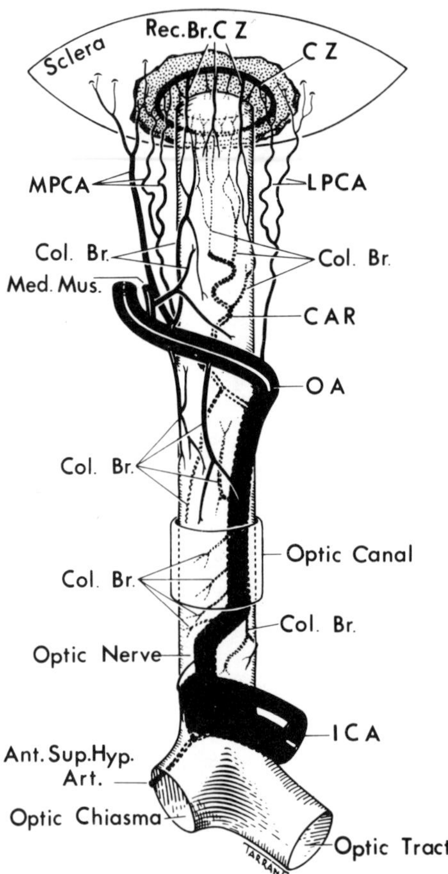

FIGURE 8–4. Diagrammatic representation of peripheral arterial supply of the optic nerve, as seen from above. [Reproduced from Hayreh SS: *Br J Ophthalmol* 1963;47:651–663.]

part of the optic nerve, because these variations exercise a profound influence on the pathogenesis and other features of AION.

Inter-Individual Variation in the Blood Supply of the Anterior Part of the Optic Nerve

The general impression that the pattern of blood supply of the anterior part of the optic nerve is almost identical in all eyes, and that all ischemic lesions are explainable from one standard vascular patterns, *is a fundamental error,* which is responsible for a good deal of confusion. The anatomic pattern of blood supply to this part of the optic nerve shows marked inter-individual variations, so that each optic nerve has a virtually unique pattern. The subject of inter-individual variation is discussed at length elsewhere (36). Briefly, the various factors which produce this variation include:

Variation in the Anatomic Pattern of the Arterial Supply

The usual anatomic pattern is described above and is shown in Figs. 8–2 to 8–4. However, there are tremendous variations in the anatomic pattern and some of the differences in the vascular anatomy reported in the literature (35) can be explained on this basis. I studied the anatomical pattern in one hundred human specimens and no two specimens had identical patterns, not even the two eyes of the same individual (40, 41). This clearly shows the fallacy of considering the anatomic vascular pattern of the optic nerve as identical in all humans.

Variations in the Pattern of PCA Circulation

From the account of the arterial supply of the optic nerve given above, it is evident that PCAs, via the peripapillary choroid or the short PCAs, are the main source of blood supply to the anterior part of the optic nerve. In view of that, the following variations in the PCAs would profoundly influence the blood supply:

(a) Variations in number of PCAs supplying an eye: There may be one to five, but the usual number is 2 to 3 PCAs supplying an eye, as discussed elsewhere (33, 42, 43).

(b) Variations in the area of supply by each PCA and in the location of the watershed zones between the various PCAs: My clinical and experimental studies have clearly demonstrated that the various PCAs act as end-arteries (44, 45). The border between the territories of distribution of any two end-arteries is called the *watershed zone*. The location of the watershed zone between the various PCAs depends upon the area of supply by each PCA. My fluorescein fundus angiographic studies in man have shown that when there are two PCAs (i.e. medial and lateral), there is a wide variation in the area supplied by the two PCAs (25, 28, 36, 44–46), and their supply in the posterior part of the fundus (including the anterior part of the optic nerve) varies accordingly (Figs. 8–5 to 8–11); also, the locations of the watershed zone between them may be anywhere between the fovea and the nasal peripapillary region (Figs. 8–8 to 8–12). Thus, the location of the watershed zone in relation to the optic nerve head varies markedly from eye to eye. Fig. 8–13 illustrates some of these locations. The importance of the location of the watershed zone lies in the fact that in the event of a fall in the perfusion pressure in the vascular bed supplied by the end arteries, the watershed zone, which is an area of comparatively poor vascularity, is most vulnerable to ischemic disorders. In our studies on patients with AION, we have found ample evidence that the area of

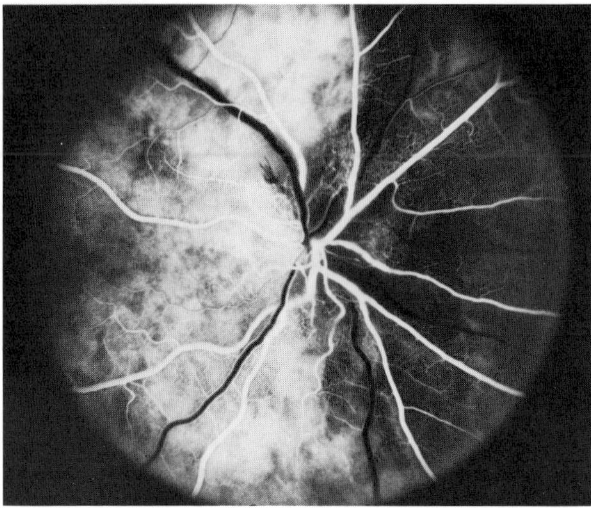

FIGURE 8–5. Fluorescein fundus angiogram of right eye of a 75-year-old man with AION (results of a temporal artery biopsy showed no arteritis), shows normal filling of the area supplied by the lateral PCA (including the temporal half of the optic disk) but no filling of the area supplied by the medial PCA. [Reproduced from Hayreh SS, 1985 (36).]

the optic nerve involved depends upon the location of the watershed zone and distribution of the PCAs in relation to the optic disk (Figs. 8–5 to 8–7 and 8–9 to 8–11). The part of the optic nerve situated in the watershed zone is highly susceptible to ischemia. If the optic nerve head is supplied by only one PCA, and that PCA has poor blood flow, the optic nerve is

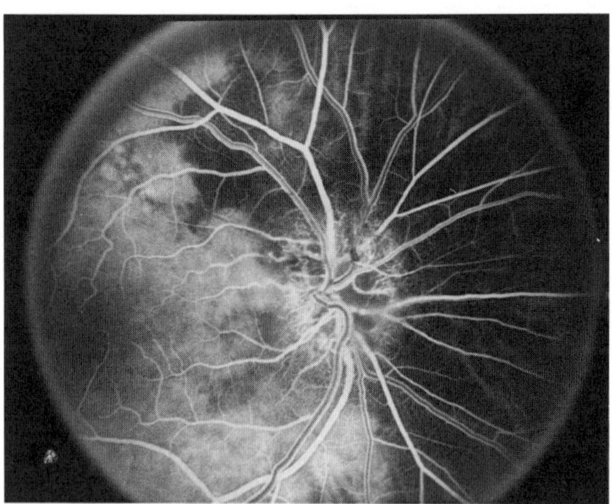

FIGURE 8–6. Fluorescein fundus angiogram of right eye of an 82-year-old man with arteritic AION shows normal filling of the area supplied by the lateral PCA (including the temporal ¼ of the optic disk) but no filling of the area supplied by the medial PCA (including the nasal ¾ of the disk). [Reproduced from Hayreh SS, 1978 (25).]

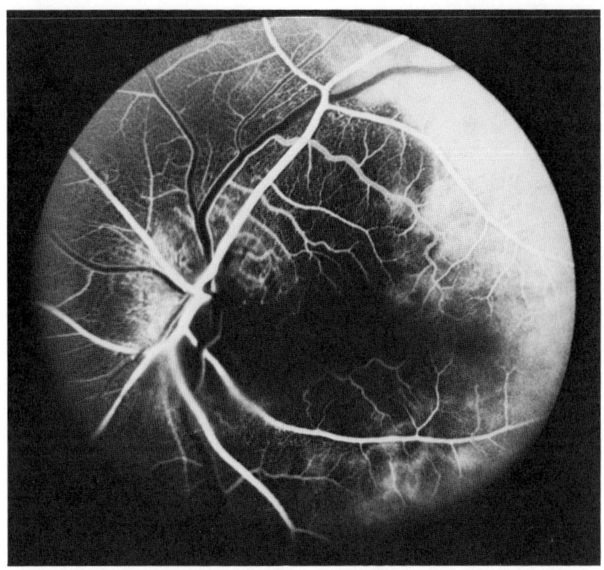

FIGURE 8–7. Fluorescein fundus angiogram of left eye of a 63-year-old woman with arteritic AION shows normal filling of the area supplied by the lateral PCA but no filling of the area supplied by the medial PCA (including the entire optic disk). [Reproduced from Hayreh SS, 1978 (25).]

susceptible to ischemia; however, if the PCA supplying the nerve has normal blood flow, in spite of the other PCAs having poor or no blood flow, the disk is not vulnerable to ischemia.

(c) Difference in blood flow in various PCAs as well as short PCAs: Our clinical and experimental studies have indicated that the mean blood pressures in the various PCAs may be different in health as well as in disease (36). In the event of a fall of perfusion pressure, the vascular bed supplied by one artery may be affected earlier and more than the others.

Variations in the Blood Flow

The blood flow in the various intraocular vascular beds, including the optic nerve head and choroidal and retinal circulations, depends upon at least the following four parameters:

(a) Intraocular pressure
(b) Mean blood pressure (= diastolic blood pressure + ⅓ of the difference between the systolic and diastolic blood pressure)
(c) Peripheral vascular resistance
(d) Presence or absence of blood flow autoregulation:

Retinal and optic nerve head circulations have autoregulation, so they

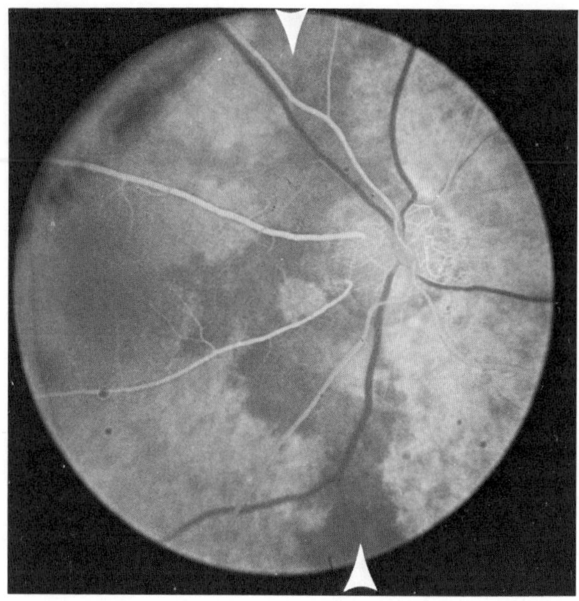

FIGURE 8–8. Fluorescein fundus angiogram of right eye of a 66-year-old man with old CRA occlusion shows nonfilling of the watershed zone (indicated by arrows) between the lateral and medial PCAs. [Reproduced from Hayreh SS, 1975 (44).]

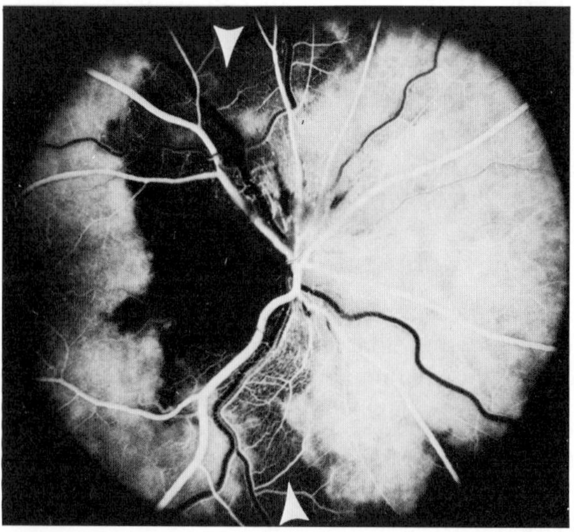

FIGURE 8–9. Fluorescein fundus angiogram of right eye of a 60-year-old man with non arteritic AION shows nonfilling of the watershed zone (indicated by arrows) between the lateral and medial PCAs. [Reproduced from Hayreh SS, 1985 (36).]

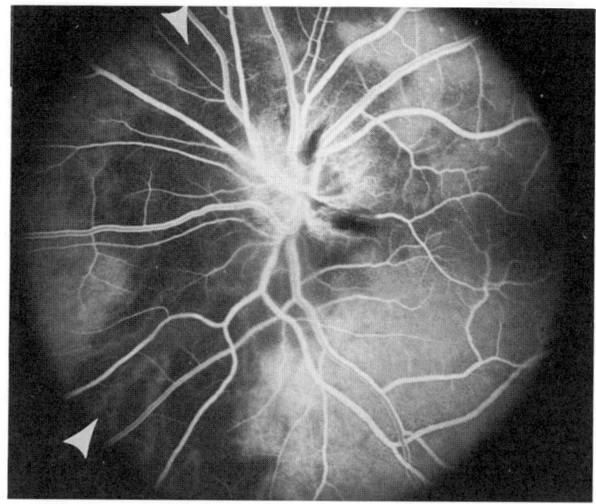

FIGURE 8–10. Fluorescein fundus angiogram of left eye of a 74-year-old man with arteritic AION shows nonfilling of the watershed zone (indicated by arrows) between the lateral and medial PCAs. [Reproduced from Hayreh SS, 1985 (36).]

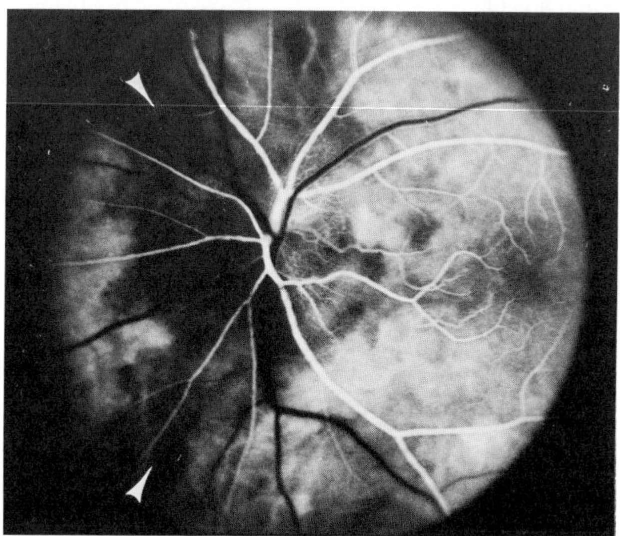

FIGURE 8–11. Fluorescein fundus angiogram of left eye of a 45-year-old woman with nonarteritic AION shows nonfilling of the watershed zone (indicated by arrows) between the lateral and medial PCAs. [Reproduced from Hayreh SS, 1985 (36).]

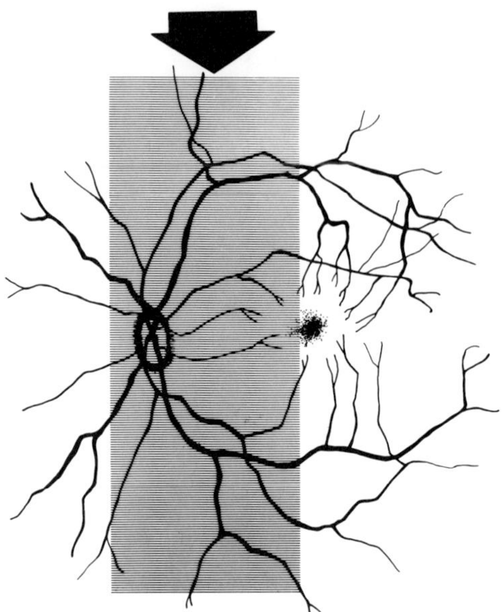

FIGURE 8–12. The watershed zone between the lateral and medial PCAs may be situated *anywhere* within the shaded area (indicated by arrow) of the choroid between the fovea and nasal peripapillary choroid.

are able to regulate the blood flow within a certain range of fluctuation of the perfusion pressure. However, the choroidal circulation has no autoregulation and it is most susceptible to changes in the perfusion pressure.

Blood flow can be calculated by the following formula:

$$\frac{\textit{Perfusion pressure (mean BP minus intraocular pressure)}}{\textit{Peripheral vascular resistance}}$$

Currently, there are no means of measuring the mean blood pressure in the capillaries of the optic nerve head, nor the peripheral vascular resistance, nor the autoregulation. Moreover, the mean blood pressure and intraocular pressure may fluctuate widely during a 24-hour day.

In conclusion, when all the variations mentioned above are combined and the various factors that influence the blood flow are considered, enormous interindividual variations exist in the blood supply of the optic nerve head, which makes the subject extremely complex. A lack of appreciation of all these complexities of the blood supply of the optic nerve in health and disease, is responsible for many of the problems in understanding the pathogenesis of ischemic disorders of the anterior part of the optic nerve.

Pathogenesis

AION is due to acute ischemia of the anterior part of the optic nerve (1, 8, 28, 36, 38, 39), whose main source of blood supply is from the PCAs.

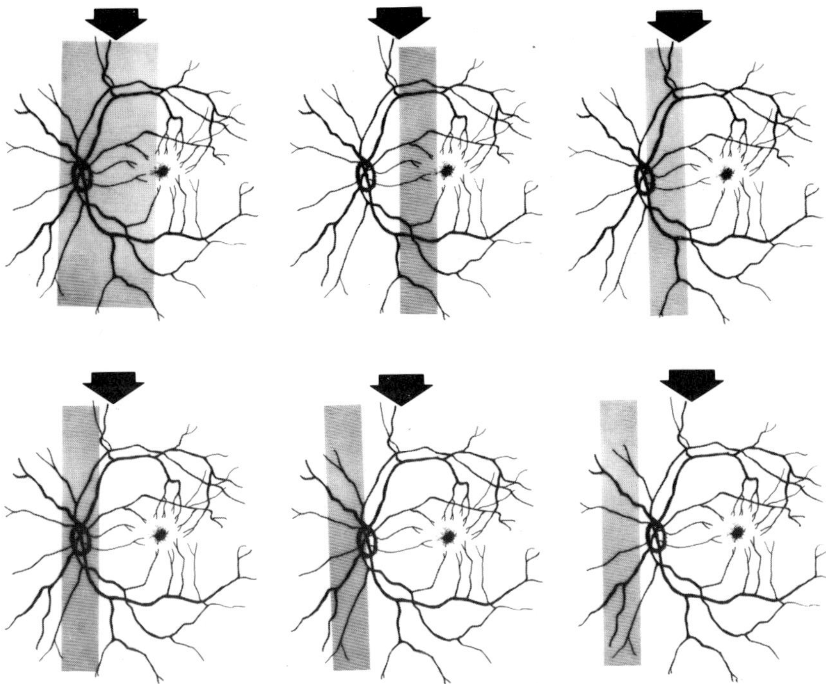

FIGURE 8–13. Schematic representations of locations of the watershed zone (shaded area) between the lateral and medial PCAs. *Top left diagram* shows total area where the watershed may be situated (as in Fig. 7–12), and *remaining five diagrams* show some examples of possible locations.

Etiologically and pathogenetically, AION cases can be broadly classified into two groups (28).

1. Group A is due to thrombotic or embolic occlusion of the PCAs or of the arterioles feeding the anterior part of the optic nerve.

(a) Thrombotic occlusion of the PCAs (Figs. 8–6, 8–7) or their subdivisions most commonly is caused by giant cell arteritis and less commonly by other types of vasculitis (e.g., polyarteritis nodosa, systemic lupus erythematosus, and herpes zoster).

(b) Embolic occlusion of the PCAs (Fig. 8–5) or of the optic nerve arterioles seems to occur much less frequently than thrombotic occlusion, but this impression may be erroneous because of our inability to see the emboli in these vessels on ophthalmoscopy, as compared with the ease with which emboli in the retinal arteries can be seen. Multiple emboli in the vessels of the anterior part of the optic nerve have been demonstrated histopathologically in AION (47).

In group A cases, there is usually massive, severe, and permanent damage to the nerve, the extent of which depends on the size of the artery involved and the area of the nerve supplied by the occluded artery.

2. Group B AION is due to transient nonperfusion or hypoperfusion of the nutrient vessels in the anterior part of the optic nerve. As discussed above, the blood flow depends upon the perfusion pressure in the vessels. A fall of the perfusion pressure below the critical level in the capillaries of the anterior part of the optic nerve may occur because of a marked fall in mean blood pressure (e.g., in shock, during sleep in susceptible persons, severe internal carotid artery and/or ophthalmic artery stenosis or occlusion (48), and other causes) or to a rise in the intraocular pressure (26), or a combination of the two (e.g., in neovascular glaucoma associated with ocular ischemia due to internal carotid artery and/or ophthalmic artery stenosis or occlusion). The optic nerve damage, which may be mild to marked, depends upon the sclerotic changes in its vessels (49, 50) and the duration and severity of the transient ischemia, but it is usually less extensive and less severe than in group A. The majority of AION cases, fortunately, belong to group B. Available clinical evidence indicates that certain segments of the optic nerve head (e.g., the upper part) are more vulnerable to ischemia than others. Because the ischemia in group B most probably is due to transient non-perfusion without an organic block in the vessels, fluorescein fundus angiography may reveal no or minimal filling defect or a delay in filling in the optic disk and/or peripapillary choroid (Fig. 8–14). In group A, by contrast, fluorescein angiography, during the first few days after the onset of AION, shows gross filling defects in the deep vessels of the optic disk and adjacent choroid, depending on the distribution pattern of the occluded artery (Figs. 8–5 to 8–7).

It is of fundamental importance to appreciate that neural ischemia is not an "all or none phenomenon"; there is a wide range of ischemia (27, 30), varying from mild subclinical hypoxia to severe ischemia producing immediate total infarction of neural tissue (as in AION due to giant cell arteritis) Thus, the clinical picture of AION can vary widely, reflecting this wide spectrum.

Risk Factors

Available evidence indicates that AION is frequently a manifestation of systemic and/or ocular disease processes (8), and these include:

1. Giant cell arteritis: This is the most important, though not the most common cause, of AION. Amaurosis fugax preceding the development of AION is seen most commonly in this condition. In every patient 60 years or older, who has a recent history of amaurosis fugax and where I cannot find an evident cause, I investigate for giant cell arteritis on a very urgent basis.

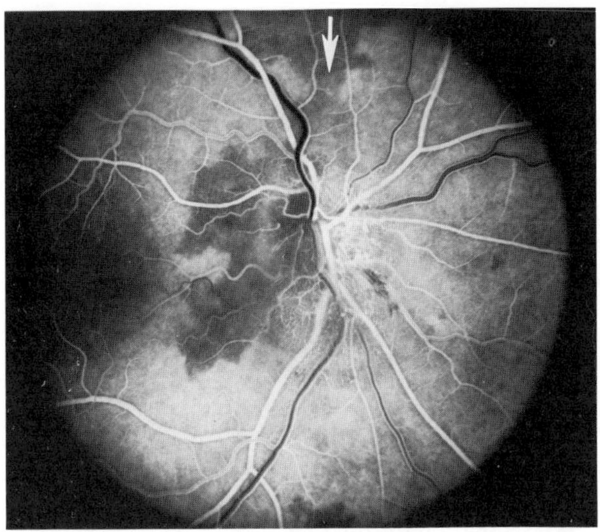

FIGURE 8–14. Fluorescein fundus angiogram of right eye of a 46-year-old man with nonarteritic AION shows nonfilling of the temporal part of the optic disk, temporal peripapillary choroid, and upper half of the watershed zone (indicated by arrow). [Reproduced from Hayreh SS, 1985 (36).]

2. Vasculitis: This may be due to systemic collagen vascular diseases (e.g., systemic lupus erythematosus and polyarteritis nodosa), herpes zoster, and other causes. AION has been seen in association with these disorders.

3. Malignant arterial hypertension: Renovascular malignant arterial hypertension, toxemia of pregnancy and renal disease can produce AION (51). Ordinary benign arterial hypertension, although seen frequently in our prospective series of about 450 patients with AION, did not emerge as a risk factor in the production of AION on statistical analyses (52); this contradicts assertions by Ellenberger (based on retrospective review of only 18 patients!) that AION "represents a direct and early complication of hypertensive arterial disease" (53).

4. Systemic arterial hypotension: I have seen a number of patients with this condition develop AION. The arterial hypotension may develop acutely, e.g., during surgical procedures, renal hemodialysis, or massive hemorrhage.

5. Atherosclerosis and arteriosclerosis: As a part of generalized atherosclerosis and arteriosclerosis, the internal carotid artery, ophthalmic artery, PCAs and other nutrient arteries to the optic nerve may be involved and contribute to the development of AION.

6. Diabetes mellitus: In our prospective series of about 450 patients with AION, this was a significantly important association, predicting a

rapid development of AION in the second eye, particularly in young diabetics (52).

7. Massive or recurrent systemic hemorrhages: AION can develop after massive or recurrent hemorrhages, which are usually from the gastrointestinal tract and uterus and less frequently from other sources (54). Such hemorrhages may or may not be associated with severe arterial hypotension.

8. Migraine: I have seen young patients with migraine develop AION and it seems reasonable to assume that there is an association between the two conditions.

9. Hematologic disorders: AION has been reported in patients with sickle-cell trait, polycythemia, thrombocytopenic purpura, leukemias and various types of anemias.

10. Ocular factors: These include:

(a) Absent or small cup in the optic disc: Recent studies have shown that eyes with nonarteritic AION have no or a very small cup in the optic disc (37,55–58), so that overcrowding of the nerve fibers in a small scleral canal may be a precipitating factor in the production of AION, although not the primary factor (56).

(b) Raised intraocular pressure: This reduces the perfusion pressure in the capillaries of the optic nerve head and is an important factor in the production of AION in susceptible individuals, e.g., in acute angle closure glaucoma, during the immediate postoperative period after cataract extraction (26), in neovascular glaucoma with ocular ischemia due to internal carotid artery and/or ophthalmic artery stenosis or occlusion (48), or in eyes with preexisting low perfusion pressure in the vessels of the optic nerve head. During surgical procedures under general anesthesia, inadvertent pressure on the eyeballs, with or without systemic arterial hypotension, can produce AION.

(c) Marked optic disc edema: When this is seen with raised intracranial pressure or other causes, transient obscuration of vision may be the presenting or a prominent feature; the attacks may be brought about by a change of posture, sudden movement, or stooping. The transient obscuration may progress to complete blindness because of the development of AION. The mechanism of development of AION in these cases has been discussed in detail elsewhere (14).

(d) Location of the watershed zone of the PCAs in relation to the optic disk: The part of the optic disk located in the watershed zone is susceptible to ischemia in the event of a fall in perfusion pressure in the choroidal vascular bed supplied by the PCAs (Figs. 8–9 to 8–13). If the optic disk is situated away from the watershed zone (as in top central and bottom right diagrams in Fig. 8–13), it is relatively safe in such an event; however, if the entire disk lies on the watershed zone (as in Fig. 8–10, and bottom left diagram of Fig. 8–13), it is most vulnerable to ischemic damage.

11. Factors influencing the prevalence of bilateral AION: We recently

analyzed our data on about 450 patients with AION, collected prospectively (52). It showed that the prevalence of second eye involvement was 36% in arteritic AION and 32% in nonarteritic AION after a median follow-up period of about 2 years. Ninety-five percent of the patients with bilateral arteritic AION had the second eye involved before the start of adequate systemic corticosteroid therapy and the rest within 48 hours of the start of the therapy; none started thereafter, which shows that systemic corticosteroid therapy is effective in the prevention of development of AION in giant cell arteritis. In non-arteritic AION, the risk of developing AION faster in the second eye is significantly greater in (a) young (<45 years old) diabetics than in older diabetics or in persons with other systemic diseases, (b) in men than in women, and (c) in younger than in older persons.

Differential Diagnosis of Arteritic AION

In elderly and late-middle-aged patients with AION, the first important step is to rule out giant-cell arteritis because of the imminent danger of bilateral total blindness. I have found the following highly suggestive of AION due to giant cell arteritis (28):

1. Systemic manifestations: The patient may complain of weight loss, malaise, "flu"-like symptoms, fever of unknown origin, anemia, polymyalgia, jaw claudication, neck pain, headache, or vague ill-health. These may be typical enough to indicate giant-cell arteritis. However, in the *occult variety* (I find that a considerable proportion of arteritic AION patients belong to this group), the patient is perfectly fit and healthy, with no symptoms at all.
2. High erythrocyte sedimentation rate: If the ESR is very high, e.g., 80 mm Westergren or higher, it is fairly suggestive of giant-cell arteritis but I have seen patients in their sixties, with ESR as low as 5 mm and confirmed giant-cell arteritis, so the so-called normal ESR does not rule out arteritis.
3. Early, massive visual loss: If from the very start the eye is totally blind or the visual acuity is reduced to bare light perception or hand motion, with almost non-recordable visual fields, this is highly suggestive of arteritic AION. However, in our series, about 25% of eyes with arteritic AION had 6/12 or better vision (29).
4. Chalky-white swollen optic disk: In about half of the cases of arteritic AION, the swollen disk has a chalky white appearance (7,8), which is almost diagnostic of arteritic AION.
5. Nonfilling of the optic disc and adjacent half of the choroid on fluorescein fundus angiography: If angiography is performed within the first few days after the onset of visual loss, one half of the choroid (usually the nasal half) shows no filling because of complete occlusion of the PCA

(Figs. 8–6, 8–7) (7, 8, 25, 28, 36). This, also, is almost diagnostic of arteritic AION. However, if angiography is performed after the first few days, the filling defect may be absent.

Thus, although none of these criteria is always present in arteritic AION, information obtained from using the various parameters collectively is extremely helpful in the diagnosis of giant-cell arteritis. To confirm the diagnosis finally, a temporal artery biopsy should be performed.

6. Temporal artery biopsy: The biopsy establishes the diagnosis. If there is a strong suspicion of giant cell arteritis from the five parameters mentioned above and temporal artery biopsy does not confirm the diagnosis, I perform a biopsy on the second side. I have seen cases where the biopsy was negative on one side but positive on the other. In every patient with suspected giant cell arteritis, it is absolutely essential to perform the biopsy before committing the patient to long-term systemic corticosteroid therapy; I find no exception to this rule.

In conclusion, I find that by using these six parameters collectively, one can establish the diagnosis of giant cell arteritis almost invariably, although none of the criteria is individually infallible.

Posterior Ischemic Optic Neuropathy

PION is due to ischemia of the posterior part of the optic nerve (2). Since the site of ischemia is farther back in the optic nerve, the optic disk is normal during the acute phase, as in retrobulbar optic neuritis. However, ischemic degeneration of the optic nerve fibers can produce descending optic atrophy, the location and severity of which would depend on the fibers involved. Because the nerve fibers from the different parts of the retina are arranged differently in various regions of the optic nerve, the degree of visual loss depends upon the site and extent of the lesion. PION has been seen with giant-cell arteritis and systemic lupus erythematosus. In other cases it is logical to presume that other factors (e.g., atherosclerosis, arteriosclerosis, collagen vascular disease, malignant arterial hypertension, diabetes mellitus, thromboembolic disorders, hematologic disorders) that produce AION could also produce PION by involving the nutrient vessels to the optic nerve.

Acknowledgments. I am grateful to my wife, Shelagh, for her help in the preparation of this manuscript, to Mrs. Ellen Ballas and Mrs. Georgiane Parkes-Perret for their secretarial help, and to the ophthalmic photography department for the illustrations. This study was supported by research grants from the British Medical Research Council, National Institutes of Health (Grant Nos. EY-1151 and 1576) and Research to Prevent Blindness Inc.

References

1. Hayreh SS: Anterior ischaemic optic neuropathy: I. Terminology and pathogenesis. *Br J Opthalmol* 1974;58:955–989.
2. Hayreh SS: Posterior ischemic optic neuropathy. *Opthalmologica* 1981;182:29–41.
3. Birkhead NC, Wagener HP, Shick RM: Treatment of temporal arteritis with adrenal corticosteroids. *Jama* 1957;163:821–827.
4. Cullen JF: Ischaemic optic neuropathy. *Trans Ophthalmol Soc UK* 1967; 87:759–774.
5. Cullen JF: Occult temporal arteritis: A common cause of blindness in old age. *Br J Ophthalmol* 1967;51:513–525.
6. Cullen JF, Coleiro JA: Ophthalmic complications of giant cell arteritis. *Surv Ophthalmol* 1976;20:247–260
7. Hayreh SS: Anterior ischaemic optic neuropathy: II. Fundus on ophthalmoscopy and fluorescein angiography. *Br J Ophthalmol* 1974;58:964–980.
8. Hayreh SS: *Anterior Ischemic Optic Neuropathy*. New York, Springer-Verlag, 1975.
9. Meadows SP: Temporal or giant cell arteritis: Ophthalmic aspects, in Smith JL (ed): *Neuro-Ophthalmology: Symposium of the University of Miami and the Bascom Palmer Eye Institute*. St Louis, The CV Mosby Co, 1968, vol 4, pp 148–157.
10. Berens C: The fundus changes and the blood pressure in the retinal arteries in increased intracranial pressure. *Assoc Res Nerv Ment Dis* 1929;8:263–309.
11. Cogan DG: Blackouts not obviously due to carotid occlusion. *Arch Ophthalmol* 1961;66:180–187
12. de Schweinitz GE: The relation of cerebral decompression to the relief of the ocular manifestations of increased intracranial tension. *Ann Ophthalmol* 1911;20:271–284.
13. Edwards CH, Paterson JH: A review of the symptoms and signs of acoustic neurofibromata. *Brain* 1951;74:144–190.
14. Hayreh SS: Optic disc edema in raised intracranial pressure: VI. Associated visual disturbances and their pathogenesis. *Arch Ophthalmol* 1977; 95:1566–1579.
15. Jackson JH: Lecture on optic neuritis from intracranial disease. *Med Times Gaz* 1871;2:241–243, 341–342, 581.
16. Jefferson A: Hypertensive cerebral vascular disease and intracranial tumour. *QJ Med* 1955;24:245–268.
17. Lyle TK: Some pitfalls in the diagnosis of plerocephalic oedema. *Trans Ophthalmol Soc UK* 1953;73:87–102.
18. Meadows SP: The swollen optic disc. *Trans Ophthalmol Soc UK* 1959;79:121–143.
19. Paton L: Optic neuritis in cerebral tumours and its subsidence after operation. *Trans Ophthalmol Soc UK* 1905;25:129–162.
20. Paton L: Optic neuritis in cerebral tumours. *Trans Ophthalmol Soc UK* 1908;28:112–144.
21. Uhthoff W: Ophthalmic experiences and considerations on the surgery of cerebral tumours and tower skull. *Trans Ophthalmol Soc UK* 1914;34:47–123.

22. Walsh FB, Hoyt WF: *Clinical Neuro-Ophthalmology,* ed 3. Baltimore, Williams & Wilkins, Co., 1969, pp 575–576, 2404.
23. West S: Sequel of a case of optic neuritis, with numerous sudden, short attacks of complete blindness. *Trans Ophthalmol Soc UK* 1883;3:136–138.
24. Hayreh SS: Anterior ischaemic optic neuropathy: III. Treatment, prophylaxis, and differential diagnosis. *Br J Ophthalmol* 1974;58:981–989.
25. Hayreh SS: Ischemic optic neuropathy. *Int Ophthalmol* 1978;1:9–18.
26. Hayreh SS: Anterior ischemic optic neuropathy: IV. Occurrence after cataract extraction. *Arch Ophthalmol* 1980;98:1410–1416.
27. Hayreh SS: Anterior ischemic optic neuropathy: V. Optic disc edema an early sign. *Arch Ophthalmol* 1981;99:1030–1040.
28. Hayreh SS: Anterior ischemic optic neuropathy. *Arch Neurol* 1981;38:675–678.
29. Hayreh SS, Podhajsky P: Visual field defects in anterior ischemic optic neuropathy. *Doc Ophthalmol Proc Ser* 1979;19:53–71.
30. Hayreh SS, Zahoruk RM: Anterior ischemic optic neuropathy: VI. In juvenile diabetics. *Ophthalmologica* 1981;182:13–28.
31. Hayreh SS: Blood supply and vascular disorders of the optic nerve. *Ann Inst Barraquer* 1963;4:7–109.
32. Hayreh SS: Blood supply of the optic nerve head and its role in optic atrophy, glaucoma and oedema of the optic disc. *Br J Ophthalmol* 1969;53:721–748.
33. Hayreh SS:Pathogenesis of visual field defects: Role of the ciliary circulation. *Br J Ophthalmol* 1970;54:289–311.
34. Hayreh SS: Anatomy and physiology of the optic nerve head. *Trans Am Acad Ophthalmol Otolaryngol* 1974;78:240–254.
35. Hayreh SS: Structure and blood supply of the optic nerve, in Heilmann K, Richardson KT (eds): *Glaucoma: Conceptions of a Disease: Pathogenesis, Diagnosis, and Therapy*. Stuttgart, Thieme, 1978, pp 78–96.
36. Hayreh SS: Inter-individual variation in blood supply of the optic nerve head: Its importance in various ischemic disorders of the optic nerve head, and glaucoma, low-tension glaucoma and allied disorders. *Doc Ophthalmol* 1985;59:217–246.
37. Hayreh SS: Pathogenesis of cupping of the optic disc. *Br J Ophthalmol* 1974;58:863–876.
38. Hayreh SS, Baines JAB: Occlusion of the posterior ciliary artery: III. Effects on the optic nerve head. *Br J Ophthalmol* 1972;56:754–764.
39. Hayreh SS, Chopdar A: Occlusion of the posterior ciliary artery: V. Protective influence of simultaneous vortex vein occlusion. *Arch Ophthalmol* 1982;100:1481–1491.
40. Hayreh SS: *A Study of the Central Artery of the Retina in Human Beings in Its Intra-orbital and Intra-neural Course,* thesis, Master of Surgery. Panjab University, India, 1958.
41. Singh S, Dass R: The central artery of the retina: II. Distribution and anastomoses. *Br J Ophthalmol* 1960;44:280–299.
42. Hayreh SS: The ophthalmic artery: III. Branches. *Br J Ophthalmol* 1962;46:212–247.
43. Hayreh SS: Arterial blood supply of the eye, in Bernstein EF (ed): *Amaurosis Fugax*. New York, Springer-Verlag, 1987.

44. Hayreh SS: Segmental nature of choroidal vasculature. *Br J Ophthalmol* 1975;59:631–648.
45. Hayreh SS: Physiological anatomy of the choroidal vascular bed. *Int Ophthalmol* 1983;6:85–93.
46. Hayreh SS: Acute choroidal ischaemia. *Trans Ophthalmol Soc UK* 1980;100:400–407.
47. Lieberman MF, Shahi A, Green WR: Embolic ischemic optic neuropathy. *Am J Ophthalmol* 1978;86:206–210.
48. Hayreh SS, Podhajsky P: Ocular neovascularization with retinal vascular occlusion: II. Occurrence in central and branch retinal artery occlusion. *Arch Ophthalmol* 1982;100:1585–1596.
49. Battistini A, Caffi M: Alterazioni vascolari del nervoottico nella senilita. *Ann Ottal* 1959;85:715–722.
50. Ellenberger C, Netsky MG: Infarction in the optic nerve. *J Neurol Neurosurg Psychiatry* 1968;31:606–611.
51. Hayreh SS, Servais GE, Virdi PS: Fundus lesions in malignant hypertension: V. Hypertensive optic neuropathy. *Ophthalmology* 1986;93:74–87.
52. Beri M., Klugman MR, Kohler JA, et al: Anterior ischemic optic neuropathy: VIII. Incidence of bilaterality and various influencing factors. Ophthalmology 1987;94:1020–1028
53. Ellenberger C: Ischemic optic neuropathy as a possible early complication of vascular hypertension. *AM J Ophthalmol* 1979;88:1045–1051.
54. Hayreh SS: Anterior ischemic optic neuropathy: VIII. Clinical features and pathogenesis of post-hemorrhagic amaurosis. Ophthalmology 1987;94:1488–1502.
55. Beck RW, Savino PJ, Repka MX, et al: Optic disc structure in anterior ischemic optic neuropathy. *Ophthalmology* 1984;91:1334–1337.
56. Beck RW, Servais GE, Hayreh SS: Anterior ischemic optic neuropathy: IX. Cup-disc-ratio and its role in the pathogenesis. Ophthalmology 1987;1503–1508.
57. Doro S, Lessell S: Cup-disc ratio and ischemic optic neuropathy. *Arch Ophthalmol* 1985;103:1143–1144.
58. Feit RH, Tomsak RL, Ellenberger C: Structural factors in the pathogenesis of ischemic optic neuropathy. *Am J Ophthalmol* 1984;98:105–108.

CHAPTER 9

Risk of Cerebrovascular Disease in Patients with Anterior Ischemic Optic Neuropathy

Peter J. Savino

Anterior ischemic optic neuropathy (AION) is a disorder that affects many patients over age 50. It is caused by infarction of the optic nerve head and is thought to be secondary to posterior ciliary artery insufficiency. A minority of patients with AION have giant-cell arteritis as an identifiable cause, but the majority fall into the idiopathic group—the so-called nonarteritic AION.

Although AION is seen frequently, the exact pathophysiologic mechanisms involved remain obscure. Few pathologic specimens are available for examination. Quigly and coworkers (1) examined three eyes from patients with AION. They addressed the question of nerve fiber layer attrition and compared this to the pattern of loss in glaucoma. However, the specimens they examined showed no unequivocal evidence of vascular occlusive phenomenon in the posterior ciliary circulation.

Despite the lack of pathologic evidence, it is assumed that the insult to the optic nerve in AION is ischemic. Ischemic lesions in this area may be due to thromboembolism or hypoperfusion. The latter is known to be a cause of AION and has been well documented in patients who have had significant blood loss (2).

Embolism is a less likely mechanism of AION. Patients with AION and substantial evidence of emboli in the retinal or ciliary circulation are rarely seen, but cases are reported occasionally (3).

Another facet of AION appears to fly in the face of it being a systemic vascular problem. Previous reports have failed to prove a significant increase in any vascular or other systemic disorder in patients with AION, possibly because of the small size of the patient populations studied. Likewise, no apparent increase in the prevalence of stroke is found in these patients. Thus, AION does not appear to be the same as amaurosis fugax or retinal artery occlusion as a potential precursor of cerebrovascular incidents.

Two studies (4,5) have addressed the question of the association of various systemic diseases with nonarteritic AION. Repka and associates (4) reviewed the experience of the Neuro-Ophthalmology Service at Wills

Eye Hospital in Philadelphia. They divided their patients into two groups (younger and older than 65 years) and discovered a significantly ($p<.5$) increased prevalence of hypertension and diabetes mellitus in the younger age group only. In patients more than 64 years of age no diseases occurred significantly more often than in the general population (Public Health Service Data).

The data on mortality rates were identical to those for the two comparable control groups for death from all causes (Fig. 9–1). However, patients with AION died of ischemic heart disease more often than expected, but this was not statistically significant (Fig. 9–2). Only 3 of 102 patients younger than 65 and 2 of 67 older than 65 had recorded cerebrovascular events. This was not different than the prevalence in the control population.

A similar study performed at the Wilmer Eye Institute (5) confirmed some of the Wills observations but also found contradictory data. The patient group was large (217 patients) with an excellent follow-up percentage (98%). The points of agreement between the studies are increased hypertension in the group younger than 65 years, the lack of increased hypertension in older patients, increased prevalence of diabetes mellitus in AION patients younger than 65, and no increase in mortality rate compared to a control group.

The Wilmer study (5) did show an increased prevalence of cerebrovascular disease. Fourteen patients had cerebrovascular accidents, and

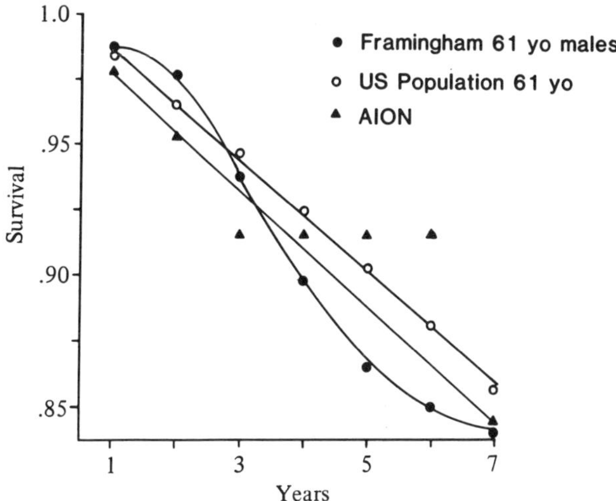

FIGURE 9–1. Fraction of patients surviving *v* time for nonarteritic anterior ischemic optic neuropathy (AION). Comparison with the two control groups shows no difference in mortality. ● = Framingham males, 61 years old; ○ = U. S. population, 61 years old; ▲ = AION.

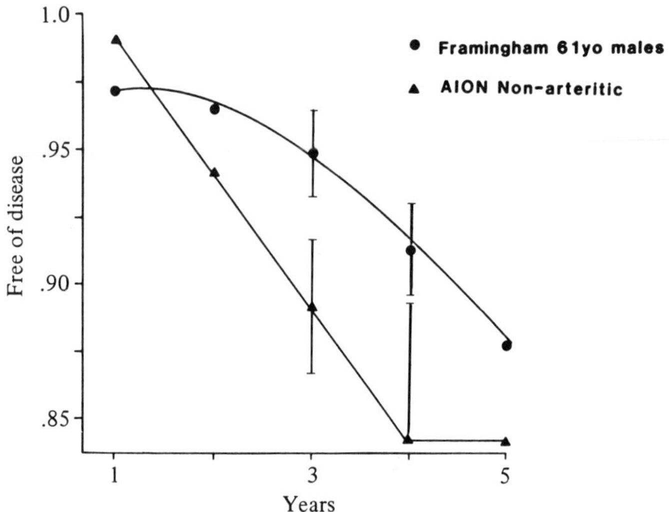

FIGURE 9–2. Fraction of patients free of ischemic heart disease *v* time for nonarteritic anterior ischemic optic neuropathy (AION). ● = Framingham males, 61 years old; ▲ AION nonarteritic.

12 had TIAs after AION. However, the types of cerebrovascular events were not described beyond the statement that the events were distributed equally between "the sides ipsilateral and contralateral to the eye in which the AION had occurred." No patient died of stroke.

The patients in the Wilmer study also had an increase in the prevalence of cardiac disease, particularly myocardial infarction. The mortality rate in these patients, however, did not differ from that of the control group.

All the differences in the findings between these two studies (4,5) are not resolved easily. The number of patients and the follow-up percentage are higher in the Wilmer study. However, the follow-up period actually was longer in the Wills study. The control groups used also were different. Guyer et al (5) also indicated that an increased prevalence of hypertension was not the critical factor as both studies had almost identical percentages of patients with systemic hypertension.

Since the suggestions by the Wilmer report, all patients with nonarteritic AION who have presented to the Neuro-Ophthalmology Service at Wills Eye Hospital have been studied by means of carotid sonography, Doppler examinations and oculoplethysmography (OPG). Twenty consecutive patients have been studied, and no patient had evidence of hemodynamically significant stenosis in the ipsilateral carotid circulation (unpublished data). Because embolism is an extremely unlikely cause of AION, the presence of an embolic focus in the carotid system also appears irrelevant.

What, then, can explain the vasculopathy of AION if the cause is not systemic? Hoyt (6) commented that patients with AION appeared to have a peculiar optic disc structure with no physiologic cupping. Beck and associates (7) reported their findings in 51 patients with AION and confirmed the absence of physiologic cupping. Wirtshaffer (8) proposed a developmentally inadequate anastomotic arterial system within the optic nerve head as the cause. This or a similar explanation that corresponds with the anomalous appearance of the optic nerve head could explain the apparent conundrum of an ocular vasculopathy that does not appear to be due to a systemic vasculopathy.

References

1. Quigley HA, Miller NR, Green WR: The pattern of optic nerve fiber loss in anterior ischemic optic neuropathy. *Am J Ophthalmol* 1985;100:769–776.
2. Drance SM, Morgan RW, Sweeney VP: Shock-induced optic neuropathy: A cause of nonprogressive glaucoma. *N Engl J Med* 1973;288:392–395.
3. Tomsak RL: Ischemic optic neuropathy associated with retinal embolism. *Am J Ophthalmol* 1985;99:590–592.
4. Repka MX, Savino PJ, Schatz NJ, et al: Clinical profile and long-term implications of anterior ischemic optic neuropathy. *Am J Ophthalmol* 1983;96:478–483.
5. Guyer DR, Miller NR, Auer CL, et al: The risk of cerebrovascular and cardiovascular disease in patients with anterior ischemic optic neuropathy. *Arch Ophthalmol* 1985;103:1136–1142.
6. Hoyt WF: Rocky mountain neuro-ophthalmology society meeting. February 1982.
7. Beck RW, Savino RJ, Repka MX, et al: Optic disc structure in anterior ischemic optic neuropathy. *Ophthalmology* 1984;91:1334–1337.
8. Wirtschaffer JD: Discussion. *Ophthalmology* 1984;91:1337.

Chapter 10

Chronic Ocular Ischemia and Carotid Vascular Disease

John E. Carter

Although most ocular manifestations of extracranial cerebrovascular disease have a strokelike temporal profile, some patients have ocular abnormalities that are most compatible with a chronic state of ocular ischemia and have evidence of severe, usually bilateral, extracranial cerebrovascular occlusive disease. Similar ocular findings may be seen in other conditions that produce chronic retinal ischemia or altered retinal blood flow, but in some situations it is difficult to dismiss the associated cerebrovascular occlusive disease as an incidental finding.

Although they represent two ends of a spectrum of pathology secondary to chronic ischemia, the ocular findings in this setting can be separated into a hemorrhagic retinopathy, which usually is referred to as venous stasis retinopathy, and a more diffuse ocular condition termed ischemic oculopathy (1,2). In the neurology literature, the term venous stasis retinopathy usually is reserved for this specific setting. In the ophthalmology literature, however, some confusion exists because the term venous stasis retinopathy has been used to describe other conditions with a similar retinopathy. No generally acceptable term specific to the findings associated with carotid vascular disease has been suggested. Discussions of patients with cerebrovascular disease in the ophthalmology literature generally use the term "venous stasis retinopathy of carotid occlusive disease". For the purposes of this review venous stasis retinopathy refers to the retinal changes described in association with carotid atherosclerotic occlusive disease.

Clinical Findings and Natural History of Venous Stasis Retinopathy and Ischemic Oculopathy

Venous stasis retinopathy, although not referred to as such, was recognized as a manifestation of aortic arch syndromes (3–5) for some years before 1963 when Hedges (6) and Kearns and Hollenhorst (7) described its association with carotid occlusive disease. The earliest changes in venous stasis retinopathy consist of microaneurysms and small dot-and-blot hemorrhages. These findings are most prominent beginning at the midperiphery of the fundus. More severe ischemia produces dilatation and darkening of the retinal veins, often with marked irregularity of the caliber of the major retinal veins. Hemorrhages in the nerve fiber layer may occur. Swelling of the optic disk is unusual but may be present to mild degree, as is sometimes seen with severe diabetic retinopathy. Fig. 10–1 illustrates these changes. If the ischemia persists, neovascularization of the retina and optic disk may develop (Fig. 10–2). More severe ischemia may produce pallor or a gray cast to the macula that is due to retinal edema. Although visual impairment and retinal edema always should coexist, the remainder of the signs of venous stasis retinopathy may be present in patients who have normal visual function. Venous stasis retinopathy may be seen in patients who recently have had a stroke (6,7), who have ongoing transient monocular or cerebral ischemic attacks (7–9), who have had known cerebrovascular disease in the past but have no recent symptoms (7), or who have symptoms limited to mild visual loss (9,10). Occasionally, the finding is incidental (11).

In ischemic oculopathy (1,2) additional changes take place in the anterior segment of the eye if the ischemic state continues. This condition also has been termed ischemic ophthalmia, ischemic ophthalmopathy, and ischemic ocular inflammation. These findings also were recognized earlier in aortic arch syndromes (4, 5). Smith (12) first called attention to the association of neovascular glaucoma and occlusion of the ICA. The spectrum of changes seen in ischemic oculopathy subsequently were described in detail by Hoefnagels (13) and Knox (14). The abnormalities include episcleral vascular congestion, a cloudy cornea, cells and flare in the anterior chamber, and neovascularization of the iris (Fig. 10–3). The pupil often is middilated and reacts sluggishly or not at all to either direct or consensual stimulation. Intraocular pressure usually is elevated but may be normal or even decreased. In most cases venous stasis retinopathy continues to be present, but the retinal arteries and veins may become markedly attenuated, with visibly sluggish blood flow through the veins. Optic atrophy may develop.

Patients with venous stasis retinopathy or ischemic oculopathy invariably have a marked reduction of the central retinal artery pressure on ophthalmodynamometry. Often pressure is so low that touching the eye produces pulsation in the central retinal artery so that pressure cannot be measured. In some cases diastolic pressure in the central retinal artery is so low that spontaneous pulsations are present (7,13,15–17).

Ischemic pain is a feature in some patients with venous stasis retinopathy and ischemic oculopathy. It is characterized as a constant aching over the orbit, upper face, and temple and may be worse when the patient is in an upright position (16,18). This pain is not related to glaucoma, which also may be a source of pain in patients with ischemic oculopathy.

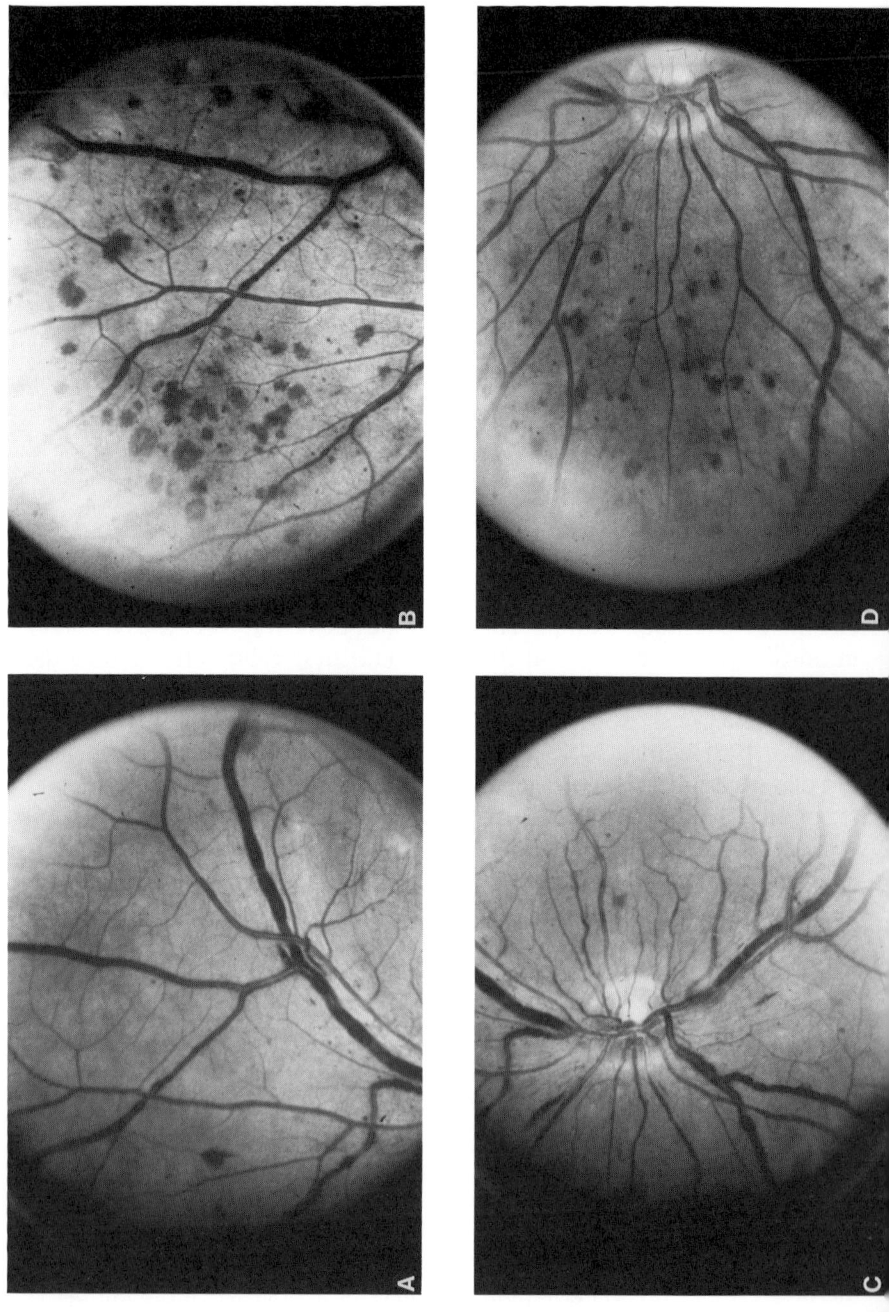
B
D
A
C

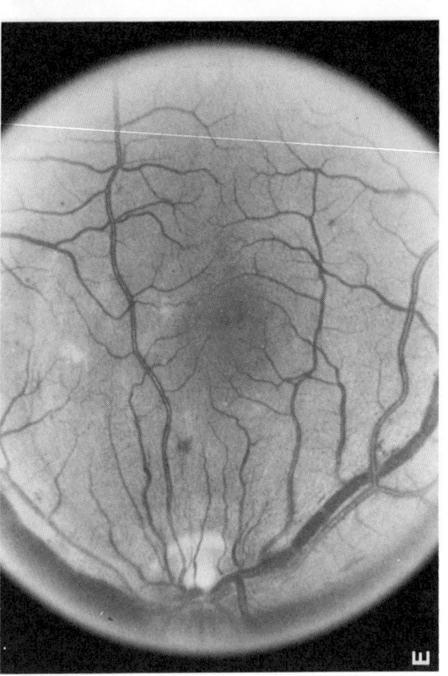

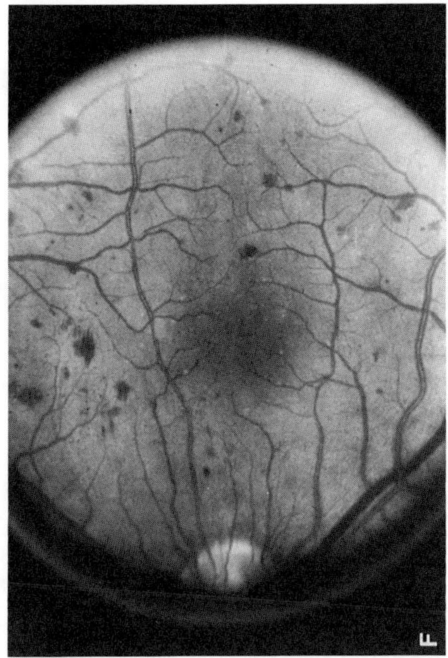

FIGURE 10–1. *Case 1*. Early and advanced venous stasis retinopathy of the left eye. A, C, and E on the left were taken 1 month after occlusion of the common carotid artery. A follows the superior vascular arcade down toward the optic disk, which is seen in B. The optic disk is minimally swollen. The major veins not only are dilated but also show striking irregularity in caliber. Several splinter hemorrhages in the nerve fiber layer and a number of small intraretinal hemorrhages are present along the vascular arcades. The macula, C, is almost unaffected. B, D, and F on the right were taken 6 months after the occlusion and show substantial worsening of the retinopathy even though the sausagelike irregularity of the major veins is not quite as prominent. Although a few hemorrhages are seen in the macular area, F, the degree of abnormality is small compared with areas outside the vascular arcades seen in B and D. The right eye was normal.

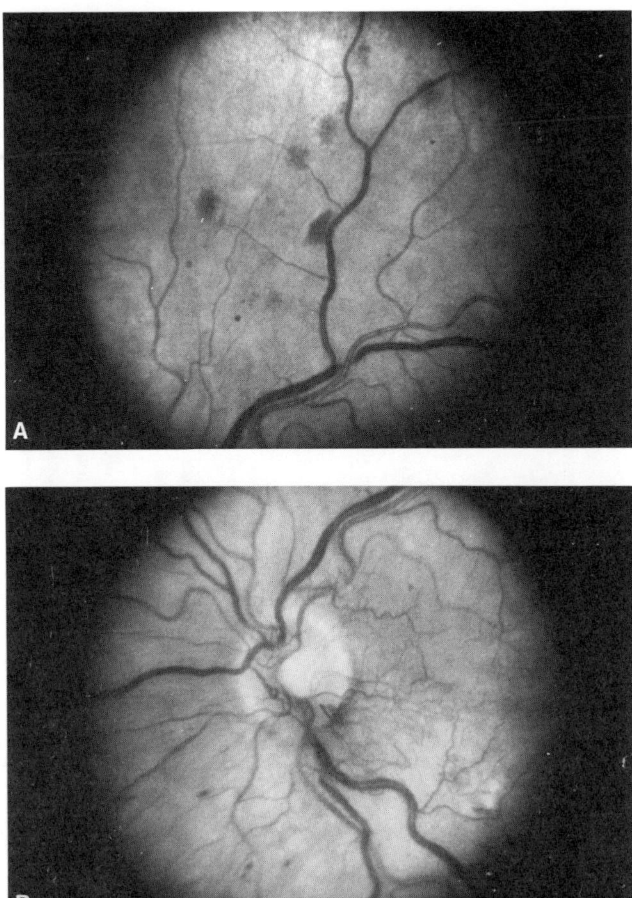

FIGURE 10–2. *Case 2*. B shows the optic disk of the left eye with a few small, scattered intraretinal hemorrhages but a prominent neovascular net covering the entire temporal quadrant of the disk and peripapillary retina from superior division of the central retinal artery to the inferior division of the central retinal vein. Involvement of the macular region, D, and midperiphery, A and C, are more equal in this diabetic, but the right eye was completely normal.

The natural history of ischemic oculopathy is not completely clear because mild degrees of venous stasis retinopathy may be seen in the setting of a presumed acute occlusion of the ICA. A patient may have experienced a TIA or stroke and be found to have venous stasis retinopathy and, on investigation, a severe stenosis or occlusion in the ipsilateral carotid system. This was the case with the patient reported by Hedges (6). This patient had an unsuccessful endarterectomy for an occlusion of the ICA, yet most of his retinal abnormalities resolved. Most subsequent reports of patients

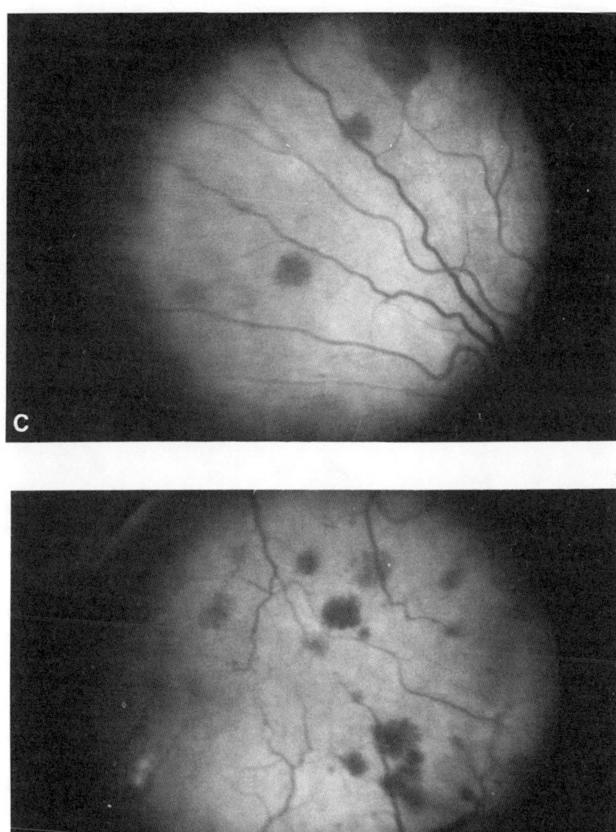

FIGURE 10–2 (*continued*)

with venous stasis retinopathy generally have been concerned with patients undergoing carotid endarterectomy for stenotic lesions or extracranial-intracranial bypass for occlusions of the carotid artery in whom the retinal changes subsequently resolved. Possibly, venous stasis retinopathy that develops in the setting of an acute occlusion in the carotid system may resolve spontaneously in some cases as collateral circulation adjusts to the new hemodynamic status. This is precisely what happened in a series of patients undergoing ICA ligation (19): a hemorrhagic retinopathy developed in many but resolved spontaneously in most. Because extracranial-intracranial bypass has not been beneficial, the natural history of venous stasis retinopathy may be defined more accurately in a group of patients with an acute neurologic event associated with venous stasis retinopathy and inoperable carotid lesions.

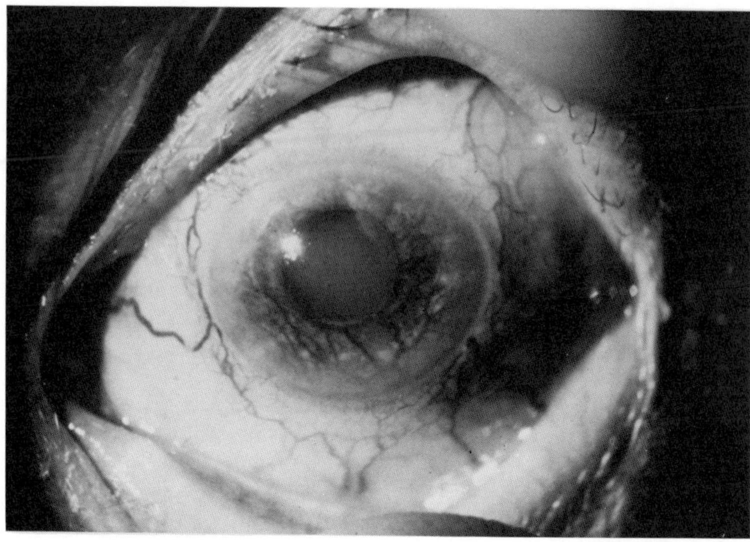

FIGURE 10–3. External photograph of a patient with neovascular glaucoma shows episcleral vascular dilatation. Blood vessels can be seen running over the surface of the iris. (Photograph courtesy of Dr. Robert Burns, reproduced by permission from *Neurologic Clinics* 1983; 1:418.)

A typical progressive course is illustrated by the following two cases (10).

Case 1

A 55-year-old man experienced sudden loss of all vision in the left eye 1 month before evaluation. Vision returned over a period of several minutes, but he was left with a persistent, subjective sense of blurring. After the initial visual loss, he also had been having episodic weakness in the right leg.

One year before admission he had had a reversible ischemic neurologic deficit in the right hemisphere that was treated by an endarterectomy of the right carotid artery. Four months before admission he underwent an aortofemoral bypass for intermittent claudication. He did not have diabetes.

The results of an examination at the time of admission were unremarkable except for the ocular findings. Visual acuity, color vision, pupil reaction, visual fields, and findings of a slit-lamp examination were normal for both eyes. The fundus examination showed a normal right eye. The left had mild disk swelling and segmental narrowing and dilatation of the major retinal veins. A few hemorrhages were present in the nerve fiber layer near the disk, and scattered intraretinal hemorrhages were present, mostly along the vascular arcades and in the nasal retina (Figs. 10–1A, C, and E).

Arteriography showed complete occlusion of the left common carotid artery. The remainder of the extracranial and intracranial vasculature was unremarkable.

It was thought that the patient had had an occlusion of the common carotid artery 1 month earlier at the time of his initial symptom, sudden visual loss. Transient ischemic attacks and persistent subjective visual blurring indicated continuing insufficiency of blood flow in the left carotid system. Complete occlusion of the common carotid artery precluded surgery, and the patient was treated with warfarin sodium.

During the first 2 weeks of therapy, the patient experienced several more TIAs; afterwards he was free of this symptom. Subjective visual blurring persisted although objectively measured visual function remained normal. Intraocular pressure was normal throughout his follow-up. The venous stasis retinopathy progressively worsened. Six months after his transient visual loss, fundoscopy showed resolution of some of the irregularity in caliber of the major retinal veins but a marked increase in the intraretinal hemorrhages (Figs. 10–1B, D, and F). Some hemorrhages were seen in the macula, but the great majority were in the midperiphery of the retina. Nine months after the onset of his symptoms, the patient was noted to have neovascularization of the optic disk and peripheral retina. One month later he was found to have iris neovascularization. At that time he underwent panretinal photocoagulation. Three months after therapy the neovascularization of the retina and optic disk had cleared, and 3 months later the iris neovascularization had resolved.

Case 2

A 63-year-old man with diabetes underwent extracapsular cataract extraction with placement of a posterior chamber intraocular lens in the right eye. Three weeks later the same procedure was done in the left eye. He had had no diabetic retinopathy before surgery. Postoperatively, vision was 20/25 in the right eye and 20/30 in the left, although the patient noted that vision in the left eye was distinctly different from that in the right. It was less sharp and bright and appeared washed out. The intraocular pressure was normal throughout his course, and the fundus on the right remained normal. The fundus on the left was normal 1 week after surgery, but 3 weeks postoperatively the left retina was noted to have dot-and-blot hemorrhages for the first time. There were no carotid bruits. The patient was followed for the next 6 months; during that time the retinopathy slowly worsened. Finally, neovascularization of the disk developed. Iris neovascularization was not present.

The patient was admitted for cerebral angiography. Except for the finding of mild diabetes, the results of the laboratory studies were normal. Angiography showed complete occlusion of the left ICA and 60% stenosis of the right ICA. An endarterectomy of the right carotid artery was performed. Because neovascularization was thought to be an indication for more aggressive management, the patient underwent panretinal photocoagulation 1 month after surgery.

Pathogenesis of Ischemic Oculopathy

Venous stasis retinopathy appears to represent a state of chronic ischemia with viable but ischemic tissue. If the ocular ischemia persists, the retinopathy progressively worsens, and neovascular changes develop in the retina and optic disk, followed by neovascularization of the iris. Neovascularization of the iris eventually produces a fibrovascular membrane that obstructs the outflow of aqueous humor through the anterior chamber angle and produces glaucoma. Iris atrophy also develops.

A similar series of events occurs in patients with diabetic retinopathy and in some patients with occlusion of the central retinal vein. In both of these conditions, the primary process is thought to occur in the retina, where ischemia results in the elaboration of a diffusable angiogenesis factor. Iris neovascularization develops when this factor circulates to the anterior chamber (20). All of the anterior segment changes in diabetes and in occlusion of the central retinal vein can be explained by the ischemic process occurring in the retina. Evidence indicates that the neovascular changes occurring in ischemic oculopathy also are secondary to the ischemia of the posterior segment rather than a direct effect of ischemia on the anterior segment (10). However, evidence also indicates a direct effect of ischemia on the anterior segment of the eye in ischemic oculopathy that is not seen in other types of neovascular glaucoma. Some patients with fully developed ischemic oculopathy and complete angle closure nevertheless have normal or low intraocular pressure. Decreased production of aqueous humor and ocular hypotony have been described in experimental (21) and therapeutic (19) ligation of the common carotid artery, presumably due to ischemia of the ciliary body. Additional evidence suggests that ischemia of the ciliary body is responsible for normal or low intraocular pressure in patients with complete angle closure due to ischemic oculopathy. Elevated intraocular pressure may develop in these patients after surgical bypass or repair of obstructive lesions in the carotid circulation (2,16).

Vascular Status of Patients with Chronic Ocular Ischemia Associated with Carotid Atherosclerotic Disease

In their original study, Kearns and Hollenhorst (7) found venous stasis retinopathy in 4% of 600 patients with symptomatic carotid artery disease, without regard to degree or location of stenosis. In a subsequent report by Kearns et al (11) of patients with occlusion of the ICA, the prevalence of venous stasis retinopathy was almost 20%. This finding suggests that occlusive lesions must be quite severe to produce ischemic oculopathy and could explain the relatively low prevalence when carotid occlusive disease in general is considered.

A review of 30 nondiabetic patients (2,10–18,22–26) and 11 diabetic patients with markedly asymmetric retinopathy (14,15,17,27,28) who had carotid arteriography and all degrees of ischemic oculopathy is summarized in Table 10-1. Table 10-2 is a compilation of the presenting complaints and ocular and arteriographic findings in the 30 nondiabetic patients. If other causes of a hemorrhagic retinopathy are excluded, the presence of venous stasis retinopathy and ischemic oculopathy in patients in the stroke-age population suggests that major, often bilateral, carotid atherosclerotic occlusive disease is present.

Differential Diagnosis in Patients with Venous Stasis Retinopathy and Ischemic Oculopathy

In patients who have classic signs and symptoms of carotid occlusive disease, such as amaurosis fugax or transient cerebral ischemic attacks, the presence of venous stasis retinopathy or fully developed ischemic oculopathy very likely is related to the carotid occlusive disease and is predictive of a high degree of occlusive disease in the carotid arteries. When associated with less specific signs and symptoms, several additional diagnoses must be considered.

Venous Stasis Retinopathy

The primary features of venous stasis retinopathy are multiple intraretinal hemorrhages and dilatation of the retinal veins. A number of systemic and ocular conditions may produce a retinopathy with these character-

TABLE 10–1. Summary of arteriographic findings in diabetic and nondiabetic patients with venous stasis retinopathy or ischemic oculopathy.

	Nondiabetic N = 30	Diabetic N = 11
At least one occlusion (CCA or ICA)	27 (90%)	9 (81%)
Bilateral occlusion (CCA + ICA or ICA + ICA)	7 (24%)	2 (18%)
At least one CCA occlusion	8 (27%)	2 (18%)

CCA, Common carotid artery; ICA, Internal carotid artery. (Reproduced by permission from Carter JE: Chronic ocular ischemia and carotid vascular disease. *Stroke* 1985; 16:721–728.)

TABLE 10–2. Arteriography in patients with chronic ocular ischemia.

Patient	Presenting problem	VSR	Ischemic oculopathy	Ipsilateral	Contralateral
1	Vitrous hemorrhage	+	+	CCAO	ICAO
2	Amaurosis fugax	+	−	CCAO	CCA stenosis
3	Amaurosis fugax	−	+	CCAO	CCA narrowed
4	Red eye	+	+	CCAO	ICA 70%
5	Neovascular glaucoma	+	+	CCAO	ICA 50%
6	Unknown		+	ICA 95%	CCAO
7	Neovascular glaucoma	+	+	CCAO	Normal
8	Blurred vision, TIA	+	−	CCAO	Normal
9	Neovascular glaucoma	+	+	ICAO	ICAO
10	Neovascular glaucoma	+	+	ICAO	ICAO
11	Incidental finding	+	+	ICAO	ICAO
12	Painful visual loss	−	+	ICAO	ICAO
13	Visual loss	−	+	ICAO	ICAO
14	Visual loss	+	−	ICAO	ICAO
15	Visual loss	+	+	ICA 99%	ICAO
16	Cerebral ischemia	+	−	ICAO	CCA narrowed
17	Visual loss	+	+	ICAO	ICA plaque
18	TIA	+	−	ICAO	Normal
19	Unknown		+	ICAO	Normal
20	Unknown		+	ICAO	Normal
21	TIA, amaurosis fugax	+	−	ICAO	?
22	TIA	+	−	ICAO	?
23	TIA	+	−	ICAO	?
24	Painful progressive visual loss	+	+	ICAO	?
25	Neovascular glaucoma		+	ICAO	?
26	Neovascular glaucoma	+	+	ICAO	?
27	Uveitis	+	+	ICAO	?
28	Neovascular glaucoma	+	+	ICA 95%	ICA 95%
29	Neovascular glaucoma	+	+	ICA 95%	ICA 75%
30	Unknown		+	ICA 75%	ICA 60%

VSR, venous stasis retinopathy; CCAO, common carotid artery occlusion; ICAO, internal carotid artery occlusion; TIA, transient ischemic attack. Percentage refers to percent stenosis of respective artery.

(Reproduced by permission from Carter JE: Chronic ocular ischemia and carotid vascular disease. *Stroke* 1985; 16:721–728.)

istics. Conditions that alter blood viscosity or oxygen-carrying capacity may cause a hemorrhagic retinopathy. These include blood dyscrasias (eg, leukemia, lymphoma, polycythemia vera, sickle cell disease) and dysproteinemias (eg, multiple myeloma, cryoglobulinemia, macroglobulinemia) and even severe anemias (usually with a hematocrit of less than 7). Advanced diabetic retinopathy may be confused with venous stasis retinopathy, but several differences distinguish the two. The retinal hemorrhages seen with diabetes are concentrated in the macular region inside the vascular arcades, whereas those of venous stasis retinopathy are most concentrated along and outside the vascular arcades. Perhaps most important, diabetes and all the systemic conditions mentioned should affect the two eyes equally and produce bilateral retinopathy. A number of reports (7,14,17,27,28) have indicated that a unilateral retinopathy (and also fully developed neovascular changes in the anterior segment of the eye) in a diabetic are likely to be associated with severe carotid occlusive disease on the same side. Any time one of the aforementioned systemic diseases appears to be producing unilateral ocular abnormalities, the clinician should suspect the presence of carotid occlusive disease.

In the absence of diabetes or the other systemic diseases mentioned, the primary differential consideration in a patient with venous stasis retinopathy is occlusion of the central retinal vein. Occlusion of the central retinal vein has been recognized for more than 100 years, and even in 1904 Coats recognized two forms of the disease: a severe form with extensive retinal hemorrhage and a poor visual prognosis, usually thought of as a complete occlusion; and a milder form with better vision and a better prognosis, which often is termed partial or impending occlusion of the central retinal vein (29). These two varieties also have been classified as ischemic and nonischemic by Hayreh (29–31), who chose to use the term venous stasis retinopathy to indicate the nonischemic variety of occlusion. Most patients in whom carotid occlusive disease has produced a retinopathy that has not yet progressed to fully developed ischemic oculopathy will maintain good vision. These patients easily are confused, both in level of visual function and in appearance of the fundus, with patients who have partial or nonischemic occlusion of the central retinal vein. This has produced considerable confusion in the literature as to which condition is under discussion and even what the difference is between the two. Hayreh (31) and Kearns (32) were given the opportunity to discuss their views of this question at a symposium of world experts on occlusion of the central retinal vein at the American Academy of Ophthalmology in 1982. Their remarks were published in adjacent articles in *Ophthalmology* in 1983. Kearns (32) admitted that the term venous stasis retinopathy might not have been the best one and proposed certain characteristics as specific for the venous stasis retinopathy of carotid occlusive disease that he and Hollenhorst (7) had described in 1963 using that term. In patients with an occlusion of the central retinal vein, the hemorrhages are prominent throughout the retina, including the area adjacent to the disk and in the macula. In patients with venous stasis retinopathy, the hemorrhages are much more marked, beginning at the vascular arcades and into the midperiphery of the retina. Patients with occlusion of the central retinal vein usually have prominent disk edema, whereas patients with venous stasis retinopathy do not. Both groups of patients have engorged retinal veins, but Kearns believes that the marked irregularity in caliber is seen only in venous stasis retinopathy. Hayreh (31) challenged not only the specificity of these retinal findings but also the existence of a direct relationship between the retinopathy and carotid occlusive disease.

The number of ways in which the eye can respond to an unlimited variety of pathologic stimuli is limited. A retinopathy with multiple retinal hemorrhages is seen with ischemia due to disease of the microvasculature, as in diabetes; with hypoxia due to decreased oxygen-carrying capacity of the blood in anemia; with hypoxia in high-altitude retinopathy; with abnormal clotting mechanisms; with increase in blood viscosity from an increase in cellular elements or abnormalities of plasma proteins; and with obstruction of the venous outflow in occlusion of the central retinal vein. Venous engorgement would be a common feature with most of these conditions. Although subtle distinctions may increase the odds of recognizing which condition is responsible for the findings in an individual patient, the similarities certainly outweigh the differences, and it would not be surprising if the accuracy in making a correct etiologic diagnosis were less than perfect. Certainly, other acknowledged experts in the field of ocular vascular disease find patients with severe carotid disease among those groups who have partial occlusion of the central retinal vein. In discussing the characteristics of "partial occlusion of the central retinal vein," Zegarra et al (33) were unable to distinguish one patient in their series with carotid occlusive disease and retinopathy except for the presence of very low pressure in the central retinal artery. They also noted the collapse of the central retinal vein along with the artery, a finding that should not be present if the venous pressure is elevated by an obstruction. Kearns et al (16) and others (28) have shown angiographic reversal of flow in ophthalmic arteries in patients with carotid occlusions and venous stasis retinopathy or ischemic oculopathy, suggesting that the ocular circulation may be compromised in this setting. The fact that diabetic patients with unilateral retinopathy are likely to have severe carotid occlusive disease on the same side (7,14,17,27,28) also supports the possibility that a low flow state in the carotid circulation can contribute to ischemia in the eye.

The most important determinant in distinguishing between the venous stasis retinopathy of carotid artery occlusive disease and other hemorrhagic retinopathies is measurement of the retinal arterial and venous pressure. In venous stasis retinopathy and ischemic oculopathy, the central retinal arterial pressure is always extremely low, and, as noted earlier, may be so low that spontaneous pulsations of the central retinal artery occur (7,13,15–17). Furthermore, pressure on the eye may be expected to collapse the veins at a very low pressure (33).

Ischemic Oculopathy

The ischemic changes in the anterior segment of the eye also are nonspecific. Gartner and Henkind (34) noted that neovascularization of the iris was associated with 41 different entities, most commonly occlusion of the central retinal vein, diabetic retinopathy, uveitis, and open-angle glaucoma, but also including systemic lupus erythematosus, sickle cell disease, retinal detachment, and giant-cell arteritis. Carotid insufficiency was responsible for only 8% of patients with iris neovascularization in Hoskins's series (35) but was still the fourth most common cause. In an evaluation of a series of patients referred with unilateral neovascular glaucoma unassociated with occlusion of the central retinal vein, retinal detachment, or intraocular tumor, Brown et al (15) found that 11 of 12 were associated with major carotid artery occlusive disease. Five were diabetic but had unilateral retinopathy. In the absence of a primary ophthalmic cause for neovascular changes, unilateral neovascularization of the retina or iris strongly suggests the diagnosis of carotid artery occlusive disease. A careful examination in conjunction with the ophthalmologist and routine laboratory studies should exclude other causes for ocular neovascularization and allow appropriate evaluation of the cervical carotid artery. Because the clinician is looking for major occlusive disease, today's sophisticated noninvasive imaging techniques and IV digital subtraction angiography should provide sufficient information with little or no risk to the patient.

Therapeutic Considerations in Patients with Chronic Ocular Ischemia

As in patients with amaurosis fugax and retinal arterial emboli, therapeutic efforts in patients with signs of chronic ocular ischemia may be directed toward two goals: preventing stroke and preserving normal visual function.

In the case of preventing stroke, the difficulty lies in the degree of occlusive disease present at the time of the diagnosis. Few would argue about performing an endarterectomy on a stenotic lesion on the symptomatic side, but this is seldom the situation. Although the conventional wisdom in cerebrovascular disease is to "operate on the symptomatic side," venous stasis retinopathy and ischemic oculopathy may be exceptions. The frequent occurrence in these patients of major bilateral carotid occlusive disease and symptoms and signs limited to the eye may indicate that intracranial blood flow is being distributed via whatever primary or collateral pathways are available at the expense of the ocular circulation. If a major source of intracranial blood flow is from the external carotid artery via maxillary and superficial temporal arteries to the ophthalmic artery, blood flow through the ophthalmic artery is reversed, and the ocular circulation may be a cul-de-sac with minimal blood flow (28). It may be reasonable to consider endarterectomy on a significant stenosis of the ICA even though it is on the opposite side, or on a significant stenosis of an external carotid artery if angiography indicates that it is a major remaining source of intracranial blood flow. Some patients will have inoperable lesions, such as an occlusion of the common carotid artery with no abnormality or even an occlusion of the ICA on the opposite side. Attempts to prevent stroke or manage cerebral ischemic symptoms by using medical management would be the most logical approach to such a patient. Extracranial-intracranial bypass surgery was ineffective in preventing stroke in a recent study (36) and is probably not a therapeutic consideration in this setting. The most accurate statement regarding stroke prevention therapy in patients with venous stasis retinopathy and ischemic oculopathy is that each case must be considered individually after careful study of the cerebral circulation.

The same statement is true when considering therapy directed at the ocular ischemia. Because the natural history is still uncertain, the efficacy of any therapy is uncertain. However, any operable carotid lesion likely will be corrected in the interest of preventing stroke in the patient. Therefore, therapy aimed specifically at correcting the ocular condition will be an issue in those patients who have inoperable lesions or in whom carotid surgery did not correct the ocular abnormalities. As noted earlier, venous stasis retinopathy may be seen in patients who are being evaluated shortly after an acute neurologic ischemic event. In this setting, the patient might be observed for a period of time after the completion of treatment aimed at preventing stroke. If the venous stasis retinopathy resolves, then no further action may be necessary. In the remainder of patients with venous stasis retinopathy, therapy probably can be started early. The presence of any neovascular changes indicates a chronic process and argues for immediate intervention. Neovascularization of the iris may regress with therapy (10,17), but this must occur before closure of the anterior chamber angle by the fibrovascular membrane if neovascular glaucoma is to be prevented.

Panretinal photocoagulation is standard therapy for conditions such as diabetic retinopathy and occlusion of the central retinal vein in which retinal ischemia results in neovascularization and is the most logical initial therapy in patients who have inoperable carotid lesions or whose symptoms and signs have persisted despite carotid surgery. Regression of the retinopathy and neovascularization of the optic disk and iris after panretinal photocoagulation has been reported in one case caused by carotid occlusive disease (10).

References

1. Walsh FB, Hoyt WF: *Clinical Neuro-ophthalmology*. Baltimore, The Williams & Wilkins Co. 1969, 1832.
2. Young LH, Appen RE: Ischemic oculopathy: A manifestation of carotid artery disease. *Arch Neurol* 1981;38:358–360.
3. Hirose K: A study of fundus changes in the early stages of Takayasu-Ohnishi (pulseless) disease. *Am J Ophthalmol* 1963;55:295–301.
4. Ostler HB: Pulseless disease (Takayasu's disease). *Am J Ophthalmol* 1957;43:583–589.
5. Tour RL, Hoyt WF: The syndrome of the aortic arch. *Am J Ophthalmol* 1959;47:35–48.

6. Hedges TR: Ophthalmoscopic findings in internal carotid artery occlusion. *Am J Ophthamol* 1963;55:1007–1012.
7. Kearns TP, Hollenhorst RW: Venous stasis retinopathy of occlusive disease of the carotid artery. *Mayo Clin Proc* 1963;38:304–312.
8. Abedin S, Simmons RJ: Neovascular glaucoma in systemic occlusive vascular disease. *Ann Ophthalmol* 1982;14:284–287.
9. Bullock JD, Falter RT, Downing JE, et al: Ischemic ophthalmia secondary to an ophthalmic artery occlusion. *Am J Ophthalmol* 1972; 74:486–493.
10. Carter JE: Panretinal photocoagulation for progressive ocular neovascularization secondary to occlusion of the common carotid artery. *Ann Ophthalmol* 1984;16:572–576.
11. Grader J: Venous stasis retinopathy: A case report. *Can J Ophthalmol* 1975;10:107–110.
12. Smith JL: Unilateral glaucoma in carotid occlusive disease. *JAMA* 1962;182:187–188.
13. Hoefnagels KLJ: Rubeosis of the iris associated with occlusion of the carotid artery. *Ophthalmologica* 1964;148:196–200.
14. Knox DL: Ischemic ocular inflammation. *Am J Ophthalmol* 1965;60:995–1002.
15. Brown GC, Magargal LE, Simeone FA, et al: Arterial obstruction and ocular neovascularization. *Ophthalmology* 1982;89:139–146.
16. Kearns TP, Siekert RG, Sundt TM Jr: The ocular aspects of bypass surgery of the carotid artery. *Mayo Clin Proc* 1979;54:3–11.
17. Kiser WD, Gonder J, Magargal LE, et al: Recovery of vision following treatment of the ocular ischemic syndrome. *Ann Ophthalmol* 1983;15:305–310.
18. Campo RV, Aaberg TM: Digital subtraction angiography in the diagnosis of retinal vascular disease. *Am J Ophthalmol* 1983;96:632–640.
19. Swan KC, Raaf J: Changes in the eye and orbit following carotid ligation. *Trans Am Ophthalmol Soc* 1951; 49:435–444.
20. Patz A: Clinical and experimental studies on retinal neovascularization. *Am J Ophthalmol* 1982;94:715–743.
21. Barany E: Influence of local arterial blood pressure on aqueous humor and intraocular pressure. *Acta Ophthalmol* 1946;24:337–387.
22. Ausman JI, Lindsay W, Ramsay RC, et al: Ipsilateral subclavian to external carotid and STA-MCA bypasses for retinal ischemia. *Surg Neurol* 1978;9:5–8.
23. Cowan CL, Butler G: Ischemic oculopathy *Ann Ophthalmol* 1983;15:1052–1057.
24. Eggleston TF, Bohling CA, Eggleston HC, et al: Photocoagulation for ocular ischemia associated with carotid artery occlusion. *Ann Ophthalmol* 1980;12:84–87.
25. Kearns TP, Younge BR, Piepgrass DG: Resolution of venous stasis retinopathy after carotid artery bypass surgery. *Mayo Clin Proc* 1980;55:342–346.
26. Neupert JR, Brubaker RF, Kearns TP, et al: Rapid resolution of venous stasis retinopathy after carotid endarterectomy. *Am J Ophthalmol* 1976;81:600–602.
27. Edwards MS, Chater NL, Stanley JA: Reversal of chronic ocular ischemia by extracranial-intracranial arterial bypass: A case report. *Neurosurgery* 1980;7:480–483.
28. Huckman MS, Haas J: Reversed flow through the ophthalmic artery as a cause of rubeosis irides. *Am J Ophthalmol* 1966;74:758–762.

29. Hayreh SS: So-called central retinal vein occlusion: I. Pathogenesis, terminology, clinical features. *Ophthalmologica* 1976;172:1–13.
30. Hayreh SS: So-called central retinal vein occlusion: II. Venous stasis retinopathy. *Ophthalmologica* 1976;172:14–37.
31. Hayreh SS: The controversy of venous stasis retinopathy, in Bernstein EF (ed): *Amaurosis Fugax*. New York, Springer-Verlag, 1987.
32. Kearns TP: Differential diagnosis of central retinal vein obstruction. *Ophthalmology* 1983;90:475–480.
33. Zegarra H, Gutman FA, Zakov N, et al: Partial occlusion of the central retinal vein. *Am J Ophthalmol* 1983;96:330–337.
34. Gartner S, Henkind P: Neovascularization of the iris (rubeosis irides). *Surv Ophthalmol* 1978;22:291–312.
35. Hoskins HO: Neovascular glaucoma. *Trans Am Acad Ophthalmol Otolaryngol* 1974;78:330–333.
36. Barnett HJM, Peerless SJ, Fox AJ, et al: Failure of extracranial-intracranial arterial bypass to reduce the risk of ischemic stroke. *N Engl J Med* 1985; 313:1191–1200.

CHAPTER 11

Chronic Ocular Ischemic Syndrome in Internal Carotid Artery Occlusive Disease: Controversy on "Venous Stasis Retinopathy"

Sohan Singh Hayreh

In 1874 Schmidt (1) reported neovascular glaucoma in a 58-year-old man who had suffered two cerebrovascular accidents—one 2.5 months before and the second 10 months after the development of glaucoma. The same year Loring (2) reported the case of a 62-year-old woman who developed central retinal artery occlusion and neovascular glaucoma, and died of cerebrovascular accident. Since then a large number of cases of chronic ocular ischemia with carotid artery disease have been reported in the literature (we have summarized and discussed the subject elsewhere (3)). The primary objective of this chapter is to deal with the controversy surrounding the "venous stasis retinopathy" attributed to carotid artery occlusive disease, and then to discuss, very briefly, various features of chronic ocular ischemic syndrome.

Venous Stasis Retinopathy

In October 1962, Hedges (4) presented *one* patient with complete occlusion of the right internal carotid artery, left hemiparesis, and the left fundus findings of dilated and tortuous retinal veins with "diffuse blotlike hemorrhages" in the macula, extending out to the equator. About 6 months later, "most of the hemorrhages and all venous dilatation had disappeared." He speculated that "these retinal findings could well be the result of retinal hypoxia induced by the carotid insufficiency." In July, 1963, Kearns and Hollenhorst (5) published findings of similar fundus changes. "In 22 of some 600 patients with intermittent insufficiency or thrombosis in the carotid arterial system" they reported dilatation of retinal veins, small "blossom-shaped" hemorrhages, microaneurysms in close proximity to the retinal veins, and "in some cases, . . . sludging of blood within the veins." These retinal lesions usually were quite mild and in the midperipheral parts of the retina. None of their patients had visual defects attributable to the retinopahy. According to them, the eye always had low central retinal artery (CRA) pressure; they further added that, "however, less than 10 percent of patients with low pressure in the retinal artery will have the retinopathy.'' In marked cases, according to them, ''the major retinal veins may become large, dark, and irregular,'' but none of their patients ''had the link-sausage veins seen in severe diabetic retinopathy or in dysglobulinemia.'' They called the condition ''Venous stasis retinopathy,'' and they stated that it was their ''impression'' that ''it probably only occurs when there is complete occlusion in the carotid system.'' They stated that this condition may be mistaken for an ''impending occlusion of the central retinal vein'' or diabetic retinopathy. Since then ''venous stasis retinopathy'' has come to be recognized as the classical and diagnostic sign of occlusive disease of the carotid arterial system, and many articles have been published promoting this concept, so it has come to be regarded as an ''established fact.'' However, none of the publications on the subject have presented any scientific evidence that internal carotid artery occlusive disease and venous stasis retinopathy have a cause-and-effect relationship, nor that chronic retinal hypoxia without appreciable visual loss can produce all these retinal vascular changes.

In 1983, Kearns (6) stated that ''It was unfortunate that Kearns and Hollenhorst (5) chose the name ''venous-stasis retinopathy.'' It is true that blood flow is slowed in the retinal veins, but the primary problem is the low perfusion pressure in the arterioles. The term 'chronic ischemic retinopathy' might have served better.''

Over the past quarter-century we have investigated the subject of central retinal vein occlusion (CRVO) experimentally in 54 eyes of rhesus monkeys (7–10) and clinically by prospective studies (11–16). In addition, for the past decade, I have continued to prospectively investigate patients with carotid artery occlusive disease and have collected data on over 200 such patients so far.

My experimental and clinical studies on CRVO were the first to indicate that CRVO consists, in fact, of two distinct entities: (i) *without ischemia* and (ii) *with ischemia,* and this has since been amply confirmed by our prospective clinical studies on over 600 patients with CRVO (7,8,11–13,15,16). It has also been confirmed by the clinical studies of a large number of other investigators. Thus the dual nature of CRVO is now a fully established fact. In our prospective studies on over 600 consecutive patients with CRVO so far, 75–80% of the patients have the nonischemic type of occlusion and 20–25% have the ischemic type. The fundus findings in nonischemic CRVO, in both experimental and clinical studies, revealed that retinopathy simply reflects a stasis of retinal venous circulation i.e., engorged retinal veins and retinal hemorrhages are always present and other secondary retinal changes occur less frequently. In view of this, I proposed the term ''venous stasis retinopathy'' for the nonischemic CRVO in 1976 (11). My studies (3,8–16) on nonischemic CRVO as well as on carotid artery occlusive disease have indicated strongly that the so-called ''venous stasis retinopathy'' attributed to carotid artery occlusive disease almost always represents nonischemic CRVO and is not a manifestation of "retinal hypoxia," as originally postulated by Hedges (4) (based on his experience with one patient!).

The following evidence indicates that a cause-and-effect relationship does not exist between internal carotid artery occlusive disease and venous stasis retinopathy.

1. The clinical picture (both symptoms and signs) of mild venous stasis retinopathy, due to CRVO, seen by us, is identical to that reported for "venous stasis retinopathy" presumed to be due to carotid artery occlusive disease. Figs. 11–1 to 11–3, showing venous stasis retinopathy due to CRVO, and Fig. 11–4 showing venous stasis retinopathy due to carotid-cavernous fistula, illustrate this.

2. Kearns and Hollenhorst (5) found *no venous stasis retinopathy* in 95% of their patients with unilateral internal carotid artery stenosis or occlusion, nor any such retinopathy in over 90% of their cases with low CRA pressure. If retinal hypoxia (secondary to internal carotid artery stenosis or occlusion) and venous stasis retinopathy were cause and effect, surely the prevalence of venous stasis retinopathy in these cases should

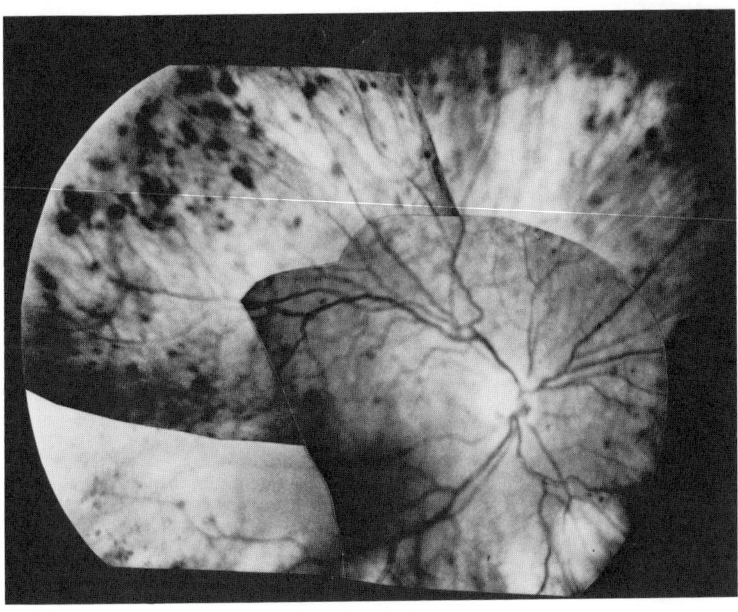

FIGURE 11–1. Composite fundus photograph of the right eye of a 73-year-old man with venous stasis retinopathy (nonischemic CRVO, and no carotid artery disease. The photograph shows mildly engorged retinal veins, retinal hemorrhages over the 360° of the equatorial and peripheral retina (most marked in the superior temporal sector), and no optic disk edema.

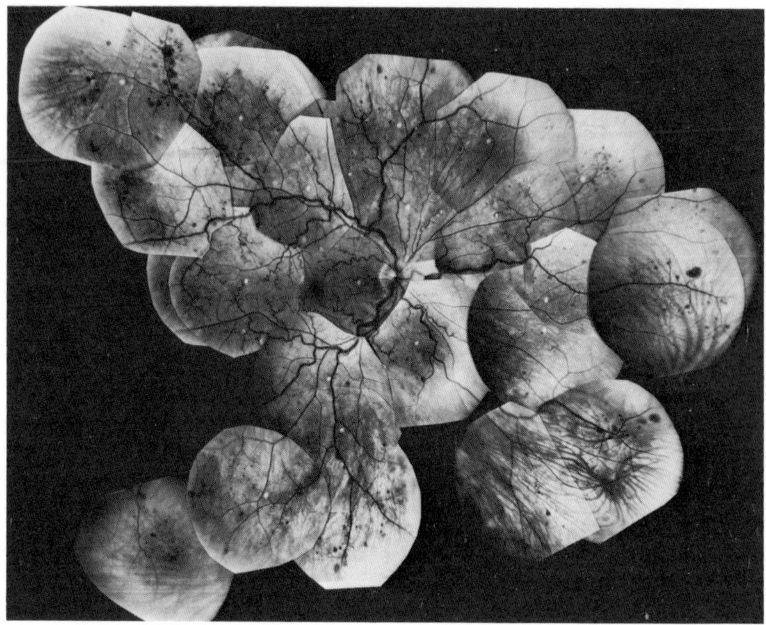

FIGURE 11–2. Composite fundus photograph of the right eye of a perfectly healthy 23-year-old man with no visual symptoms and no carotid artery disease. During a routine eye examination, he was found to have venous stasis retinopathy, with no optic disk or macular edema, a visual acuity of 6/6, normal visual fields, and no abnormality on fluorescein fundus angiography. The retinal hemorrhages were located mainly in the peripheral retina, best seen by indirect ophthalmoscopy. The retinopathy resolved completely within 1 year and the eye was never symptomatic. [Reproduced from Hayreh SS, 1983 (13).]

have been much higher. Other reports in the literature claiming venous stasis retinopathy is due to retinal hypoxia are essentially anecdotal in nature, with no systematic prospective study on the subject. My prospective studies on over 200 consecutive patients with carotid artery occlusive disease also show that venous stasis retinopathy is rare with this disease.

3. In my studies, some of the patients with unilateral internal carotid artery occlusive disease had venous stasis retinopathy only on the side with a normal internal carotid artery, and a normal fundus on the side with the internal carotid artery occlusive disease.

4. In my studies, I found no correlation between the severity of internal carotid artery disease and the presence and/or severity of venous stasis retinopathy.

5. Resolution of venous stasis retinopathy: Over recent years Kearns and his colleagues (17–19), have claimed in anecdotal case reports that

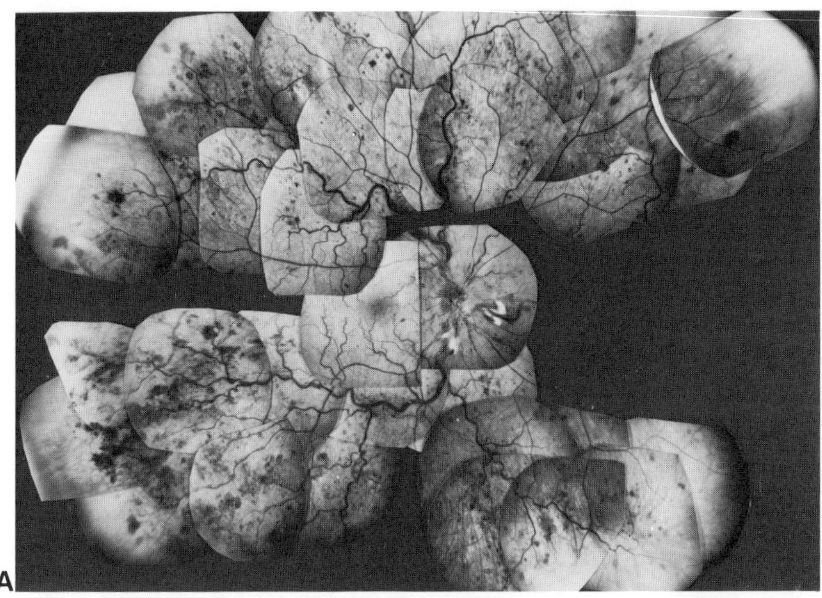

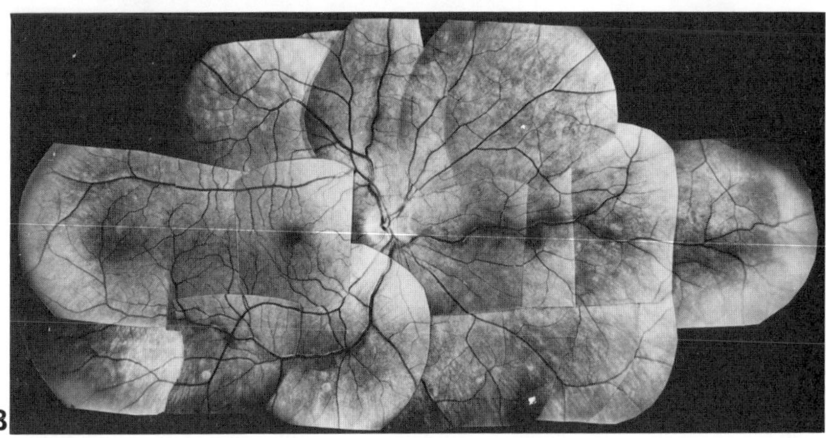

FIGURE 11–3. Composite fundus photographs of the right eye of a 31-year-old perfectly healthy man with venous stasis retinopathy and no carotid artery disease. Progressive blurred vision had developed 6 weeks before the examination; the visual acuity was 6/21. (A) Photograph taken at the initial visit shows engorged retinal veins, peripheral retinal hemorrhages, and mild edema of the macula and optic disk. The retinopathy resolved completely within 1 year (B) [Reproduced from Hayreh SS, 1983 (13).]

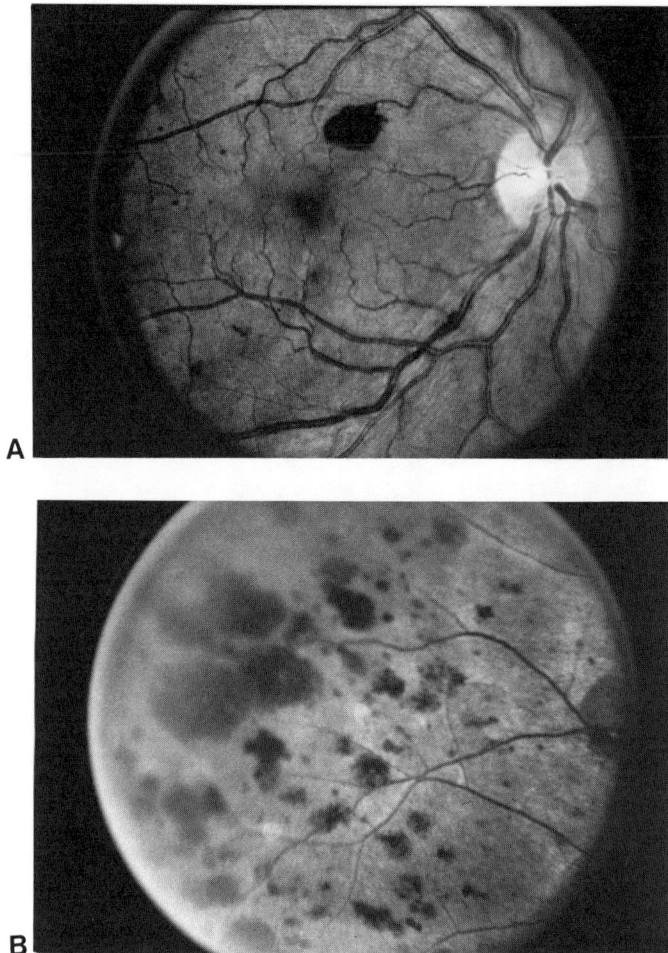

FIGURE 11–4. Fundus photographs of (A) posterior pole and (B) temporal periphery of the fundus of a 38-year-old woman who had carotid-cavernous fistula and secondary venous stasis retinopathy with engorged retinal veins and retinal hemorrhages, mostly in the peripheral retina. The retinopathy resolved on surgical closing of the fistula. (Reproduced courtesy of Dr. James Corbett, University of Iowa.) Hospitals and Clinic.

carotid endarterectomy (19) or bypass surgery (17,18) has produced resolution of venous stasis retinopathy, by improving arterial supply to the eye. In contrast, I have had at lease four patients in whom venous stasis retinopathy developed 2 weeks, 2 months, 2 years, and 3½ years after carotid endarterectomy and with normal retinal blood flow. One patient presented in my clinic with bilateral venous stasis retinopathy and bilateral marked stenosis of internal carotid artery, who would have been considered a typical example of this entity by the persons supporting it. Soon after his first visit, he had a carotid endarterectomy on one side; 3 months later the retinopathy had resolved not only on the operated side but also on the unoperated side, with CRA pressure equal and still very low on both sides. My studies on the natural history of nonischemic CRVO have shown that mild venous stasis retinopathy resolves within 6 months in one third (as quickly as 2 to 3 months in many instances) and within one year in two thirds of the cases, without any treatment (Fig. 11–1 to 11–3). Thus, my studies indicate that the resolution of retinopathy attributed to various therapeutic modalities may represent nothing more than natural resolution of venous stasis retinopathy. If retinal hypoxia were the sole cause of venous stasis retinopathy in patients with internal carotid artery occlusive disease, it is inconceivable that the retinopathy would resolve spontaneously within a few months (as has also been reported in many anecdotal reports in the literature) when the presumed retinal hypoxia still persists. It could be argued that this spontaneous resolution is due to establishment of collateral circulation to the eye and improved circulation. In a follow-up of patients with extremely low CRA pressure for years, I have observed neither any appreciable improvement in the CRA pressure nor development of venous stasis retinopathy, although a few patients progressed to develop signs of anterior segment ischemia.

Thus, it can be concluded that internal carotid artery occlusive disease and venous stasis retinopathy are most probably not cause-and-effect. Naturally the question arises, what *is* the relationship between the two, and what is responsible for all this confusion?

In patients with severe generalized atherosclerosis, arteries all over the body are involved by atherosclerotic lesions, including the carotid arteries, the coronary arteries, the CRA and the limb arteries. Atherosclerotic narrowing of coronary arteries results in myocardial infarction; of carotid arteries in cerebrovascular accidents; and of limb arteries in ischemic disorders of the limbs. Histopathologic studies have shown that the CRA and CRV lie side by side within the optic nerve, enclosed by a common envelope of fibrous tissue. Atherosclerosis and arteriosclerosis of the CRA within the optic nerve (as demonstrated by multiple histological studies) would mechanically compress the adjacent CRV; aging sclerosis of the connective tissue around the central retinal vessels further constricts the CRV (20). In addition, irritative endothelial proliferation occurs in the CRV due to compression (21,22). These changes collectively produce marked narrrowing of the lumen of the CRV within the optic nerve and endothelial proliferation ultimately occludes the vein (20). In addition, Leber (23) emphasized the role of arterial insufficiency and consequent circulatory stasis in the production of thrombosis of the CRV. Klien (21) called it stagnation thrombosis. Klien (24) further considered that hemodynamic disturbances, such as a sudden fall of blood pressure from any cause, might be a factor in the production of CRVO by causing stagnation of the circulation and primary thrombus formation. We have discussed the subject of pathogenesis of CRVO at length elsewhere (8,12). Thus, our studies have indicated that CRVO is a multifactoral process, and that slowing down of the arterial circulation and/or fall of blood pressure in the CRA contributes to the production of CRVO in susceptible individuals, although these hemodynamic changes per se may not do so. In 118 patients with retinal vein occlusion, Paton et al (25) found a high prevalence of atherosclerotic disease (as judged from a history of ischemic heart disease, cerebrovascular disease, or intermittent claudication) and carotid artery disease; hypertension and/or atherosclerotic disease were present in 81% of their cases. The majority of patients with severe atherosclerosis of the internal carotid artery (and consequent occlusion of the carotid artery) eventually succumb to myocardial infarction (26). This does not mean that carotid artery disease and myocardial infarction are cause and effect because the carotid artery has no role in the blood supply to the heart—the common underlying cause is the severe generalized atherosclerosis. The same logic must apply to carotid artery disease and venous stasis retinopathy (due to CRVO). So, carotid artery disease, myocardial ischemia and venous stasis retinopathy are three independent manifestations of severe generalized atherosclerosis, as is severe peripheral arterial ischemia. The available evidence strongly indicates that venous stasis retinopathy and carotid artery disease are usually not cause and effect but are independent manifestations of severe generalized atherosclerosis. However, hemodynamic disturbances due to carotid artery occlusive disease may make these patients more susceptible to CRVO than those patients with normal retinal hemodynamics.

Kearns (6) recently pointed out several ocular differentiating characteristics between "the retinopathy of carotid occlusive disease" and CRVO, and these were as follows:

1. *Optic disc:* Kearns claimed that in retinopathy of carotid artery disease, the disk never develops edema, which is a major feature of vein occlusion along with hemorrhages on the disk. My studies on CRVO have shown that a mild degree of nonischemic CRVO (or venous stasis retinopathy) may have neither disk edema nor hemorrhage on it (Fig. 11–1,11–2). If an eye has optic disk edema along with retinal venous engorgement and retinal hemorrhages, it is nonischemic CRVO and *not* retinopathy secondary to carotid artery occlusive disease (Fig. 11–3).
2. *Retinal veins:* In both conditions, according to Kearns (6), the retinal veins are engorged and dark. He stressed that in carotid artery disease the veins often have an irregular caliber that is "never seen" in CRVO. My experience with CRVO does not agree; I have seen irregular retinal veins with vein occlusion, although this was not a very common finding.
3. *Type and location of lesions:* According to Kearns (6): "The hemorrhages, microaneurysms, and capillary dilatation of central retinal vein

occlusion tend to be generalized. Usually, they are found distributed evenly over the entire retina. These same lesions are located usually in the mid-periphery of the retina of the patient with carotid disease.'' My studies have demonstrated clearly that in mild and even some moderate venous stasis retinopathy cases due to CRVO, the earliest hemorrhages and lesions are essentially in the peripheral retina (13) (Fig. 11–1 to 11–4) and in a fair proportion of them the condition may resolve without ever involving the posterior pole (Fig. 11–2). Figures 11–1 to 11–4 clearly show the peripheral location of the retinal hemorrhages in venous stasis retinopathy due to CRVO; these have been described as characteristic of ''venous stasis retinopathy'' due to carotid artery disease. During resolution of retinopathy of CRVO, in all patients (even in severe cases), the peripheral retinal hemorrhages are the last to disappear and may be the only hemorrhages seen for a long time. Sometimes I have come across patients with diabetic retinopathy with hemorrhages, microaneurysms, and capillary nonperfusion in the midperiphery of the retina mistakenly thought to have retinopathy due to carotid artery disease. Similarly, I have observed patients with old ischemic CRVO, who have a few hemorrhages, microaneurysms and capillary nonperfusion in the midperiphery, and are erroneously diagnosed as having retinopathy due to carotid artery disease because they happen to have the latter as well. In an occasional patient a few transient retinal hemorrhages may be seen in the fundus, particularly in the periphery, with no detectable carotid disease, or any other abnormality. Thus, the type and location of lesions have no diagnostic importance in labeling a retinopathy as due to carotid artery disease; unfortunately, this criterion has come to be regarded as a diagnostic feature of carotid artery disease. In a recent publication, Brown (27) claimed that macular edema can develop in carotid artery disease; however, a careful review of his paper indicates that his cases most probably were nonischemic CRVO (according to the criteria used by Kearns (6) and me), and I have a large collection of similar cases in my studies on CRVO. In 5 of 7 eyes in his study, visual acuity was 6/7.5 to 6/15, in one 6/21 and in another 6/60. Such good visual acuity in the majority of his cases speaks against retinal ischemia severe enough to produce retinal vascular leakage and consequent macular edema. There is no scientific evidence that low pressure in the CRA can produce macular edema indistinguishable from that seen in mild cases of nonischemic CRVO. If the perfusion pressure in the retinal arterial circulation falls very low in patients with carotid artery occlusive disease, the macular region can develop infarction, which is totally different from the genuine macular edema.

4. *Visual symptoms:* According to Kearns (6). ''In both conditions, patients may have blurred vision. The blurring of vision with central retinal vein occlusion is usually stable and does not fluctuate as it does in the retinopathy of carotid disease.'' Patients with venous stasis retinopathy due to CRVO can have ''fluctuating vision,'' because they may complain

of transient blurring of vision every morning, lasting for a few hours and gradually clearing up. This is due to transient mild macular edema that develops during sleep and resolves or improves once the patient has been up and about for some time.

5. *Associated ocular findings:* Kearns (6) stated that "a cholesterol embolus or a fibrin-platelet embolus may be present in the retinopathy of carotid occlusive disease." However, he commented, "Nevertheless, such emboli are seen more often in retinopathy of carotid disease than they are in retinopathy of retinal vein occlusion." I have seen such emboli in the retinal arteries in some cases of retinopathy of CRVO, which further indicate the presence of carotid artery disease, although Kearns dismissed this as purely "coincidental."

6. *Ocular hypotony:* Kearns (6) stated that the intraocular pressure on the affected side was usually 1 to 3 mm Hg lower than it was on the normal unaffected side in patients with venous stasis retinopathy due to carotid artery disease, and he attributed the ocular hypotony to the carotid artery disease. We, however, have demonstrated in a large prospective study that ocular hypotony (with intraocular pressure 1 to 3 mm Hg lower in the involved eye) is actually a characteristic feature of CRVO (14). No doubt ocular hypotony does occure in some of the eyes with marked ocular ischemia due to any cause, including carotid artery occlusive disease, and it is usually more marked than that seen in eyes with CRVO.

7. *Retinal artery pressure:* According to Kearns (6) a low retinal artery pressure is present in all eyes with retinopathy due to carotid artery disease "since the mechanism of production of the retinopathy of carotid disease is dependent on a low perfusion pressure and its resultant ischemia and anoxia." He stressed that low retinal artery pressure is "by far the most important" differentiating feature. As discussed in the early part of this chapter, almost 90% of patients seen by Kearns and Hollenhorst (5) with low CRA pressure associated with carotid artery disease did *not* have venous stasis retinopathy, which they claimed is due to retinal "ischemia and anoxia." It is very hard for me to understand why only a very small minority should have the "venous stasis retinopathy" when "ischemia and anoxia" are claimed to be its cause! Thus, the vast majority of the eyes with very low CRA pressure do not suffer any retinal vascular damage, as indicated by my studies.

Fundus findings in anecdotal cases of pulseless disease have been cited to prove that venous stasis retinopathy is due to low CRA pressure (28–31). The fundus findings in patients with pulseless disease vary widely. Uyama and Asayama (32), based on 79 cases of pulseless disease (Takayasu's disease), classified the disease into three types—(1) disease predominantly involving the aortic arch (38 cases), (2) thoracic or abdominal aorta (16 cases), and (3) a mixture of the previous two types (25 cases). In the first type there is cerebral hypotension, and in the second hypertension in the upper half of the body. Thus, the fundus changes should depend upon the type of disease. In the second type, these would be hypertensive, while in the first type they would be due to hypotension—and relevant to our present discussion. In eyes with low pressure in the CRA, there is dilatation of small vessels of the retina and in advanced cases there is sludging of circulation in the retinal veins. The microaneurysms, which are seen only in advanced stages of the disease (and are an important sign of this stage), have been described by Uyama and Asayama (32) as quite different in nature from those seen in diabetic retinopathy. In very advanced cases, arteriovenous anastomoses develop progressively from the periphery towards the posterior pole. *No retinal hemorrhages were seen* by Uyama and Asayama (32) in their patients, which has also been the experience of others (28,31). This fact refutes the argument that retinal hemorrhages in eyes with low retinal artery pressure in carotid occlusive disease are due to retinal ischemia. Moreover, one must be very careful not to carry over findings from one disease to another when their basic disease process is so different. Finally, an elderly patient with pulseless disease or low retinal artery pressure due to other causes is not immune from getting CRVO.

Retinal Hypoxia or Ischemia as a Cause of Retinal Vascular Changes

Usually, a stereotyped description blames retinal hypoxia/ischemia for retinal vascular changes (e.g., hemorrhages, microaneurysms, and other intraretinal microvascular abnormalities). The following evidence refutes this concept.

Experimental Acute Ischemia of the Retina

We conducted studies to find out the effects of acute ischemia on the retina after CRA occlusion in rhesus monkeys (9,10,33). These studies revealed a differential susceptibility to ischemia by the various retinal elements. Among the cytoplasmic organelles, the mitochondria were the most susceptible, with microtubules and endoplasmic reticulum less so in descending order. The nuclei were the least susceptible of all. Among the retinal cells, the ganglion cells were more susceptible than the bipolar cells; the Müller cells and astrocytic glia were less susceptible, and the pericytes and endothelial cells of the vessels were relatively resistant to ischemia (33). Our studies also revealed that among the retinal vascular cells, pericytes were more sensitive to acute ischemia than the endothelial cells (9,10). Thus, from these and other studies it is clear that the neural elements of the retina are far more sensitive to retinal ischemic damage than the retinal vessels, which are comparatively far more resistant. Therefore, retinal neural damage must precede the retinal vascular lesions. This is probably true of chronic ischemia as well.

Experimental Occlusion of the Carotid Artery

Experimental carotid artery occlusion resulted in development of dilatation and tortuosity of retinal veins and other evidence of acute retinal ischemia, but it produced no other apparent retinal lesions (e.g., hemorrhages, microaneurysms, or neovascularization (34, 35). The fundus changes had resolved completely by 1 week. This experimental study failed to produce the so-called venous stasis retinopathy due to retinal ischemia or hypoxia.

Low CRA Pressure

The other important fact to be borne in mind is that low CRA pressure does not necessarily mean retinal ischemia. We have ample clinical proof of this, because eyes of patients with carotid occlusive disease and with very low pressure (where the CRA starts to pulsate at a touch) most often do not suffer detectable inner retinal visual deficit during years of follow-up, nor do they have any other retinal lesions. In my fluorescein fundus angiographic studies of eyes with very low CRA pressure in patients with carotid artery disease, no microvascular abnormality was detected unless the eye had clinical evidence of CRVO.

Diabetic Retinopathy

Diabetic retinopathy is always put forward as evidence that retinal ischemia produces retinal vascular changes. In diabetic retinopathy, available evidence indicates that the primary change is in the pericytes and also probably in the endothelial cells of the retinal capillaries, resulting from diabetes. These changes produce secondary capillary closure and nonperfusion, resulting in retinal ischemia and, finally, the development of secondary associated neovascularization. Thus, in diabetic retinopathy, retinal ischemia and associated changes are a secondary phenomenon, whereas the retinal vascular changes are primary.

Ischemic CRVO

Our experimental and clinical studies showed that in this disease retinal neuronal damage precedes the retinal capillary damage by weeks, if not months, and that it requires a severe ischemia to produce secondary retinal capillary changes (8–10,12,13).

Thus, the statement that low CRA pressure produces ischemia is based on little scientific evidence and purely on "armchair philosophy." In fact, we have precious little scientific evidence that simple low CRA pressure with normal retinal function can produce any significant retinal or retinal vascular pathology. This discussion reveals that the whole theory that venous stasis retinopathy in patients with carotid artery disease is due to retinal ischemia or anoxia has little scientific basis. Retinal hypoxia of a marked degree, however, can produce simple dilatation of the retinal veins (most probably due to the effect of elevated carbon dioxide concentration) and no other retinal lesion.

While I question the validity of the concept and use of term "venous stasis retinopathy" for retinal changes mistakenly attributed to carotid artery occlusive disease, I have seen, in some patients with the latter disease, low CRA pressure, irregular caliber and stasis of circulation in the retinal vascular bed, including arterioles and venules, and, occasionally, neovascularization (see details below in chronic ocular ischemia). However, this fundus picture is very different from that seen in venous stasis retinopathy. I think that the cases reported in the literature as "venous stasis retinopathy due to carotid artery occlusive disease" are actually two very different types of retinopathy—most represent nonischemic CRVO (which I called venous stasis retinopathy), and a minority represent the second type (mentioned above and discussed below) in chronic ocular ischemia. Thus, lumping these two types of retinopathy under the title of "venous stasis retinopathy" is the cause of confusion.

Patients with severe carotid artery stenosis or occlusion, however, probably have a higher risk of CRVO, as discussed above, and they may suffer from ischemia.

Having said all that, one should "never say 'never' " in medicine. It *is* possible that hemorrhages, aneurysms and other retinal vascular changes may very rarely occur due to chronic retinal ischemia without apparent neuronal damage. If such a condition exists, it must indeed be extremely rare. We still await scientific proof.

Chronic Ocular Ischemia

In contrast to venous stasis retinopathy, the fundus of patients with carotid artery occlusive disease initially may present with signs of posterior segment changes secondary to ocular ischemia. The following case report represents a frequent presentation and course:

A 61-year-old man was seen in our clinic complaining of intermittent blurring of vision in his right eye for 6 months. At his first visit to our clinic, his visual acuity was 6/300 in that eye, with relative afferent pupillary defect. Examination of the anterior segment revealed extensive neovascularization of the iris and angle of the anterior chamber with total peripheral anterior synechiae, and intraocular pressure of 26 mm Hg (intraocular pressure in the fellow normal eye was 19 mm Hg). Examination of the fundus revealed slightly engorged retinal veins and a couple of very tiny retinal hemorrhages (Fig. 11–5A), with no other abnormality. Fluorescein fundus angiography revealed extremely slow filling of the retinal, choroidal and optic disk circulation, with no retinal microvascular abnormality, except for an occasional microaneurysm. The CRA at the disk did not start to fill till 22 seconds (Fig. 11–5B) (normally 10–12 seconds)

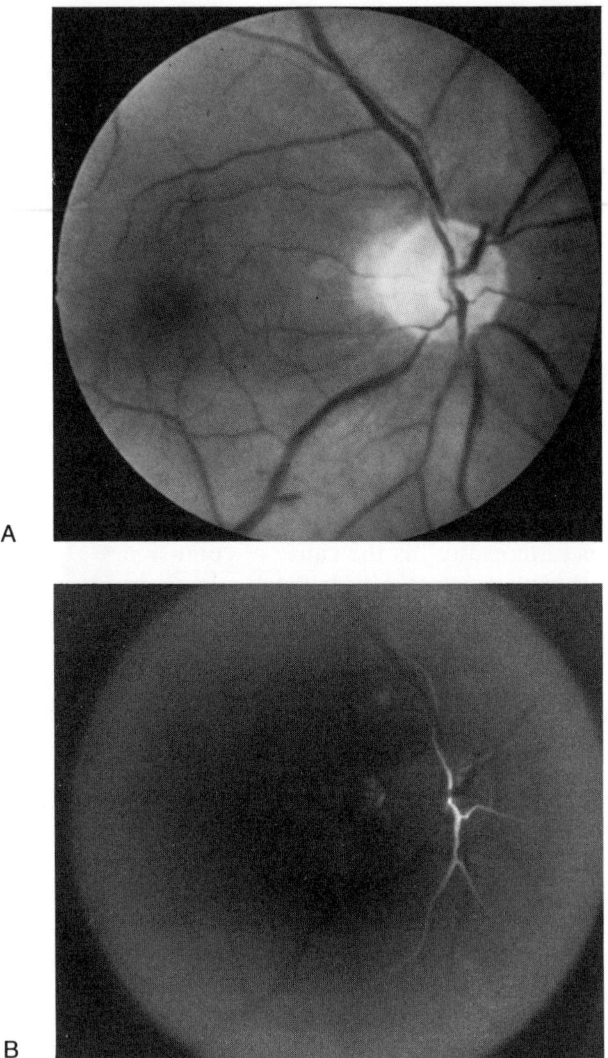

FIGURE 11–5. Fundus photograph (A) and fluorescein fundus angiograms (B to F) of the right eye of a 61-year-old man with occlusion of the right ICA and chronic ocular ischemia (see text for detailed description). Time after injection of fluorescein: (B) 22 seconds, (C) 26 seconds, (D) 43 seconds, (E) 82 seconds, and (F) about 15 minutes. [Reproduced from Hayreh SS, Podhajsky P: *Archives of Ophthalmology*, 100:1585–1596. Copyright 1982, American Medical Association. (3)]

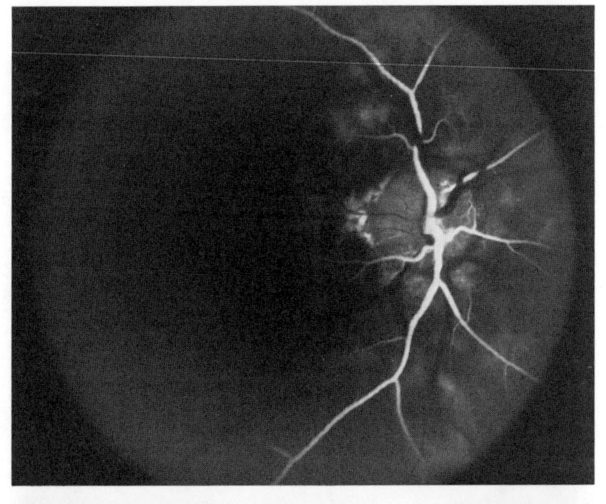
C

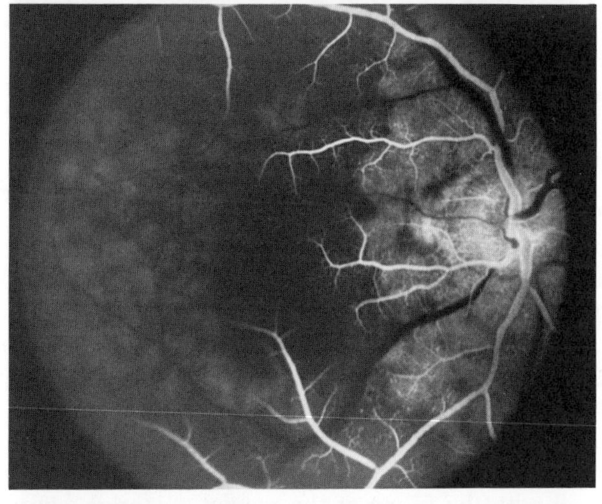
D

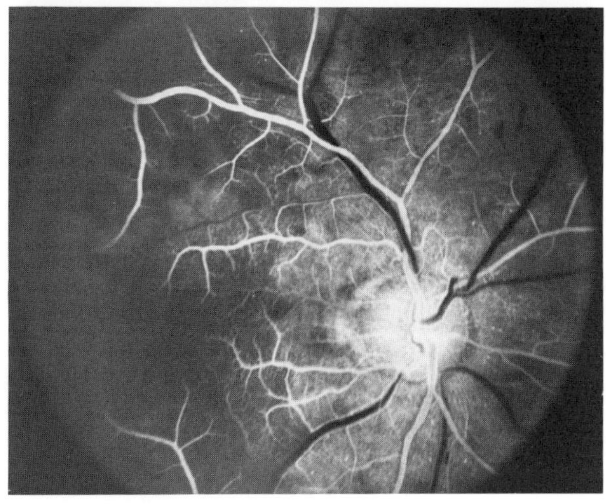
E

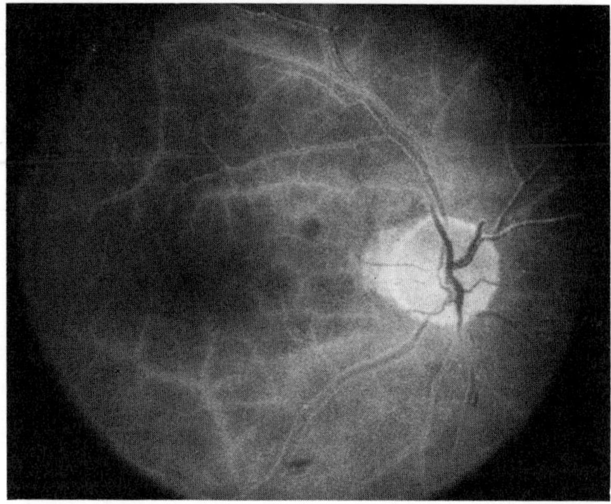

FIGURE 11–5. *Continued*

after the injection of the dye, and the retinal arterioles did not fill completely, even 60 seconds later (Fig. 11–5E) (normally within 1 second). Nasal choroid (i.e., in the distribution of the medial posterior ciliary artery) did not start to fill till 26 seconds after the injection of the dye (Fig. 11–5C)—normally it should start filling just before or simultaneously with the start of CRA filling on the disk. The nasal choroid filled completely in about 20 seconds (normally less than a second), while the temporal choroid (i.e., in the distribution of the lateral posterior ciliary artery) showed no filling till about 43 seconds after the injection of the dye (normally it should fill synchronously with medial posterior ciliary artery). The optic disk started to fill with the filling of the medial posterior ciliary artery (Fig. 11–5C) which supplied the entire disk. The retinal veins had not filled even 82 seconds after the injection of the dye (Fig. 11–5E) (normal retinal arteriovenous circulation time is only 2–3 seconds). Thus, there was a gross delay in the entire circulation of the posterior segment. By the late phase (i.e., about 15 minutes after the injection of the dye—Fig. 11–5F), the retinal and choroidal vascular bed had filled completely and the main retinal vessels leaked fluorescein and showed staining. Carotid arteriography revealed a total occlusion of the right internal carotid artery.

On follow-up, 3 months after the initial visit, the right eye had a visual acuity of bare hand motion, intraocular pressure of 25 mm Hg, cupped optic disk, and pulsating CRA on the disk. Three months later, the visual acuity in that eye was no light perception, intraocular pressure 19 mm Hg, almost complete obliteration of the retinal vessels, and evidence of old peripheral choroidal infarcts over the 360° of the fundus (identical to those seen in Fig. 11–6).

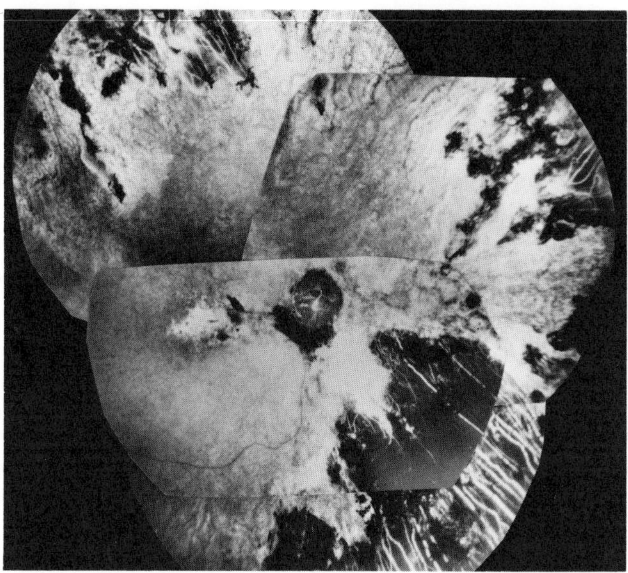

FIGURE 11–6. Composite late fluorescein angiogram of the right eye of a 54-year-old man with right ICA occlusive disease and chronic ocular ischemia (with marked ischemia of the anterior and posterior segments of the eye). It shows nonperfusion of the retinal vessels, optic disk atrophy and cupping, and peripheral chorioretinal degeneration from choroidal infarcts.

There can be no disagreement that such fundus changes are due to chronic ocular ischemia secondary to carotid artery occlusive disease. These eyes have not only sluggish circulation in the retinal vascular bed but also have as poor or poorer circulation in the choroid, optic disk and iris. We have discussed this subject in detail elsewhere (3).

The *blood flow in the intraocular vascular bed* depends upon (1) *mean blood pressure* (mean blood pressure = diastolic blood pressure + ⅓ the difference between the systolic and diastolic blood pressures) in the feeding arteries, (2) *intraocular pressure,* (3) *peripheral vascular resistance,* and (4) *presence or absence of autoregulation* in the vascular bed. *Perfusion pressure* is equal to mean blood pressure minus the intraocular pressure. The blood flow in any part of the ocular vascular bed can be calculated by dividing perfusion pressure by peripheral vascular resistance.

In the retinal vascular bed, in addition to these, the blood flow also depends on the difference in blood pressure between the CRA and CRV at the optic disk; since the pressure in the CRV depends upon the intraocular pressure, it remains fairly stable so long as the intraocular pressure is within normal limits. Thus a fall in the CRA pressure (due to carotid artery occlusive disease) with normal CRV pressure would produce marked stasis in the blood flow in the retinal vascular bed. Uyama and

Asayama (32) postulated that in pulseless disease, blood pressure in the retinal arterioles in the peripheral part of the retina may be reduced to such an extent that the peripheral retinal vessels may not be perfused, resulting in the development of arteriovenous anastomoses and capillary nonperfusion.

While retinal and optic nerve head circulations have autoregulation, the choroidal circulation does not have any autoregulation. In the event of a fall in perfusion pressure, this makes the choroidal circulation more vulnerable to ischemic disorders than the retinal or optic nerve head circulations. In electrophysiological studies in eyes of 7 patients with carotid artery occlusive disease and fundus changes of the so-called "venous stasis retinopathy", Ross Russell and Ikeda (36) showed in scotopic electroretinography, a delay in the recovery of the b wave after exposure to bright light, and in electro-oculography, significantly lower and slower light rise than in normal eyes. (This is similar to the photo-stress test in these patients.) According to them, these studies suggested that the physiologic lesion in these eyes is present at the interface between the choroid, pigment epithelium, and outer segments of the photoreceptors—the tissues supplied by the choroidal circulation only. These findings indicate that the defect is due to choroidal vascular ischemia with no evidence of retinal vascular ischemia in these eyes presumed to have retinopathy due to retinal ischemia. This also is supported by my fluorescein fundus angiographic studies in eyes where the choroidal circulation showed much more abnormality than seen in the retinal circulation. Unfortunately, the retinal vascular bed always has been the center of attention in these eyes and all ocular lesions have been attributed to retinal lesions. This is obvious from the fact that over recent years multiple terms have been used to describe fundus changes in carotid artery occlusive disease, including "venous stasis retinopathy," "hypoperfusion retinopathy," "hypotensive retinopathy," "low pressure retinopathy," (36) or "chronic ischemic retinopathy" (6)—the entire stress has been on "retinopathy," which represents only a part of the entire spectrum of changes seen in this condition. The reason is that the subject has been studied mostly by persons with almost no in-depth knowledge of ocular circulation in general and of CRVO in particular, who have based their opinions essentially on ophthalmoscopic appearance and not on routine use of fluorescein fundus angiography, which is a far more reliable and sensitive test to evaluate ocular circulatory disorders. Fluorescein angiography shows that there is impaired circulation not only in the retina but also in the choroid, optic nerve head, and iris.

The eyes of some patients with chronic ocular ischemia secondary to carotid occlusive disease also develop disk neovascularization, which has been presumed to be due to retinal ischemia by previous authors (under the mistaken assumption that the mechanism is similar to that in diabetic retinopathy or retinal vein occlusion). Panretinal photocoagulation, similar to that used to treat diabetic retinopathy, has been advocated in these eyes (37,38) because of this presumptive pathogenesis of disk neovascularization. On doing fluorescein fundus angiographic studies in a few patients with disk neovascularization and carotid artery occlusive disease, I have *not* been able to document any angiographic abnormality in the retina nor any evidence of retinal ischemia in any of them. These findings cast serious doubt on the presumed mechanism of disk neovascularization in these eyes, and on the validity of proposed panretinal photocoagulation as a treatment for these patients.

Anterior segment neovascularization in carotid artery occlusive disease: Anterior segment ischemia, due to impaired circulation in the iris and the rest of the anterior uveal circulation, is a definite clinical entity secondary to carotid artery occlusive disease. It is manifested as flare and an occasional cell in the anterior chamber (due to leakage from the ischemic iris vessels and much more so from the neovascularization of the iris and angle); these changes in the anterior chamber and iris erroneously have been diagnosed as uveitis.

Iris and angle neovascularization, with or without development of neovascular glaucoma, are well-known complications of carotid artery occlusive disease (3). Anterior segment neovascularization in these cases universally and quite wrongly has been attributed to retinal ischemia. This is because eyes with diabetic retinopathy, ischemic CRVO and other retinopathies with extensive retinal capillary nonperfusion may develop similar anterior segment neovascularization. In these conditions, it is hypothesized that retinal ischemia is the culprit in the production of anterior segment neovascularization by the release of a vasoproliferative factor, the nature and origin of which is still controversial. Clinical and experimental studies on anterior segment ischemia (e.g., in experimental studies on monkeys of cutting the various recti (39), and of vortex vein occlusion (40), and in patients with strabismus surgery or retinal detachment surgery) have indicated that anterior segment ischemia by itself does produce iris and angle neovascularization and neovascular glaucoma, and that the neovascularization does not always have to have retinal ischemia to explain it. In the literature, there are a large number of reports giving evidence of the presence of angiogenic factors in a variety of tissues (other than the retina) and agents. We have reviewed the subject elsewhere (41). In eyes with severe carotid artery occlusive disease, we have seen gross filling defects and delays on iris angiography (3), indicating iris vascular insufficiency and ischemia; which in itself can cause neovascularization of the anterior segment, without any retinal pathology. Also, it is important to remember that the anterior segment is supplied mainly by the anterior ciliary arteries (branches of the muscular arteries in the recti), while the posterior segment is supplied by the CRA and posterior ciliary arteries. Thus, anterior segment ischemia (and associated anterior segment neovascularization) and posterior segment ischemia may be two unrelated manifestations of ocular ischemia, and may not show identical severity of ischemia. The erroneous concept that in carotid artery occlusive disease neovascularization of the anterior segment is primarily due to retinal ischemia has led to advocating panretinal photocoagulation (as in diabetic retinopathy) in the management of carotid artery disease.

Management

The major complication of chronic ocular ischemia for which treatment (both prophylactic and curative) has been proposed is ocular neovascularization. As discussed above, the commonest site of neovascularization in these eyes is the anterior segment and, much less frequently, the optic disk. It has been universally accepted as fact, quite mistakenly, that the ocular neovascularization in these eyes is always secondary to retinal ischemia. In diabetic retinopathy and other types of retinopathies with extensive capillary nonperfusion seen on fluorescein fundus angiography, it has been postulated that the ischemic retina (secondary to retinal capillary nonperfusion) liberates a vasoproliferative factor that is responsible for the development of both anterior segment and posterior segment neovascularization. However, as mentioned above, fluorescein fundus angiographic studies conducted by me in patients with carotid artery occlusive disease and with very low CRA pressure, and even in those with anterior segment or disk neovascularization, have not revealed retinal capillary nonperfusion. Therefore, to postulate that the ocular neovascularization seen in carotid artery occlusive disease is pathogenetically identical to that seen in diabetic retinopathy or retinal vein occlusion is totally unwarranted. Hence, the use of panretinal photocoagulation in such eyes is illogical. There are only a couple of dubious anecdotal case reports claiming a beneficial influence from panretinal photocoagulation in these eyes (37,38). However, a review of these two cases leaves many unanswered questions about the claims. I have seen a patient who was treated by an outside ophthalmologist for disk neovascularization in an eye with mild ocular ischemia from carotid artery occlusive disease, without any beneficial influence. Dr. G.C. Brown from the Wills Eye Hospital, Philadelphia reported (at the Macula Society meeting a couple of years ago) one patient with ocular ischemia secondary to carotid artery occlusive disease in whom panretinal photocoagulation was performed and the next day the patient was totally blind from the development of severe anterior ischemic optic neuropathy. This occurred because panretinal photocoagulation (as is well-known) produces a transient rise in intraocular pressure in about one third of patients (42). In an eye with very low perfusion pressure, that rise in intraocular pressure often may be enough to shut down the circulation in the optic nerve head and cause an infarction of the optic nerve head. Thus panretinal photocoagulation in ocular ischemia secondary to carotid occlusive disease has no scientific basis and may even be a dangerous procedure. There is no hard evidence that it has any beneficial effect in these eyes.

If an eye shows evidence of poor circulation secondary to carotid occlusive disease, the most logical treatment is to try to improve the ocular circulation by relieving the carotid artery occlusion. Internal to external carotid artery bypass does not seem to help ocular ischemia appreciably. Carotid endarterectomy or surgical measures to improve the blood flow in the internal carotid artery may prove helpful. If the ocular ischemia is due to stenosis at the origin of the ophthalmic artery (as was seen by me in my anatomical studies on the ophthalmic artery in man), surgery on the carotid artery may not be of much help.

Conclusions

From this discussion the following points emerge:

1. Patients with severe generalized atherosclerotic disease may develop nonischemic CRVO (venous stasis retinopathy) and carotid artery occlusive disease as two independent manifestations of the systemic atherosclerotic disease, with no cause-and-effect relationship between the two.
2. In patients with marked generalized atherosclerosis and arteriosclerosis, sluggish retinal arterial circulation and fall of blood pressure in the retinal circulation, secondary to carotid artery occlusive disease, may produce hemodynamic changes in the retinal circulation and contribute to the production of CRVO in susceptible individuals.
3. Ocular ischemia is a well-established complication of carotid artery occlusive disease. As a result of hypoperfusion of the posterior ocular vascular bed (including the retinal, choroidal, and optic disk), the fundus may develop changes, such as sluggish circulation in the retinal arterioles (and secondarily in the retinal venous circulation), pulsating retinal arteries (if the intraocular pressure is about the level of the diastolic blood pressure in the retinal arteries), signs of optic disk ischemia (anterior ischemic optic neuropathy in acute ischemic insults, and optic disk atrophy and cupping in chronic cases), and choroidal infarcts (mainly in the peripheral fundus). Fluorescein fundus angiography (Fig. 11–5, 11–6) may reveal marked circulatory abnormalities when routine ophthalmoscopy may not reveal much change.
4. Thus, venous stasis retinopathy is not a manifestation of carotid artery occlusive disease, but chronic ischemic fundus changes (involving the retina, choroid and optic disk) are due to the carotid artery occlusive disease. Mixing of these two types of fundus changes in patients with carotid artery occlusive disease has resulted in confusion—in the former, the cause lies in obstruction to venous outflow from the retina, whereas in the latter there is impaired arterial inflow.
5. Anterior segment ischemia is a well-established complication of carotid artery occlusive disease. It may be manifested simply as flare and occasional cells in the anterior chamber (erroneously called uveitis) and/

or as iris and angle neovascularization, with or without neovascular glaucoma. We have no scientific evidence that anterior segment neovascularization is secondary to retinal ischemia in these eyes because there is evidence that anterior segment ischemia per se can cause iris and angle neovascularization and neovascular glaucoma.

6. In the management of the ocular neovascularization seen in chronic ocular ischemia, secondary to carotid artery occlusive disease, there is no definite or logical evidence that panretinal photocoagulation has a beneficial influence. On the contrary, there is evidence that it can be dangerous for the eye. Surgical measures to improve the ocular circulation, (e.g., carotid endarterectomy or other reconstructive procedures of the internal carotid artery), may be helpful in some of these eyes if performed before serious complication have developed.

In discussing the controversy on "venous stasis retinopathy due to carotid artery occlusive disease." I once wrote: "The field of medicine is littered with myths, originally drawn from simple clinical impressions, anecdotal reports, personal biases, defective experiments, erroneous interpretations, and temporary lapses of famous physicians. These myths come to be regarded as 'established facts.' Any attempt to weed out myths is met with severe resistance and even ridicule." I hope this chapter, with all the available evidence cited, will help weed out the myths from the facts, and provide a clearer perspective on the whole subject.

Terminology

The currently proposed terms to denote the fundus changes seen in eyes with chronic ocular ischemia secondary to carotid artery occlusive disease, e.g., "venous stasis retinopathy," "chronic ischemic retinopathy," "hypotensive retinopathy," "hypoperfusion retinopathy," and "low pressure retinopathy," do not reflect correctly the entire spectrum of findings in these eyes, because fluorescein fundus angiography shows impaired circulation in the retina, choroid and optic disk, and fluorescein iris angiography shows impaired circulation in the iris (3). Thus, a simple term such as "chronic ocular ischemic syndrome" may represent the pathogenetic as well as clinical features of the ocular syndrome seen in carotid artery occlusive disease. The use of the term "ischemic ocular inflammation" (43) is misleading, since the essential process is not inflammatory but ischemic.

Acknowledgments

I am grateful to my wife, Shelagh, for her help in the preparation of this manuscript, to Mrs. Ellen Ballas and Mrs. Georgiane Parkes-Perret for their secretarial help, and to the ophthalmic photography department for the illustrations. This study was supported by research grants from the British Research Council, National Institutes of Health (Grant Nos. EY-1151 and 1576) and Research to Prevent Blindness Inc.

References

1. Schmidt H: Beitrag zur Kenntniss der Embolie der Arteria Centralis Retinae. *Albrecht Von Graefes Arch Klin Exp Ophthalmol* 1874;20:287–307.
2. Loring EG: Remarks on embolism. *Am J Med Sci* 1874;67:313–328.
3. Hayreh SS, Podhajsky P: Ocular neovascularization with retinal vascular occlusion: II. Occurrence in central and branch retinal artery occlusion. *Arch Ophthalmol* 1982;100:1585–1596.
4. Hedges TR: Ophthalmoscopic findings in internal carotid artery occlusion. *Am J Ophthalmol* 1963;55:1007–1012.
5. Kearns TP, Hollenhorst RW: Venous-stasis retinopathy of occlusive disease of the carotid artery. *Mayo Clin Proc* 1963;38:304–312.
6. Kearns TP: Differential diagnosis of central retinal vein obstruction. *Ophthalmology* 1983;90:475–480.
7. Hayreh SS: Occlusion of the central retinal vessels. *Br J Ophthalmol* 1965;49:626–645.
8. Hayreh SS, vanHeuven WAJ, Hayreh MS: Experimental retinal vascular occlusion: I. Pathogenesis of central retinal vein occlusion. *Arch Ophthalmol* 1978;96:311–323.
9. Jaurez CF, Tso MOM, vanHeuven WAJ, et al: Experimental retinal vascular occlusion: II. A clinico-pathologic correlative study of simultaneous occlusion of central retinal vein and artery. *Int Ophthalmol* 1986;9:77–87.
10. Juarez CF, Tso MOM, vanHeuven WAJ, et al: Experimental retinal vascular occlusion: III. An ultrastructural study of simultaneous occlusion of central retinal vein and artery. *Int Ophthalmol* 1986;9:89–101.
11. Hayreh SS: So-called "central retinal vein occlusion": I. Pathogenesis, terminology, clinical features. *Ophthalmologica* 1976;172:1–13.
12. Hayreh SS: Central retinal vein occlusion, in Mausolf, FA (ed.): *The Eye and Systemic Disease,* ed 2. St Louis, The CV Mosby Co, 1980, pp 223–275.
13. Hayreh SS: Classification of central retinal vein occlusion. *Ophthalmology* 1983;90:458–474.
14. Hayreh SS, March W, Phelps CD: Ocular hypotony following retinal vein occlusion. 1978;96:827–833.
15. Hayreh SS, Rojas P, Podhajsky P, et al: Ocular neovascularization with retinal vascular occlusion: III. Incidence of ocular neovascularization with retinal vein occlusion. *Ophthalmology* 1983;90:488–506.
16. Servais GE, Thompson HS, Hayreh SS: Relative afferent pupillary defect in central retinal vein occlusion. *Ophthalmology* 1986;93:301–303.
17. Kearns TP, Siekert RG, Sundt TM: The ocular aspects of bypass surgery of the carotid artery. *Mayo Clin Proc* 1979;54:3–11.
18. Kearns TP, Younge BR, Piepgras DG: Resolution of venous stasis retinopathy after carotid artery bypass surgery. *Mayo Clin Proc* 1980;55:342–346.
19. Neupert JR, Brubaker RF, Kearns TP, et al: Rapid resolution of venous stasis retinopathy afer carotid endarterectomy. *Am J Ophthalmology* 1976;81:600–602.
20. Scheerer R: Theorie des Blutumlaufs in der Netzhaut. *Ber Deutsch Ophthalmol Ges Heidelberg* 1925;45:59–62.
21. Klien BA: Obstruction of the central retinal vein: A clinico-histopathologic analysis. *Am J Ophthalmol* 1944;27:1339–1354.
22. Klien BA: Occlusion of the central retinal vein: Clinical importance of certain histopathologic observations. *Am J Ophthalmol* 1953;36:316–324.

23. Leber T: *Graefe-Saemisch Handbuch der Gesamten Augenheilkunde*, ed 2. Leipzig Engelmann, 1915.
24. Klien BA: Side lights on retinal venous occlusion. *Am J Ophthalmol* 1966;61:25–35.
25. Paton A, Rubenstein K, Smith VH: Arterial insufficiency in retinal venous occlusion. *Trans Ophthalmol Soc UK* 1964;84:559–593.
26. Toole JF, Yuson CP, Janeway R, et al: Transient ischemic attacks: A prospective study of 225 patients. *Neurology* 1978;28:746–753.
27. Brown G: Macular edema in association with severe carotid artery obstruction. *Am J Ophthalmol* 1986;102:442–448.
28. Dowling JL, Smith TR: An ocular study of pulseless disease. *Arch Ophthalmol* 1960;64:236–243.
29. Hirose K: A study of fundus changes in the early stages of Takayasu-Ohnishi (pulseless) disease. *Am J Ophthalmol* 1963;55:295–301.
30. Ostler HB: Pulseless disease (Takayasu's disease). *Am J Ophthalmol* 1957;43:583–589.
31. Tour RL, Hoyt WF: The syndrome of the aortic arch: Ocular manifestations of "pulseless disease" and a report of a surgically treated case. *Am J Ophthalmol* 1959;47:35–48.
32. Uyama M, Asayama K: Retinal vascular changes in Takayasu's disease (pulseless disease): Occurrence and evolution of the lesion. *Doc Ophthalmol Proc Ser* 1976;9:549–554.
33. Hayreh SS, Kolder HE, Weingeist TA: Central retinal artery occlusion and retinal tolerance time. *Ophthalmology* 1980;87:75–78.
34. Slakter JS, Spertus AD, Weissman SS, et al: An experimental model of carotid occlusive disease. *Am J Ophthalmol* 1984;97:168–172.
35. Spertus AD, Slakter JS, Weissman SS, et al: Experimental carotid occlusion: Fundoscopic and fluorescein angiographic findings. *J Ophthalmol* 1984;68:47–57.
36. Ross Russell RW, Ikeda H: Clinical and electrophysiological observations in patients with low pressure retinopathy. *Br J Ophthalmol* 1986;70:651–656.
37. Carter JE: Panretinal photocoagulation for progressive ocular neovascularization secondary to occlusion of the common carotid artery. *Ann Ophthalmol* 1984;16:572–576.
38. Eggleston TF, Bohling CA, Eggleston HC, et al: Photocoagulation for ocular ischemia associated with carotid artery occlusion. *Ann Ophthalmol* 1980;12:844–887.
39. Virdi PS, Hayreh SS: Anterior segment ischemia after recession of various recti: An experimental study. Ophthalmology 1987;94:1258–1271.
40. Hayreh SS, Baines JAB: Occlusion of the vortex veins: An experimental study. *Br J Ophthalmol* 1973;57:217–238.
41. Hayreh SS, Lata GF: Ocular neovascularization: Experimental animal model and studies on angiogenic factor(s). *Int Ophthalmol* 1986;9:109–120.
42. Mensher JH: Anterior chamber depth alteration after retinal photocoagulation. *Arch Ophthalmol* 1977;95:113–116.
43. Knox DL: Ischemic ocular inflammation. *Am J Ophthalmol* 1965;60:995–1002.

CHAPTER 12

Role of Vascular Spasm and Ocular Migraine

Donald J. Dalessio

Amaurosis infers blindness occurring without an apparent lesion of the eye, an extraocular cause, if you will. The term amaurosis fugax has come to be associated with vascular disease, but it could just as well apply to the visual phenomena that accompany migraine. Hence, a discussion of migrainous visual auras and their possible pathogenesis is appropriate here.

Migraine is not a disease but rather a series of complex vasomotor events that may be neurogenically induced (ie, initiated by cerebral activity). Many distinguished physicians have attempted to define migraine, not always very successfully.

For example the Research Group on Migraine and Headache of the World Federation of Neurology produced the following (1): "A familial disorder characterized by recurrent attacks of headache widely variable in intensity, frequency, and duration. The attacks are commonly unilateral and usually associated with anorexia, nausea and vomiting. In some cases the headaches are preceded or accompanied by or associated with neurological and mood disturbances."

If this definition were definitive, this chapter could stop here, for little mention is made of the migrainous visual auras, and the nonpainful features of migraine which are so common, are barely recognized.

Prodromal features of migraine are variegated and multiple and include changes in mental status and mood, among others. The preheadache phenomena are extremely variable and conspicuous. Some patients with migraine headache never have clearly defined prodromes. Many have feelings of mounting tension, hunger, and wakefulness, often followed by profound sleep just preceding the attack. Still others are aware of declining energy and drive; and a few, of extreme buoyance, talkativeness, and well-being just before the attack.

The mood disorders that accompany the headache are often outstanding. Patients complain of feeling prostrated, dejected, and, often, seriously depressed. At such times they are unsocial, rejecting companionship or the presence of others; irritable and irascible; and often unwilling to assume their usual responsibilities, especially rejecting any demand to make a decision. Their judgment is poor, and they are impulsive, hostile, and sometimes destructive, often directing hostility at those who are dependent upon them. Memory, attention, concentration, and retention are usually poor during the headache, and cooperation is denied.

A small group predictably have visual and other sensory disturbances immediately before the onset of the headache. Some patients have visual disturbances not always followed by headache, and another group have headache frequently, with visual disturbances perhaps only three or four times during a lifetime.

These visual disturbances precede the headache and last a few minutes to an hour. Rarely, they may persist for hours. When they are short-lived, they usually terminate before the onset of the headache, and between the visual disturbance and the headache phase, a symptom-free phase occurs when the patient feels relatively well. Then, however, the headache begins and becomes gradually worse. On the other hand, if the visual disturbances have been of 30 to 60 minutes duration, they may dwindle off only gradually, overlapping the beginning of the headache and persisting for a few minutes or even hours during the headache phase.

The preheadache visual disturbances may be blind spots arranged in quadrants of the visual field or may be isolated areas of blindness. Field defects may be homonymous, quadrantic, or hemianoptic. Such defects are usually contralateral to the side of the headache.

Also, patients may experience areas of bright flashes of light, geometric designs, wavy visions, golden balls, stars, tessellations, serrations, and so-called fortification phenomena. Most of these visual hallucinations are mobile and interfere with vision. These disturbances are not to be confused with visual difficulties, such as photophobia, large pupil with blurred vision, focusing difficulties, increased lacrimation, or edema of the lids, or with the ophthalmoplegic phenomena that accompany the headache itself and usually occur later in its course after the headache is well established or receding.

Other prodromes occurring along with but independent of these disturbances, and sometimes occurring as isolated events, are paresthesias of the face and hand and even of the foot on the contralateral side. Rarely, aphasia or anomia occurs. Another relatively common preheadache phenomenon is vertigo. This may begin suddenly as a violent spinning with nausea, vomiting, sweating, prostration, and even syncope, followed by intense headache and further nausea and vomiting.

Specific Visual Auras

Several specific visual auras occur during migraine, and some of these may be related to pathophysiologic, vasospastic changes.

The classical scintillating scotomata or fortification spectra have been described since antiquity, often by physicians observing their own visual abnormalities; among these are included Sir William Gowers (2), Hubert

Airey (3), K.S. Lashley (4), and Walter Alvarez (5). Most begin with a small area of visual loss, centrally located, which then expands in a typical arc across the field of vision. At the periphery jagged lines often appear, fortificationlike in appearance and suggesting the ancient walled cities of Europe, such as Carcassonne. In general these attacks last 20 to 30 minutes, eventually moving beyond the periphery of the visual field, and normal vision returns. It can be postulated that the visual loss represents an inhibitory process and that the spectral appearances are excitatory. Often both phenomena occur during a single attack, but either may appear separately.

These effects are presumably due to some change in the occipital cortex, and some observers, by plotting the movement of their own scotomas, have estimated the scotomas move across the visual fields at the rate of 3 mm/min. This figure comes close to the velocity of spreading depression (SD) of Leao (6); Milner (7) was first to make this association in 1958. The concept of spreading depression as it relates to migraine is discussed subsequently.

Usually the scotomas are bilateral and symmetrical, but sometimes the patient does not recognize this, if they are homonymous, and more striking in one eye than the other. Even Airey (3), who described his own visual loss in such detail, was unable to say "with certainty whether the disease really affects both eyes."

The problem is further complicated by the description of ocular migraine. Transient monocular disturbances may occur, accompanied by changes in retinal circulation of one eye, as documented by fundus photography by using fluorescein angiography (8). Such a case was described in a patient with cluster headaches (8). It is hoped that such events are rare; it is easy to see how confusion would arise in trying to understand this symptom and its possible relationship to amaurosis fugax.

Hedges (9) described a group of patients who had what was termed isolated ophthalmic migraine. These were visual abnormalities that occurred in patients over the age of 50 years, many of whom (one third) had had a history of migraine but were then quiescent. Some patients had single or recurring scintillating scotomas that might be homonymous and were not followed by headache. These patients had a relatively benign prognosis. Another group had monocular visual changes, and in this subset almost half had vascular disease. Many probably were describing amaurosis fugax. These findings reinforce the concept that monocular visual loss is often atheroembolic in origin and must be considered so by the treating physician.

Other Visual Phenomena

Other visual disturbances associated with migraine often are classified as perceptual disturbances (10). Some patients report alterations in size and shape of objects, termed metamorphosia by Critchley (11). He suggested that alterations in the shape of objects might occur when the migrainous process involves structures adjacent to the occipital lobes and the geniculate-striate radiations. In 1955 Todd (12) described the Alice In Wonderland syndrome, perhaps related to Lewis Carroll's migrainous visions. In the story Alice changes from very tall (macropsia) to very short (micropsia). She has moments of dissociation, addresses herself as two persons, and has feelings of levitation. Teichopsia may occur, with luminous lights before the whole field of vision, as well as the aforementioned metamorphosia, which implies a more fanciful cortical expression of the migraine process. Mosiac vision can be suitably so classified as well.

Migraine Accompaniments or Equivalents

Fisher (13) has introduced the concept of migrainous accompaniments (of the aged) to characterize those patients who, after age 40, have what appear to be transient ischemic attacks (TIAs), but who, after appropriate investigation, including angiograms, are found to be normal. Fisher also excluded those patients with evidence of "cerebral thrombosis, embolism and dissection, epilepsy, thrombocytopenia of various types, and polycythemia." His patients had "scintillations or other visual displays in the spell, next in order, paresthesias, aphasia, dysarthria and paralysis; build up of scintillation (9); march of paresthesias; progression from one accompaniment to another often without a delay; the occurrence of two or more similar spells; headache in the spells; episodes lasting fifteen to twenty-five minutes; characteristic mid-life flurry; and a generally benign course."

Probably, most clinicians would be reassured by the "benign course," and almost all would remain suspicious that the cause of these spells might be atheroembolic despite the negative findings on the diagnostic workup.

Migraine Etiology and Visual Observations

Migraine is a complex physiologic process. Like Boris Karloff's icicle, the perfect murder weapon that would kill, melt, and leave no trace, migraine produces great disability but is basically a benign process, a distressing but not dangerous affliction.

Most who study migraine agree on some things. It seems clear that the painful part of migraine represents vascular dilatation combined with sterile inflammation; dilation by itself is often nonpainful. I have proposed (14), with others, that migraine is a syndrome of self-limited neurogenic inflammation and that multiple vasoactive substances, including serotonin, vasodilator polypeptides, substance P, prostaglandins, catecholamines, and histamine, interact in ways not completely understood, at least in the periphery. All these substances have potent biologic properties, particularly on vascular smooth muscle.

Some or all of these same vasoactive materials also may be active centrally as neurotransmitters and have been suggested as important in migraine pathogenesis. Moskowitz (15) described nervous connections containing substance P between the trigeminal ganglia and cerebral blood vessels in animals and inferred that the existence of a similar system in humans could be presumed. Lance and his colleagues (16,17) have shown that stimulation of the locus coeruleus in the cat and monkey can induce a series of vascular events similar to migraine. The relationships of encephalin levels to migraine and headache in general has been considered by Mosnaim and colleagues (18), among others, who found that plasma levels of methionine enkephalin (MET), an endogenous peptide with opiodlike effects, increased with the migraine attack.

But what of the central processes of migraine, which presumably produce the visual phenomena being discussed here? It generally has been held that the prodromes of migraine are associated with a reduction in blood flow to the cerebral cortex that is sometimes focal and sometimes generalized.

Edmeads (19) has studied cerebral blood flow in migraine. His work in part has confirmed Wolff's hypothesis that cerebral blood flow is decreased during auras and increased during headaches. However, some findings were unexpected. The distribution in time and spacc of the blood flow changes did not always correlate with clinical features of the attack. Autoregulation of the cerebral blood vessels may be impaired in aura and in headache, and this is a key factor in intensifying and prolonging attacks.

Sakai and Meyer (20) used a noninvasive method of inhalation of xenon-133 and showed that blood flow in the gray matter (Fg) was increased during migraine, only slowly returning to baseline values after several days. These authors described "marked cerebral dysautoregulation" during the migraine episode, with recovery as the headache subsided. They further noted significant regional reductions in Fg during the prodromes of classical migraine.

Invasive Studies of Regional Cerebral Blood Flow

In contrast, findings obtained by using the regional cerebral blood flow (rCBF) method of Olesen and Lauritzen (21,22) has cast doubt on Wolff's old but useful and heuristic theory. These authors injected xenon-133 into the carotid artery and studied induced migraine produced after arteriography in a series of patients. They described a type of "spreading oligemia" that generally began in the occipital region and spread anteriorly. This oligemia advanced at a speed of 2 mm/min over the hemisphere but did not cross the rolandic or sylvian sulci. Typically, the spreading oligemia reached the primary sensorimotor area after symptoms produced from that region had begun, and the oligemia persisted there long after the focal symptoms had ceased. Olesen and Lauritzen (21,22) suggested, therefore, that the painless preheadache phenomena of classical migraine were not secondary to observed oligemia but that they might be secondary to SD as described by Leao (6). Stated in another way, the spreading oligemia may be an epiphenomenon that accompanies SD, with the focal migraine symptoms understood as a manifestation of the prolonged inhibition of cortical neurons evoked by SD.

The striking oligemia observed by Olesen and Lauritzen (21,22) in classical migraine did *not* appear in those patients with common migraine studied in a similar manner. In these patients, no significant changes occurred in regional or general cerebral blood flow between the resting state, the onset of common migraine, and the fully developed attack. Olesen and Lauritzen therefore suggested that classical and common migraine were different, at least with respect to studies of cerebral blood flow.

Doppler Studies

Dynamic noninvasive studies by means of Doppler sonography cannot be used to measure cerebral blood flow but are invaluable in surveying the extracranial vascular tree. They pose no risk to the patient and can be repeated with impunity. Furthermore, by applying anatomic principles, the clinician can infer changes intracranially in patients so studied. In migraine, which is, after all, a benign syndrome, that type of inference is perhaps sufficient.

Schroth and colleagues (23) described ultrasonic Doppler flow in migraine and in cluster headache. They found a characteristic increase in flow velocity in the common, internal, and external carotid arteries during spontaneous migraine attacks; flow was reduced in the ophthalmic artery on the ipsilateral headache side. This was in contrast to the findings in cluster headache, during which a marked increase in blood flow was seen in the ophthalmic artery during painful episodes. The authors suggested that the reduced blood flow in the migrainous ophthalmic artery might represent a passive steal, produced by intracranial vasodilatation, but this remains a supposition only. Schroth et al (23) did not differentiate between classical and common migraine in their observations.

Arteriographic Studies

The results of clinical observations suggest that the degree of cerebral vasospasm that occurs in migraine is more severe and asymmetrical than that suggested by the experimental studies of Olesen and his group (21,22). Only a few angiograms showing migrainous vasospasm are available, but these are impressive. The latest angiographic study, published by Lieberman et al (24) described a 39-year-old woman with a history of migraine who developed bilateral cervical carotid and intracranial vasospasm during a migraine attack. This patient was entirely well and had no history of heart disease, diabetes, hyperlipidemia, or problems with her neck. Her only medication before admission was acetaminophen. She was not taking ergot compounds, amphetamines, illicit drugs, or oral contraceptives and had no history of smoking. The arteriogram of the right common carotid artery, obtained by using the digital subtraction imaging technique the day after the patient developed hemiplegic migraine, showed a complete occlusion of the cervical portion of the right ICA approximately 3 cm distal to the common carotid bifurcation. The next day the right common carotid artery was open, but the caliber of the cervical ICA was decreased, and the proximal segment of one of the branches of the right middle cerebral artery was narrowed. At this time, also, the left common carotid artery had focal narrowing involving the left cervical ICA.

Similar related observations have been published sporadically over the last 20 years. These cannot be ignored, nor can the striking hemispheric changes in blood flow that have been reported by others. It is clear that some patients with migraine have marked vasospastic alterations in intracranial blood flow that are, for the most part, benign and that leave no residual neurologic abnormality.

Finally, occasionally a patient with "complicated migraine" will have a permanent neurologic deficit and presumably has suffered a vasospastic stroke (25). Here the boundary between benign vasospasm (migraine) and stroke would seem to have been completely erased.

In closing, a brief mention should be made of some recent studies on visual function and migraine that may pertain to the topic at hand. Electrophysiologic studies, especially evoked responses, are consistently reliable. Furthermore, they are noninvasive and well tolerated, and they are often quickly done and not offensive to the person being studied.

Gawel, Connolly, and Rose (26) reported in 1983 that visual evoked responses (VER) were abnormal in migraine patients as contrasted with normal controls. Several VER abnormalities were seen in patients, including variation in amplitude and delays, and even a hemispheric abnormality was suggested.

Our current study (27), which concludes this chapter, was designed to assess several specific electrophysiologic variables in women who have migraine. Spectral analysis of the EEG, pattern-shift, VERs, and a visual "odd-ball" P300 paradigm were obtained from women who reported a history of migraine and were compared with age-matched control subjects who were free of severe headache complaints. Preliminary data suggested that the migraine patients showed an overall higher EEG frequeny in the alpha band and greater variance of frequency and power relative to control subjects. Full-field VERs showed no substantial differences between the patients and controls for either latency or amplitude of the P2 component. Half-field VERs also yielded normal response patterns for both groups, although some tendency of longer latency P2 components was obtained for temporal compared with nasal stimulation recordings. The visual P300 components showed normal variation in latency and amplitude for both groups.

Thus, though migraine patients may report strange and wondrous objects in the visual fields, their visual apparatus appears to be normal.

The close relationship between migraine and amaurosis fugax is self-evident and perhaps confusing. Nonetheless, the differences between migraine, especially as manifested in its visual auras, and amaurosis fugax associated with atherosclerotic disease are also evident and are of importance to the physician who deals with the visual obscurations of whatever sort.

References

1. World Federation of Neurology Research Group on Migraine and Headache: Definition of migraine, in Cochrane AL (ed): *Background to Migraine*. London, William Heinemann Ltd, 1970, pp 181–182.
2. Gowers WR: *A Manual of Diseases of the Nervous System,* ed 2. London, J & A Churchill, 1893.
3. Airey H: On a distinct form of transient hemiopsia. *Philos Trans R Soc Lond [Biol]* 1870;160:247–264.
4. Lashley KS: Patterns of cerebral integration indicated by the scotomas of migraine. *Arch Neurol Psychiatry* 1941;46:331–339.
5. Alvarez WC: The migrainous scotoma as studied in 618 persons. *Am J Ophthalmol* 1960;49:489–504.
6. Leao AP: Spreading depression of activity in the cerebral cortex. *J Neurophysiol (London)* 1944;7:359–390.
7. Milner PM: Note on possible correspondence between the scotomas of migraine and spreading depression of Leao. *Electroencephalogr Clin Neurophysiol* 1958;10:705.
8. Kline LB, Kelly CB: Ocular migraine in a patient with cluster headaches. *Headache* 1980;20:253–257.
9. Hedges TR: An ophthalmologist's view of headache. *Headache* 1979;19:151–155.
10. Wilkinson M, Robinson D: Migraine art. *Cephalalgia* 1985;5:151–158.
11. Critchley M: Metamorphopsia of central origin. *Trans Ophthalmol Soc UK* 1949;69:111.
12. Todd J: The syndrome of Alice in Wonderland. *Can Med Assoc J* 1955;73:701–706.
13. Fisher CM: Late-life migraine accompaniments as a cause of unexplained transient ischemic attacks. *Can J Neurol Sci* 1980;7:9–17.
14. Dalessio DJ: The relationship of vasoactive substances to vascular permeability and their role in migraine, in *Research and Clinical Studies in Headache* Basel, Karger, 1976, vol 4, pp. 76–84.
15. Moskowitz MA: The neurobiology of vascular head pain. *Ann Neurol* 1984;16:157–158.
16. Goadsby PJ, Lambert GA, Lance JW: Differential effects on the internal and external carotid circulation of the monkey evoked by locus coeruleus stimulation. *Brain Res* 1982;249:247–254.

17. Lance JW, Lambert GA, Goadsby PJ, et al: Brainstem influences on the cephalic circulation: Experimental data from cat and monkey of relevance to the mechanism of migraine. *Headache* 1983;23:258–265.
18. Mosnaim AD, Wolf ME, Chevesich BJ, et al: Plasma methionine encephalin levels: A biological marker for migraine? *Headache* 1985;25:259–261.
19. Edmeads J: Cerebral blood flow in migraine. *Headache* 1977;17:148–152.
20. Sakai F, Meyer JS: Regional cerebral hemodynamics during migraine and cluster headache measured by the ^{133}Xenon inhalation method. *Headache* 1978;18:122–132.
21. Olesen J, Larsen B, Lauritzen M: Focal hyperemia followed by spreading oligemia and impaired activation of rCBF in classic migraine. *Ann Neurol* 1981;9:344–352.
22. Lauritzen M, Olesen TS, Lassen NA, et al: Changes in regional cerebral blood flow during the course of classic migraine attacks *Ann Neurol* 1983;13:633–641.
23. Schroth G, Gerber WD, Langohr HD: Ultrasonic Doppler flow in migraine and cluster headache. *Headache* 1983;23:284–288.
24. Lieberman AN, Jonas S, Hass WK, et al. Bilateral cervical carotid and intracranial vasospasm causing cerebral ischemia in a migrainous patient: A case of "diplegic migraine." *Headache* 1984;24:245–248.
25. Spaccavento LJ, Solomon GD: Migraine as an etiology of stroke in young adults. *Headache* 1984;24:19–22.
26. Gawel M, Connolly JF, Rose FC: Migraine patients exhibit abnormalities in the visual evoked potential. *Headache* 1983;23:49–52.
27. Dalessio DJ, Polich J, Ehlers C: Endogenous and psychic determinants of migraine, in Amery WL, Wauquier A (eds): *The Prelude to the Migraine Attack*. London, Balliere Tindall/WB Saunders Co, 1986, pp 3–8.

Chapter 13

Nonembolic Sources of Amaurosis Fugax

Marjorie E. Seybold

A number of causes of transient visual loss are not related to carotid-based disease. Some of these, such as the prodromal events of AION and ocular migraine are discussed in other chapters. Others are described here (Table 13–1) to alert the reader to their existence and, when possible, to describe the differences from embolic amaurosis fugax.

Intraocular Sources

Intraocular sources of amaurosis fugax frequently go unrecognized. All are uncommon, and some may be unsuspected if not seen during the acute episode. One of the least often reported causes is recurrent hyphema. Episodes of hemorrhage into the anterior chamber may occur spontaneously, with iris vascular anomalies or after intraocular surgery. In the latter case, the hemorrhage may occur months or even years after uncomplicated surgery, especially surgery for cataracts. Generally, the visual loss lasts for days or weeks, but, occasionally, it may be quite brief, lasting only a few hours (1). The bleeding may be so minimal that it is detected only by gonioscopy (2). Clues to the diagnosis include a duration of several hours, occurrence on awakening, slow onset and clearing of the vision loss, history of past intraocular surgery, and blood in the inferior anterior chamber or deep in the chamber angle.

Narrow-angle glaucoma usually is characterized by severe pain. Thus, when it occurs without significant pain, its occurrence often goes unrecognized. The episodes of loss of vision may be relatively brief, lasting seconds or minutes (3,4). Narrow anterior chamber angles, pain (if present, though minor), and repetition of attacks under certain lighting conditions are useful clues to diagnosis. Elevated IOP is helpful for diagnosis but is not always present between attacks.

Patients with optic nerve head drusen may report visual obscurations that last seconds to hours (5). Drusen usually are recognized on optic disk inspection, although they also may appear as pseudopapilledema.

TABLE 13–1. Sources of amaurosis fugax.

Intraocular
- 1. Recurrent hyphema
- 2. Glaucoma
- 3. Drusen
- 4. Congenital anomaly of the optic disk
- 5. Anterior ischemic neuropathy
  - a. Arteritic
  - b. Nonarteritic
- 6. Choroidal insufficiency secondary to periarteritis nodosa

Intraorbital
- 1. Hemangioma
- 2. Osteoma

Intracranial
- 1. Papilledema
- 2. Arteriovenous malformation
- 3. Tumor

Carotid
- 1. Dissection
- 2. Thrombosis
- 3. Embolism

Other
- 1. Hematologic causes
  - a. Anemia
  - b. Polycythemia
  - c. Sickle cell disease
  - d. Thrombocytosis
- 2. Hypertension
- 3. Hypotension
- 4. Cardiac causes
  - a. Arrhythmia
  - b. Embolism
  - c. Mitral valve prolapse
- 5. Migraine
- 6. Raynaud's phenomenon
- 7. Fat embolism
- 8. Unknown

Congenital anomalies of the optic disk are a well-described cause of transient visual loss that lasts seconds to minutes, rarely hours, without accompanying symptoms (6–8). Some episodes may seem to be precipitated by bright light (6–8), a symptom similar to that described in patients with carotid artery occlusive disease (9). Cases have been observed in which the amaurosis coincides with dilatation of the retinal veins (7,8). In these cases, which were associated also with disk anomalies, intermittent venous obstruction may lead to arterial obstruction that, in turn, induces amaurosis (10). Judging from the cases reported, amaurosis fugax with disk anomalies appears to be benign.

Transient visual loss may occur hours or days before permanent visual loss in patients with AION (10). This phenomenon is said to be more common with the arteritic form of AION (11). The optic disk is said to be "always edematous, although the swelling may be slight and involve only a segment of the disk." (11)

Newman et al (12) reported a case of a patient with "macula-sparing monocular blackouts." The patient, who had known periarteritis nodosa, had four- to five-minute episodes of monocular peripheral loss of vision in either eye, although never both simultaneously. Between attacks the fundi appeared normal. Direct visualization during an episode, fluorescein angiography, and autopsy findings indicated a selective loss of choroid perfusion. The transient attacks may have been precipitated by minor changes in ophthalmic or systemic arterial pressure in the already impaired choroidal system.

Intraorbital Sources

Intraorbital masses have been associated with transient gaze-evoked loss of vision. In both a woman with a cavernous hemangioma of the orbit (13) and a boy with an osteoma arising from the ethmoid (14), transient loss of vision occurred with downgaze and remained until primary position was resumed. Both patients had proptosis and a swollen disk on the side of the visual episodes.

Intracranial Sources

Patients with papilledema frequently have very brief (1 to 2 seconds) episodes of monocular or binocular loss of vision. These often are triggered by head or body movement, especially leaning over. The cause of the episodes is unknown but may be related to transient fluctuations in subarachnoid pressure that are transmitted to the optic nerve or its vasculature.

Walsh and Hoyt (10) reported episodes of amaurosis fugax in patients with "massive ipsilateral arteriovenous malformation." They speculated that the "attacks were ischemic in nature and were related to changes in blood flow in other areas supplied by the internal carotid artery."

Cogan (15) described two patients with tumors (patients 1 and 2) who had episodes of amaurosis fugax presumably due to direct involvement of visual pathways by the tumor. One patient who had a glioma of the frontal lobe, directly involving the optic nerve, experienced frequent 10-minute episodes of unilateral loss of vision over an 8-month period. The second patient developed transient unilateral loss of vision and was found to have a pituitary tumor with a homonymous hemianopia. Removal of the tumor was followed by cessation of the blackouts.

Carotid Sources

Mokri et al (16) reported that 1 of the 36 patients they studied who had spontaneous dissection of the ICA developed amaurosis fugax as the initial manifestation of the dissection. A second patient also developed amaurosis fugax, but apparently this occurred in conjunction with cerebral events.

Carotid embolic and occlusive disease as a cause of amaurosis fugax is discussed in other chapters of this book.

Other Sources

Transient loss of vision has been described in various hematologic abnormalities, including polycythemia (17), severe anemia (18), sickle cell disease (18), and thrombocytosis (19). Hypoxia and sludging are the likely sources of amaurosis fugax in the first three disorders, whereas presumed platelet emboli have been observed in the patients with thrombocytosis (20).

Hypertensive crises can produce TMB that lasts from minutes to hours (10). Angiospasm is thought to be the mechanism that induces the blindness in these patients.

Hypotension is a well-recognized cause of amaurosis fugax. Hoyt (21) described several characteristics he thought were useful in differentiating hypotensive from embolic amaurosis fugax. Hypotensive episodes are likely to begin with a constriction of the visual field and to resolve with return of central vision first. Rapid onset and clearing with sector or altitudinal characteristics suggest embolism as the cause of the episode. Hypotensive amaurosis fugax may occur with unilateral pain and may be related to change in body position (21).

Focal neurologic deficits, including amaurosis fugax, may occur because of cardiac abnormalities. A fall in cardiac output, as may occur with an arrhythmia, is thought to cause transient focal visual symptoms rarely (10). Embolic material may originate from cardiac as well as carotid sources, either as an aftermath to myocardial infarction, from valvular disease, from myxoma, or in association with atrial fibrillation. Episodes of amaurosis fugax also have been reported in patients with mitral valve prolapse (22,23). Carotid angiography in some of these patients (22) failed to reveal a carotid source for the visual events.

Migraine as a source of amaurosis fugax is considered in chapter 12.

Raynaud's phenomenon has been implicated as a rare cause of transient loss of vision (10). The assumed source of the visual change is spasm of the CRA.

Fat embolism after crushing injuries, usually to the legs, may cause transient loss of vision. Given the clinical setting in which it occurs, it is unlikely to be mistaken for other causes of amaurosis fugax.

The cause of amaurosis fugax is not always recognized. This is particularly true when the loss of vision occurs in relatively young, otherwise healthy individuals. Eadie et al (24) described 12 patients, including eight who had cerebral angiography, in whom no cause could be detected. None had experienced any permanent visual loss or generalized disability at the time of followup (mean 1.8 years).

References

1. Watzke RC: Intraocular hemorrhage from vascularization of the cataract incision. *Ophthalmology* 1980;87:19–23.
2. Swan KC: Hyphema due to wound vascularization after cataract extraction. *Arch Ophthalmol* 1973;89:87–90.
3. Ravits J, Seybold ME: Transient monocular visual loss from narrow angle glaucoma. *Arch Neurol* 1984;41:991–993.
4. Fisher CM: Some neuro-ophthalmological observations. *J Neuro Neurosurg Psychiatry* 1967;30:383–392.
5. Glaser JS: Topical diagnosis: Prechiasmal visual pathways, in Glaser JS (ed): *Neuro-ophthalmology*. Hagarstown, MD, Harper & Row Publishers Inc, 1978, p 79.
6. Seybold M, Rosen PN: Peripapillary staphyloma and amaurosis fugax. *Ann Ophthalmol* 1977;9:1139–1141.
7. Graether JM: Transient amaurosis in one eye with simultaneous dilatation of retinal veins. *Arch Ophthalmol* 1963;70:342–345.
8. Longfellow DW, Davis FS Jr, Walsh FB: Unilateral intermittent blindness with dilation of retinal veins. *Arch Ophthalmol* 1962;67:554–555.
9. Furlan AJ, Whisnant JP, Kearns TP: Unilateral visual loss in bright light: An unusual symptom of carotid artery occlusive disease. *Arch Neurol* 1979;36:675–676.
10. Walsh FB, Hoyt WF: *Clinical Neuro-Ophthalmology,* ed 3. Baltimore, The Williams & Wilkins Co, 1969, vol 2, pp 1707, 1807, 1869, 1870, 1882, 1890, 1915.
11. Lessell S: Nonarteritic anterior ischemic optic neuropathy (AION). Presented at the UCSF Update in Neuro-ophthalmology, San Francisco, Dec 11–12, 1986.
12. Newman NM, Hoyt WF, Spencer WH: Macula-sparing monocular blackouts: Clinical and pathologic investigations of intermittent choroidal vascular insufficiency in a case of periarteritis nodosa. *Arch Ophthalmol* 1974;91:367–370.
13. Brown GC, Shields JA: Amaurosis fugax secondary to presumed cavernous hemangioma of the orbit. *Ann Ophthalmol* 1981;13:1205–1209.
14. Wilkes SR, Trautmann JC, DeSanto LW, et al: Osteoma: An unusual cause of amaurosis fugax. *Mayo Clin Proc* 1979;54:258–260.
15. Cogan DG: Blackouts not obviously due to carotid occlusion. *Arch Ophthalmol* 1961;66:180–187.
16. Mokri B, Sundt TM Jr, Houser OW, et al: Spontaneous dissection of the cervical internal carotid artery. *Ann Neurol* 1986;19:126–138.
17. Johnson DR, Chalgren WS: Polycythemia vera and the nervous system. *Neurology* 1951;1:53–67.

18. Hoyt WF: Ocular symptoms and signs, in Wylie ES, Ehrenfeld WK (eds): *Extracranial Occlusive Cerebrovascular Disease: Diagnosis and Management*. Philadelphia, WB Saunders Co, 1970, pp 64–95.
19. Levin J, Swanson PD: Idiopathic thrombocytosis: A treatable cause of transient ischemic attacks. *Neurology* 1968;18:711–713.
20. Cogan DG: Occlusive arterial disease in the eye, In *Ophthalmic Manifestations of Systemic Vascular Disease. Major Problems in Internal Medicine*. Philadelphia, WB Saunders Co, 1974, vol 3, p 123.
21. Hoyt WF: Retinal ischemic symptoms in cardiovascular diagnosis. *Postgrad Med* 1972;52:85–90.
22. Wilson LA, Keeling PWN, Malcolm AD, et al: Visual complications of mitral leaflet prolapse. *Br Med J* 1977;2:86–88.
23. Kimball RW, Hedges TR: Amaurosis fugax caused by a prolapsed mitral valve leaflet in the midsystolic click, late systolic murmur syndrome. *Am J Ophthalmol* 1977;83:469–470.
24. Eadie MJ, Sutherland JM, Tyrer JH: Recurrent monocular blindness of uncertain cause. *Lancet* 1968;1:319–321.

CHAPTER 14

Natural History of Amaurosis Fugax

Ralph W. Ross Russell

Pathogenesis

Amaurosis fugax (TMB) is a common symptom in a number of disorders and is caused by an abrupt and transient reduction in ocular perfusion to one eye (1). The visual loss is sudden and complete as if a curtain were drawn over the eye. Loss of vision may involve the whole field or sometimes may be restricted to the upper or lower half. Positive visual phenomena are unusual. Recovery usually occurs after a few minutes, and restoration of vision is complete. Occlusions of the central retinal artery by an embolus that causes a partial or temporarv blockage of the vessel is considered the probable explanation for most cases for the following reasons:

1. Ophthalmoscopic observations have been made of emboli traversing the retinal circulation during attacks of visual loss (2,3). Indirect evidence suggests that these are composed of fibrin-platelet aggregates (4).
2. Cholesterol emboli may be lodged in the retinal circulation and may persist for days or weeks after an attack (5).
3. About one third of the patients have a likely source of arterial embolus in the internal carotid artery or in the heart (6).

Embolism is not, however, the only cause of amaurosis fugax. Patients with other conditions, such as giant-cell arteritis, polycythemia or macroglobulinaemia, or raised ICP, may suffer similar loss of vision. Also, many observations of patients during attacks have shown no abnormality in the retinal arteries. In some patients with typical amaurosis fugax, usually in younger age groups, all routine investigations may show no evidence of abnormalities. In these patients the symptoms have been ascribed to vasospasm or to migraine (7). A qualitative platelet abnormality that causes spontaneous aggregation may be a factor in some of this group. Other underlying systemic disorders include accelerated hypertension, thrombocythemia, and lupus erythematosus.

Occasionally patients describe a type of amaurosis fugax characterized by a blurring or fragmentation of vision in one eye without profound visual loss. This symptom may occur in patients who have glaucoma, retinal venous occlusion, or retinal hypoperfusion secondary to extracranial artery disease (retinal insufficiency) (8).

Age Profile

The age profile compiled from published series from the United Kingdom is shown in Fig. 14–1. In patients less than 40 years old, the prevalence of amaurosis fugax is low (6%) and apparently equal for men and for women. In the 40 to 80 age group, men outnumber women at a ratio of 2.3:1. Prevalence is highest in the 60 to 70 age group; one third of patients fall into this bracket.

Associated Features

Elevated blood pressure (110 mm Hg, diastolic) and ischemic heart disease (treated or untreated angina or history of myocardial infarction) each occur in 20% of cases. Intermittent claudication is present in 15%, and impaired glucose tolerance in 6%. Heavy cigarette smoking is a feature in 55%. Ipsilateral carotid bruit is detected in 30%.

Diagnostic Evaluation

The initial examination of a patient with amaurosis fugax is designed to detect the presence of an underlying disease or a carotid arterial abnormality that could either obstruct blood flow to the eye or provide a source

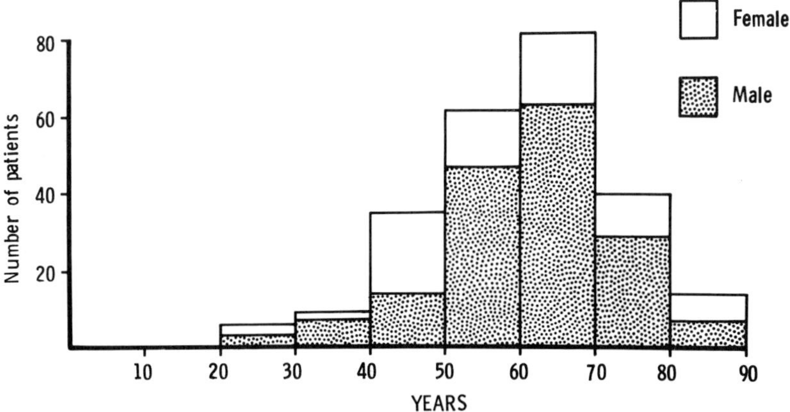

FIGURE 14–1. Age and sex distribution in 248 patients with amaurosis fugax.

of retinal embolism. Raised ICP or glaucoma is detected readily on clinical examination. In those patients with attacks secondary to hematologic disorders such as polycythemia or thrombocytosis, this can be detected on routine investigations and by the characteristic retinal appearances of retardation of blood flow, vasodilatation, and retinal hemorrhages. Patients with giant-cell arteritis may show focal ischemic changes in the retina (cotton-wool spots). The ESR usually elevated. Patients with a cardiac source for embolism usually have clinical evidence of valvular disease; less common varieties such as endomyocardial fibrosis or mitral valve leaflet prolapse may require echocardiography for diagnosis.

The place of carotid angiography in the detection of surgically treatable lesions of the carotid artery has been evaluated in a number of reports (6,9). Angiography shows carotid stenosis in 25%–30% and occlusion in 10%. These figures are probably too high as angiography has not been used often. Realistic figures for atheromatous carotid disease is approximately 20%–25% of the total. The combination of clinical signs and risk factors (carotid bruit, history of transient cerebral ischemia, systemic hypertension, intermittent claudication, or age greater than 50 years) has been useful in predicting the presence of a surgically accessible lesion (6). If three of these factors are present, 85% of cases have surgically treatable carotid lesions; and if four factors are present, the percentage is 100. Conversely, if none of the risk factors is present, the usefulness of angiography is so low as to make it unnecessary.

Unusual types of carotid disease that occasionally cause embolism include fibromuscular dysplasia, carotid buckling or looping, dissection, and saccular aneurysm.

Modern sonographic techniques that combine a velocity profile of the vessel with B-mode imaging correlate closely with angiography. These techniques have a major role as screening procedures for the detection of carotid artery disease in those patients who have arterial symptoms at other sites.

Natural History

The demonstration by Fisher (1) that amaurosis fugax may herald stroke or TIA has generated much interest in both medical and surgical treatment in the hope of preventing cerebral ischemia.

Before embarking on therapy, it is essential to gather some information on the natural history of the disease. This will make it possible to calculate the number of patients and the probable time necessary to achieve a statistically significant result in any clinical trial. Few natural history studies of patients with amaurosis fugax are available.

Marshall and Meadows (10) did a retrospective review of 80 patients and a follow-up study that lasted 20 years in some cases. They found only five patients who had suffered a permanent hemiplegia, five who had had a transient cerebral ischemia, and nine who had lost the sight in one eye from CRA occlusion. Although most of the patients in this series were middle-aged men, the authors did identify a group of young women who had a favorable prognosis.

A report from Paris (11) published shortly after Marshall's and Meadows' paper had different results. Sixty-six patients similar in age and sex distribution to those in the previous study (10) had follow-up examinations for a period of up to 4 years. Of these, 22% had a cerebral TIA, 40% had a permanent stroke, and 7.5% lost vision in one eye. A more recent report (12) included 56 patients with amaurosis fugax who had follow-up examinations for a mean of 4.9 years after the first symptom. During the study period, either transient or permanent cerebral ischemia developed in 34% of those who had had no previous cerebral vascular symptoms. Permanent visual loss occurred in three.

These three papers indicate the uncertainty that surrounds the natural history of amaurosis fugax. Some discrepancies can be explained by the retrospective nature of the studies and by differences in criteria for entry and follow-up. The ways in which patients are selected for inclusion is critical and is not always described. The high prevalence of cerebral vascular symptoms in the French study may have been caused by the inclusion of patients who came to the hospital because of cerebral symptoms and gave a history of having had amaurosis fugax in the preceding days or weeks. The completeness of the follow-up study in the 1968 British paper suggests that untraced patients had not been included, and because such patients may have died or suffered a stroke, this is a factor that may distort the results towards a more favorable outcome.

A definitive natural history study ideally should be prospective. The patients should be unselected and should be a consecutive series of those exhibiting the symptom. The patients should be representative of the disease as a whole, and their selection should not be biased by the sources of referral (eg, the natural history of patients at an ophthalmic unit will probably be quite different from those in a hospital for cardiac diseases). Finally, every effort must be made to make the follow-up study complete and to extend it over some years.

Sample Studies

The following study (13) meets only some of the aforementioned criteria: It was retrospective and consisted of 110 medically treated patients with amaurosis fugax who were selected from a number of different sources and considered to be representative of the disease as a whole. The age range at the time of presentation was wide, and men outnumbered women at a ratio of 2.2:1.0. Most of the patients were more than 55 years old, but 13% were under the age of 45, and 5% were in the 15–24 age range (Table 14–1).

TABLE 14–1. Distribution of amaurosis fugax by age and sex.

Age (yr)	Male (N = 76)	Female (N = 34)	Total (N = 110)
15–24	3	2	5
25–34	2	0	2
35–44	6	1	7
45–54	9	4	13
55–64	29	11	40
65–74	21	10	31
>75	6	6	12

Risk factors such as heavy smoking, hypertension, and ischemic heart disease possibly accounting for embolism were present in 8%. Patients with repeated attacks of amaurosis fugax in the same eye were examined by carotid angiography. Findings were normal in 60%, carotid stenosis or atheroma was present in 25%, carotid occlusion was present in 10%, and other lesions such as kinking or looping occurred in 5%. Patients with carotid abnormalities have a significantly greater risk of stroke (5% per year) than those with normal carotid arteries.

Follow-up studies of these patients were done after an interval of 0 to 19 years (mean, 8 years). Results were expressed as survival curves. (Fig. 14–2) so comparisons could be made with an age- and sex-matched control

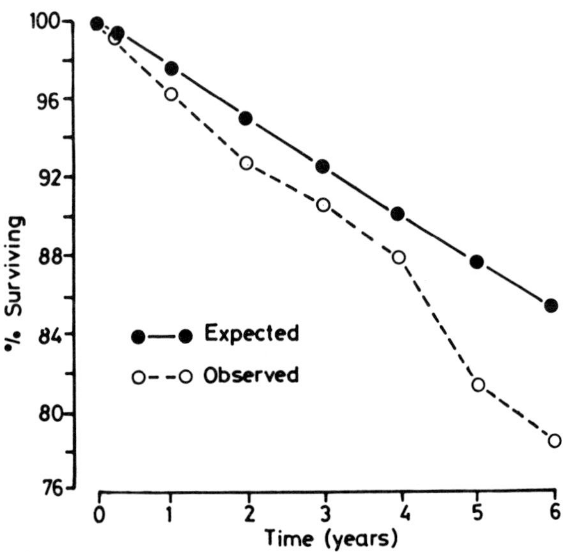

FIGURE 14–2. Survival curve for males and females combined after one or more attacks of amaurosis fugax compared with the expected survival for a population of equivalent age and sex in England and Wales, 1975.

TABLE 14–2. Cause of death following amaurosis fugax.

Cause	No.	% of total group
Cardiac disease	17	15.5
Stroke	5	4.5
Cancer	5	4.5
Respiratory disease	3	2.5
Other	1	1.0
Total	31	28.0

group. A major finding was an increased mortality rate compared with the control population series derived from the figures of the Registrar General of the United Kingdom for the same period. After 6 years, the mortality rate in the amaurosis fugax group was 21% compared with an expected mortality rate of 15%. This was due primarily to an increased death rate in men (26%) compared with an expected 17%. The most common cause of death was myocardial infarction or cardiac failure (Table 14–2). Survival free of fatal ischemic heart disease occurred significantly less frequently in the amaurosis fugax group (Fig. 14–3). Fatal and nonfatal stroke occurred in 13% of the amaurosis fugax group over a 6-year period compared with an expected 3% (the latter figure was derived from the

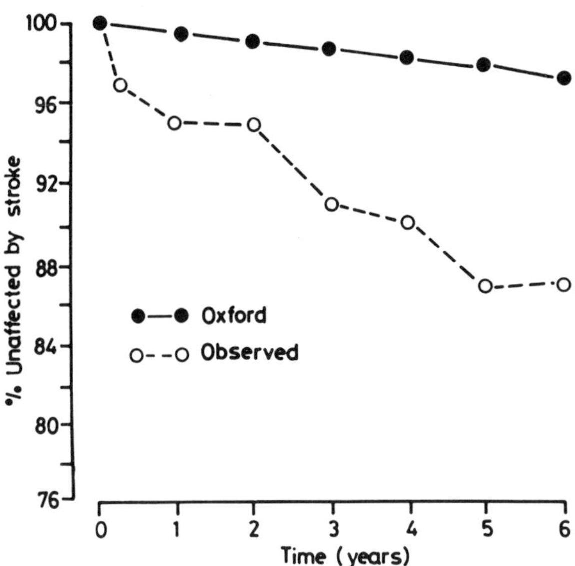

FIGURE 14–3. Survival free from stroke for males and females combined after one or more attacks of amaurosis fugax compared with the expected stroke rate for a population of equivalent age and sex in Oxfordshire, 1981–1983.

Oxford Community Stroke Project 1979). All those patients who experienced strokes were 57 years or older at presentation. During the 6 years of follow-up, 4.5% of patients suffered a cerebral TIA, 3% had a nonfatal myocardial infarction, and 6% suffered permanent loss of vision in one eye.

Patients with amaurosis fugax had a shortened life span; their mortality rate was 1.4 times greater than expected. This was caused by an increase in heart disease; the prevalence was four times that in the general population. Mortality rate was constant over the 6 years of follow-up. There was no evidence cf an increase in death rate in the early months after amaurosis fugax. Patients with amaurosis fugax also had an increased risk of stroke. The rate was four times that expected, but the absolute risk was still small, about 2% per year. Little evidence of variation in this stroke rate was seen during the follow-up period, and no indication was seen of an increased risk in the first year after the development of symptoms, such as was suggested by Whisnant et al (14) who studied patients with transient cerebral ischemia. Patients with carotid stenosis or occlusion showed a higher risk of stroke (5% per year). The risk of permanent visual loss was approximately 1% per year.

Amaurosis fugax is a marker or risk factor for atherosclerosis indicating generalized arterial disease. The risk of stroke is low and is probably less than in patients with transient cerebral ischemia for whom most studies have shown a stroke rate of 5% to 10% per year (14). In our study no strokes occurred in patients less than 55 years old. Patients with amaurosis fugax probably should not be subjected to carotid endarterectomy unless a highly experienced vascular surgical unit with a record of low morbidity and mortality in their patients is available. Similarly, it is not justifiable to perform carotid angiography in patients who are less than 55 years old.

A similar natural history (15) recently has been completed on patients observed to have cholesterol emboli in retinal arteries. As pointed out by Pfaffenbach and Hollenhorst (16), these may occur in the absence of any visual symptoms, but they also may cause either permanent or temporary visual loss. The explanation for this seems to lie in the flat configuration of the crystals of cholesterol esters. If they are lodged with the long axis parallel to the long axis of the vessel, they may cause minimal obstruction to flow; however, if they are rotated about 90°, they may block the lumen. All the patients in this study (15) have had episodic or permanent visual loss. More than 58 patients were in follow-up studies of from 0–12 years (mean, 4.5 years). All patients received medical treatment, but none had carotid surgery.

In this group of patients life expectancy again was significantly shortened in men when compared with an age- and sex-matched control group (Fig. 14–4). Stroke rather than heart disease was the most common cause of death, and there was also an increase in nonfatal cerebral vascular disease. In a 6-year period, stroke developed in 25% as compared with an expected 3% (Fig. 14–5). This is a greater increase than that found in patients with

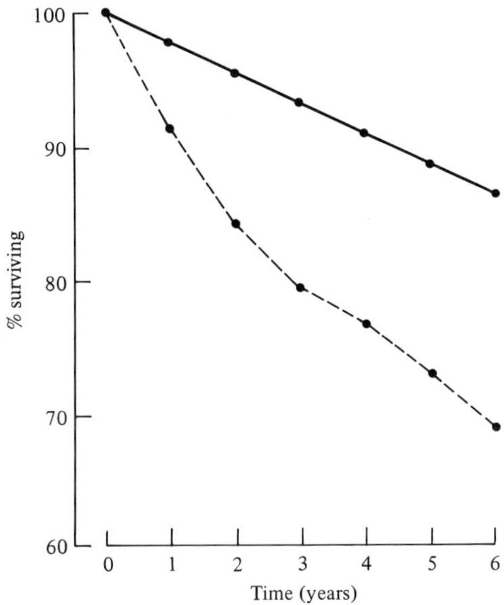

FIGURE 14–4. Survival curve for males and females combined after visual loss due to cholesterol emboli compared with expected survival for a population of equivalent age and sex in England and Wales, 1979.

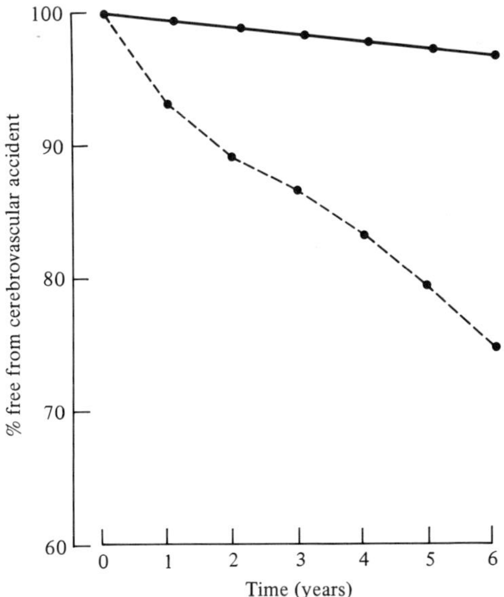

FIGURE 14–5. Survival free from stroke (fatal and nonfatal) for males and females combined after visual loss due to cholesterol emboli compared with the expected stroke rate for a population of equivalent age and sex in Oxfordshire, 1981–1983.

amaurosis fugax. No significant increase in myocardial infarction was found, although this has been documented by other studies (16) that included asymptomatic patients.

These two retrospective natural history studies are complementary. They point to the conclusion that (with the exception of a group of young patients who appear to have a benign, nonprogressive variety) amaurosis fugax is a powerful indicator of vascular disease in the coronary and cerebral circulations. Detection of cholesterol emboli by ophthalmoscopy has an even greater predictive value.

Therefore, amaurosis fugax should be regarded as an important symptom that requires the immediate attention of both ophthalmologist and internist. Only after careful evaluation of each individual patient can informed advice be given on prognosis and possible treatment.

References

1. Fisher CM: Transient monocular blindness associated with hemiplegia. *Arch Ophthalmol* 1952;47:167–203.
2. Fisher CM: Observations of the fundus oculi in transient monocular blindness. *Neurology* 1959;9:333–347.
3. Ross Russell RW: Observations on the retinal blood vessels in monocular blindness. *Lancet* 1961;2:1422–1428.
4. McBrien DJ, Bradley RD, Ashton N: The nature of retinal emboli in stenosis of the internal carotid artery. *Lancet* 1963;1:697–699.
5. Ross Russell RW: The source of retinal emboli. *Lancet* 1968;2:789–793.
6. Wilson LA, Ross Russell RW: Amaurosis fugax and carotid artery disease: Indications for angiography. *Br Med J* 1977;2:435–437.
7. Eadie MJ, Sutherland JM, Tyrer JM: Recurrent monocular blindness of uncertain cause. *Lancet* 1968;1:319–321.
8. Ross Russell RW, Page NGR: Critical perfusion of brain and retina. *Brain* 1982;106:419–434.
9. Hooshmand H, Vines FS, Lee HM, Grindal A: Amaurosis fugax: Diagnostic and therapeutic aspects. *Stroke* 1974;5:643–647.
10. Marshall J, Meadows SP: The natural history of amaurosis fugax. *Brain* 1968;91:419–434.
11. Morax PV, Aron Rosa D, Gautier JC: Symptomes et signes ophthalmologique des stenoses et occlusions carotidiennes. *Bull Soc Ophthalmol Fr* 1970; suppl 1, p 169.
12. Parkin PJ, Kendall BE, Marshall J, et al: Amaurosis fugax: Some aspects of management. *J Neurol Neurosurg Psychiatry* 1982;45:1–6.
13. Poole CJM, Ross Russell RW: Mortality and stroke after amaurosis fugax. *J Neurol Neurosurg Psychiatry* 1985;48:902–903.
14. Whisnant JP, Matsumoto N, Elveback LR: Transient cerebral ischaemic attacks in a community. *Mayo Clin Proc* 1973;48:194–198.
15. Howard RS, Ross Russell RW: Prognosis in retinal embolism. *J Neurol Neurosurg Psychiatry* 1987; in press.
16. Pfaffenbach DD, Hollenhorst RW: Morbidity and survivorship of patients with embolic cholesterol crystals in the ocular fundus. *Am J Ophthalmol* 1973;75:66–72.

Chapter 15

Noninvasive Vascular Examination in Amaurosis Fugax

Shirley M. Otis

Amaurosis fugax, also known as TMB, has been recognized as an important manifestation of carotid artery disease since early medical literature. Extracranial carotid disease is estimated to account for up to half of all cerebrovascular accidents (1–6). Transient ischemic attacks are the most common manifestation of carotid disease, and amaurosis fugax is a form of transient ischemia.

Amaurosis fugax long has been recognized to carry a significant risk of stroke, although somewhat less than classic TIAs (7). Prevalence of carotid arterial disease in amaurosis fugax has been estimated at between 50% and 78% (7,8). The carotid arteries long have been implicated as the source of retinal arterial emboli; the internal, common, and, rarely, external carotids have been demonstrated as sources (9).

In 1914, Hunt (10) reported a probable clinical relationship between transient ocular symptoms and carotid artery disease. In the early 1950s, Fisher (11–13) confirmed an association between monocular visual loss and contralateral hemiplegia and observed retinal artery emboli. Millikan et al (14) suggested that cerebral ischemia may be transient because of emboli lodging in arteries and subsequently fragmenting. Hollenhorst (15) reported that CRA occlusion occurred in 7% of patients with carotid disease. In 1966, Ehrenfeld et al (16) found irregular intimal surfaces with ulceration in 18 of 32 patients who underwent carotid endarterectomy and had symptoms of amaurosis fugax.

In 1972, Kollarits et al (17) showed the association between carotid atheroma and arterioretinal emboli. Of 45 patients who underwent carotid arteriography for suspected carotid disease, 43 (96%) were found to have a probable carotid source for the emboli. Further angiographic studies were undertaken in patients with amaurosis fugax by Theile et al (18). They concluded that amaurosis fugax was a highly specific symptom for disease of the carotid bifurcation and that potential embolic lesions were more common than hemodynamically significant lesions.

The hospital frequency cooperative study (19) also noted that when ipsilateral monocular visual loss was analyzed as a single symptom, it was usually a symptom for carotid artery disease. A study of the correlation between the presence of carotid plaques, occurrence of TIAs, and findings on CT scanning was performed by Zukowski et al (20). It provided further evidence and support for the embolic theory by revealing the association between macroscopic ulceration of atheromatous carotid plaques and evidence of cerebral infarction on preoperative CT brain scans of patients having carotid endarterectomy for TIAs, including amaurosis fugax.

Arteriographic studies of patients with amaurosis fugax and CRA occlusion were reported by Sheng et al (21). Over half of all patients with CRA occlusion who underwent angiography had significant lesions in the ipsilateral carotid artery. Sheng et al emphasized that carotid atheromatous disease was an important cause of CRA occlusion and that CRA occlusion could be considered a significant marker for extracranial carotid disease. They further emphasized that this should be an indication for complete carotid evaluation.

In an earlier report of amaurosis fugax and the results of arteriography, Adams et al (22) pointed out and concluded that patients with TMB should be assumed to have carotid artery disease. However, they also noted that their patients with amaurosis fugax were a heterogeneous group, that emboli may arise from several sites, that the visual symptoms should not be considered a specific indicator of stenosis of the ICA. They, and a number of other authors (18,20,21), have emphasized the need to systematically evaluate these patients by performing a full diagnostic workup of the extracranial carotid system and for other causes.

A number of noninvasive vascular studies have been developed for the evaluation of extracranial vascular disease and show both specificity and sensitivity for the detection of atheromatous carotid plaques and ulcerations. Noninvasive vascular studies should be the initial diagnostic procedure of choice for patients with amaurosis fugax.

Vascular Physiology

When the aforementioned facts are considered, vascular workup becomes imperative for the proper care and management of the patient with amaurosis fugax. However, an understanding of the various possible vascular mechanisms of amaurosis fugax is required before its causes can be investigated appropriately.

Ischemic attacks in the brain and in the eye are similar, particularly because the ophthalmic, middle cerebral, and anterior cerebral arteries all originate from the ICA. The retina derives blood from two sources: the CRA and the ciliary arteries; both of these sources arise from the ophthalmic artery. The outer retinal layers are supplied by the short ciliary arteries, which also supply the optic disk and optic nerve, and the inner retina is supplied by the CRA. Temporary reduction in ocular blood supply in either of these arteries or emboli may produce amaurosis fugax or TMB (9).

The two separate circulatory systems aid in supplying circulation to the retina, which has the greatest rate of oxygen consumption per gram of tissue in the body. The blood flow in the CRA is approximately 28 ml/min, and that in the choroid circulation is 150 ml/min. The retinal circulation is similar to that of the brain; both are autoregulated and responsive to changes in P_{CO_2} (23).

Embolism is the most common single cause of amaurosis fugax; however, ischemic oculopathy, although less frequent, is a serious cause. It may be related to stenosis of the ophthalmic artery (which reduces OAP), CRA thrombosis, or chronic ocular hypoxia. Obstruction in the carotid or ophthalmic artery or the CRA caused by thrombosis, embolus, or spasm may result in retinal ischemia secondary to reduction of pressure to the retinal circulation (23–24). A large series of patients with ischemic oculopathy at the Cleveland Clinic showed a significant correlation with ipsilateral carotid artery disease; however, a host of other pathologic conditions may be associated with such oculopathy (25).

An extensive review of chronic ocular ischemia by Carter (26) found that venous stasis retinopathy and ischemic oculopathy were less frequent manifestations of cerebrovascular disease than TMB was. However, they were readily recognizable and highly specific for major, often bilateral, carotid disease (26). These findings then may act as a warning and prompt the clinician to perform a vascular evaluation. Noninvasive vascular studies may show insufficient blood flow in the carotid system. Low retinal artery pressure is the most specific distinguishing feature. Because carotid stenoses are a hemodynamically significant problem, noninvasive studies such as OPG, Doppler ophthalmic tests, and other indirect studies are very reliable in indicating disease. In addition, Doppler ophthalmic tests may indicate a change in flow from the external carotid artery via the collaterals to the ophthalmic artery, with reversed ophthalmic artery flow secondary to stenosis or occlusions. This is opposed to emboli that may or may not originate from hemodynamically significant carotid lesions and, therefore, may not be readily evaluated by indirect, noninvasive measures. Significant carotid lesions should, however, be identified easily by the direct, noninvasive vascular studies of duplex Doppler scanning and spectral frequency analysis.

Noninvasive Methods

Although contrast angiography still is considered the best choice for evaluation of carotid artery disease, it has significant risks, costs, and discomfort. These considerations have led to a search for safe, widely applicable, easily repeatable, and accurate noninvasive methods of evaluating carotid artery disease.

The techniques used for noninvasive diagnosis are separated readily into indirect and direct. Indirect methods test for hemodynamic changes at some point removed from the site of involvement. More advanced lesions produce changes in pressure and flow, resulting in the development of collateral pathways that can be evaluated by indirect methods.

Indirect Noninvasive Tests

The ophthalmic artery is the first branch of the ICA, and obstructive lesions at the carotid bifurcation may produce pressure and flow changes in the orbital branches of the ophthamic artery and its periorbital ramifications. Indirect tests are the most common noninvasive techniques used today. They include Doppler ophthalmic examination, pressure OPG, pulse-delayed OPG, and thermography. Only the first two techniques are discussed here.

Doppler Ophthalmic Examination

Doppler ophthalmic examination as initially described by Brockenbrough (27) and modified by Barnes (28) uses a directional-sensing Doppler system to evaluate flow dynamics in the frontal or supraorbital branches of the ophthalmic artery. Reversed flow in the frontal artery indicates extracranial collateral flow in the presence of significant stenosis. Compression studies of selected branches of the external carotid artery may produce a decrease, obliteration, or reversal of flow in the medial frontal artery if the medial frontal artery is the source of collateral flow to the brain. Compression of the common carotid artery can confirm decreased or retrograde flow in the ophthalmic artery.

This method alone, however, is an unsuitable diagnostic test for the patient with focal symptoms, such as amaurosis fugax, because the periorbital Doppler examination relies on the hemodynamically significant change in ophthalmic flow and the subsequent development of collateral pathways. Nonobstructive carotid lesions would not be detectable by this method. The Doppler ophthalmic examination is 87% accurate in detecting hemodynamically significant lesions when this method is compared with angiography (60).

The greatest disadvantage of the periorbital Doppler examination is that it cannot differentiate between very high-grade stenosis and occlusion or location of the disease (ie, significant siphon disease *v* carotid disease). However, one of the major strengths is its versatility in direct evaluation of the external carotid artery as a major collateral to the eye.

Evidence for the clinical importance of external carotid collaterals as sources of embolization is derived from several studies and has been reviewed by Burnbaum et al (29). Their findings confirmed that in the presence of ICA occlusion, atheromatous disease of the external or common carotid arteries is a potential source for retinal emboli. Doppler ophthalmic examination can be very helpful in evaluating these collateral systems; however, direct evaluation of the external carotid artery by means of duplex Doppler scanning must be used to show nonhemodynamically significant stenosis of the external carotid artery.

Oculoplethysmography by Pressure Methods

Pressure OPG is performed essentially by measuring ocular blood pressure in much the way blood pressure conventionally is measured by using the brachial artery. In the technique developed by Gee (30,31), suction cups are placed on the sclerae of both eyes and held in place by negative pressure between 300 and 500 mm Hg. This pressure is sufficient to obliterate ocular pulsations, and the point at which they return as the vacuum is slowly reduced indicates the systolic pressure in the retinal artery. Comparisons are made of ocular pulse amplitudes bilaterally as well as of specific pressure differences. A difference of 5 mm Hg between the eyes is thought to indicate significant disease.

The OPG has a number of diagnostic limitations. The most notable is that it cannot be performed in the presence of ocular disease. The sensitivity of the technique is again a result of the hemodynamic collateral effects, and tests are not indicative of carotid pathology unless a lesion reduces the diameter of the ICA by 50% or more. Use of OPG to measure ophthalmic pressure directly can be very helpful in the evaluation of chronic ocular ischemic diseases that result in low retinal artery pressure. This method is most helpful when performed in conjunction with other direct methods, such as duplex Doppler scanning and spectral frequency analysis. The findings of OPG cannot be used to differentiate high-grade stenosis from complete occlusion or to determine where the problem lies (ie, ophthalmic or siphon disease). If OPG is performed in conjunction with direct methods, and no significant stenosis is found in the carotid artery, abnormal findings may indicate siphon disease or significant ophthalmic artery disease. Although siphon disease does not carry the same risk of stroke as TIAs and disease of the carotid bifurcation, a significant risk exists, as pointed out in a study on the natural history of isolated stenosis of the carotid siphon by Borozan et al (32).

Amaurosis fugax associated with stenosis of the ophthalmic artery can occur independent of any disease in the carotid artery (33). Gross et al (33) described local stenosis of the ophthalmic artery as a cause of falsely abnormal findings on OPG, and Weinberger et al (34) documented a significant stenosis at the origin of the ophthalmic artery in a patient with two episodes of amaurosis fugax. Reduced OAP was found on noninvasive testing of the carotid artery by OPG, and no lesion was evident in the carotid artery by cerebral angiography (34).

Pressure OPG is an accurate method for detection of high-grade lesions; however, the method cannot detect lesions that do not reduce flow, which may be the cause of emboli. The method also cannot differentiate between a high-grade stenosis and total occlusion, a finding of significant clinical importance.

Baker et al (35) compared pressure OPG in 227 patients who underwent arteriography. The overall accuracy was 93% when the lumen reduction was more than 60%. Blackshear (36) found 80% to 97% overall accuracy with the same lumen reduction. Eikelboom (37) reported results of 106 patients who had hemodynamically significant stenosis (greater than 65%) on angiograms and found a sensitivity of 89% and a specificity of 84%.

Direct, Noninvasive Tests

A number of reliable, direct, noninvasive tests are available, including velocity wave form analysis, carotid phonoangiography, phonoangiographic spectral analysis, continuous or pulse-wave ultrasonic arteriography, B-mode imaging, and ultrasonic duplex Doppler scanning. Although all the methods have been helpful in the direct, noninvasive evaluation of carotid artery disease, duplex Doppler scanning has been the most valuable in the direct evaluation in patients with amaurosis fugax.

Duplex Doppler Scanning

The combination of high-resolution B-mode imaging with Doppler flow analysis is a significant advancement in the noninvasive vascular carotid evaluation. The duplex system uses the physiologic information derived from Doppler examinations to evaluate blood velocities within the artery visualized and the two-dimensional imaging to define the walls of the vessels and evaluate plaque deposits.

This concept was first integrated into a duplex system by Barber et al (38,39). The original two-dimensional imaging of peripheral blood vessels was first performed by Olinger (40), who used a pulsed echo system. He noted important limitations of the systems. Total occlusion of the ICA appeared to be patent by B-mode imaging, and absorption characteristics of plaques varied widely, depending upon the absence or presence of calcifications. Because of these limitations, development of a duplex scanner that combined real-time B-mode imaging with Doppler sonography was undertaken. The duplex concept incorporates both anatomic and physiologic information, which were integrated into the duplex scanner system described by Barber et al (38,39). The B-mode instrument used highly sensitive components, specifically designed for near-field work, such as that required for carotid evaluation. Sonographic transducers usually use frequencies of either 5 to 10 MHz, and real-time imaging is used in all the available duplex systems. The Doppler components may be pulsed or continuous wave, or both, depending on the manufacturers.

Doppler signal processing varies widely between manufacturers; however, all modern duplex devices use fast Fourier transform (FFT) frequency spectral analysis for processing information from Doppler frequency shifts. In addition, many instruments also are able to measure the volume of blood flow, spectral broadening, and flow velocity.

A systematic evaluation of the patient is made with the patient supine. Blood vessels are identified by their characteristic B-mode images, and systematic studies of the common carotid, internal carotid, and external carotid arteries are done sequentially. Both longitudinal and transverse evaluation of each individual artery is undertaken. However, frequently, it is difficult to obtain satisfactory transverse scans of the internal and external carotid branches because of their location and because it is possible to image only those surfaces of a vessel that are essentially perpendicular to the emitting sound beam.

Experienced sonographers recognize a number of problems in B-mode scanning, particularly evaluation of atheromatous lesions in longitudinal sections. In a fair number of patients, the bifurcation of the common carotid artery is not seen in one plane, and it is necessary to reposition the transducer at the bifurcation and shift back and forth between the branches several times to identify the appropriate artery and to locate the atheromatous lesion (41). This can be further complicated when the carotid bifurcation is high in the neck where the field of view may be significantly restricted because of the mandible. Severe atherosclerotic lesions may interfere with imaging when shadowing from a plaque on the near wall of the vessel may obscure large portions of the artery and make them difficult to delineate. Transverse scans can be very helpful with these problems, particularly in identifying small plaques not otherwise seen on the longitudinal view.

A number of problems are encountered when the ICA is occluded. In this instance, one of the external carotid branches may be mistaken for the ICA. If the examination shows branches arising from this artery, then the results clearly distinguish the artery as the external carotid. Doppler sampling is, of course, necessary to help identify arteries properly. The high resistance signal in the external carotid artery is clearly distinguishable from the low-resistance, pulsatile features seen in the ICA. These differences in Doppler signals and the identification of branches are the most important method of distinguishing between the ICA and the external carotid artery (40). In addition, correspondence between gentle, rapid tapping of the superficial temporal artery and oscillation seen in the external carotid artery on the Doppler sample may be used (42). Doppler sampling should be done systematically throughout the common carotid, internal carotid, and external carotid arteries, and the frequency spectra should be recorded.

Certain normal imaging appearances of the extracranial arteries can be recognized by the sonographer. The common carotid artery has a uniform diameter until the bifurcation, where widening is usually significant. A circumscribed area of widening also occurs at the origin of the ICA. The arterial walls of the common internal and external carotid arteries are similar, with fairly uniform thicknesses of the vessel walls and the presence of echogenic lines along the luminal surfaces. The echogenic line has been studied histologically by Wolverson et al (43). It most probably arises from strong reflections at the intimal surface, but it does not specifically describe an anatomic structure other than probably the surface of the intima (43). The lumen of all the carotid vessels should be echo-free. Plaques generally can be distinguished from artifactual echos; plaques have synchronous pulsations with the arterial wall and usually are seen in one or more planes of investigation.

Generally, satisfactory images of the vessels in one plane are obtained in almost all the patients studied and in two planes in 65% to 70% of patients. B-mode imaging in itself is inadequate for measuring the severity of carotid obstruction. The hemodynamic status of the vessels evaluated by Doppler signals is more relevant than the anatomic measurements that can be made with B-mode visualization. Measurement of lumen narrowing can be made by transverse section, but the Doppler assessment is clearly the most accurate evaluation (41,44).

Analysis of audible signals has been performed for years by sonographers, and an experienced sonographer can recognize the different flow signals in the internal carotid and common carotid arteries and can identify increased velocity, turbulence, and other flow disturbances (42). However, these methods are subjective and require considerable experience. All modern duplex units now use the FFT spectral analysis for real-time study of the Doppler-shifted signals. Frequency spectrum analyzers usually display time on the X-axis (in seconds) and the Doppler frequency shift (represented in kHz or cm/s) on the X-axis. Blood flow away from the transducer usually is indicated in upward deflections and flow toward the transducer in deflections below the baseline. Amplitudes are expressed by shades of gray, which are related directly to the portion of blood cells moving at specific velocities during specific time. A normal Doppler spectrum, therefore, consists of systolic peak frequency and a narrow band of frequencies during systole resulting in a clear region beneath the systolic peak (window). Spectral changes occur with spectral broadening during the deceleration phase of systole with minimal stenosis, and further stenosis generally results in increased spectral broadening until the entire window beneath the systolic peak is filled, followed by an increase in peak systolic and diastolic frequencies. With significant turbulence, flow becomes distributed more uniformly across a wide range of frequencies, and with severe turbulence, flow may be concentrated at lower frequencies (45).

Doppler instruments may be either continuous wave or pulsed wave. Both methods have proponents, and both have advantages and disadvantages. The pulsed Doppler is range-gated such that Doppler shifts are recorded only from a specific location, allowing a small sample volume. A small sample volume directly in the center of the vessel may identify abnormal flow more accurately in that a wide variety of normal velocities occurs across the arterial lumen. Pulsed Doppler systems are limited, however, by the maximum frequency shift that can be recorded accurately. When this maximum is exceeded, a condition termed *aliasing* occurs (44).

Typical abnormalities in flow are found in areas of stenoses. Laminar flow is seen in normal vessels and in the prestenotic area. In areas of stenoses, velocities are increased, and as the stenotic jet reaches the poststenotic area, the flow stream spreads out rapidly, producing disturbed flow patterns with turbulence. These disturbances in flow have been evaluated in detail by Spencer (42). With severe lesions, poststenotic turbulence may cause arterial wall vibration with high-amplitude, low-frequency signals in the Doppler spectrum; a loss of definition of the upper border of the spectrum; bidirectional flow; and a bruitlike sound in the audible Doppler output. One or two centimeters beyond the stenosis this turbulence subsides; however, some spectral broadening continues, with a bubbling or fluttering quality to the audible signals. Laminar flow usually is reestablished within 3 cm of the stenosis; however, this is variable. The relationship of velocity, Doppler frequency shift, lumen narrowing, and flow has been evaluated by Spencer (Fig. 15-1). As the lumen is reduced, flow velocity must increase for the same volume of blood to transverse the narrowed segment. Increases in stenotic velocity do not continue to

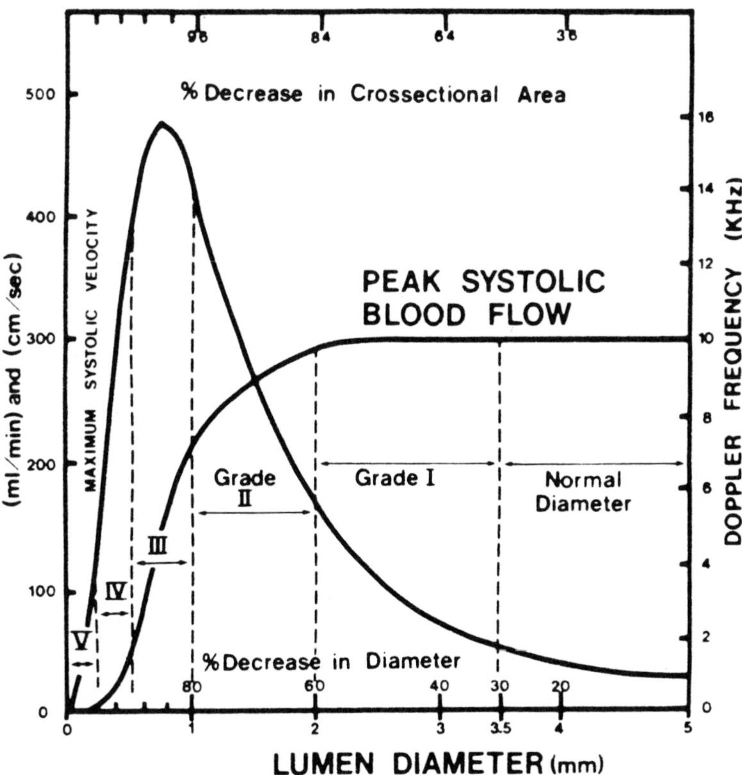

FIGURE 15–1. Relationship of velocity, Doppler frequency shift, lumen narrowing, and flow. [From Spencer MP, 1981 (42). Reprinted with permission of the publisher.]

the point of occlusion. Peak systolic velocities occur with a lumen of 1 to 1.5 mm in diameter, and as stenoses progress beyond this point, velocity falls off rapidly. A 50% reduction in diameter corresponds to a reduction in area of 75%, and reduction of blood flow remains stable until the reduction in diameter approaches 60%. Beyond this level of obstruction, flow decreases precipitiously. As the diameter of the lumen decreases, flow velocity and Doppler-shifted frequency rise inversely, and peak velocities occur at approximately the point at which flow begins to fall off.

It should be remembered that velocities in stenotic zones are influenced by blood pressure, cardiac output, arterial compliance, peripheral resistance, and the presence of significant contralateral carotid obstruction. Because of these influences, a number of methods have been devised to evaluate peak stenotic velocity shifts. Spencer and Reid (46) and Ritgers et al (47) found that comparing internal-to-internal peak systolic velocity ratios increased accuracy. Whereas Blackshear et al (48) used internal carotid stenotic zone to common carotid ratios, other ratios also have been reported (44).

As useful as Doppler techniques are, they may not be useful for detecting nonstenotic carotid disease that does not produce flow effects (48). The coupling with B-mode imaging, however, permits evaluation of nonstenotic plaque.

Plaque Identification

It is generally accepted that ulcerated plaque is the underlying cause for most TIAs and, specifically, amaurosis fugax (17,49,50). The exact sequence of events leading to the ischemia are unclear, but emboli of fibrin, atheromatous debris, and cholesterol crystals may be released from these ulcerated areas. If so, it would be advantageous to detect such ulcerated lesions by noninvasive methods. Traditionally duplex Doppler scanning has been used principally to identify obstructed lesions, but more recently, the interest has turned toward characterization of the appearance and composition of plaque.

Javid (51,52) has identified three specific types of atherosclerotic plaque formation. Type I is the fatty streak that appears to be of no clinical significance. These plaques that contain a large amount of lipid material are the least echogenic type of plaque and may be difficult to identify sonographically. Type II, the fibrous plaque, is atherosclerotic plaque extending into the vessel lumen that may or may not cause flow abnormalities. Uniformly, fibrous plaque is homogeneous in echogenicity; however, large focal deposits of lipid material or thrombus may be seen. Thrombus deposition on plaque surfaces or in the lumen is of considerable interest because of the hazard of embolization. However, the ability to recognize a thrombus within the vascular lumen is extremely difficult and the thrombus often is missed. Type III plaque is a complicated plaque with endothelial ulceration, mural hemorrhage, necrosis, and calcification. High-resolution imaging is very sensitive for detection of calcifications, and small areas may be detected. Large areas of calcific deposits may obscure the other atheromatous areas and part of the wall of the vessel because of shadowing and also may prevent adequate evaluation of flow.

All three types of plaque can be identified by using B-mode carotid imaging and have been reported in detail by Wolverson et al (43) and Lusby et al (53). Lusby et al found that the presence of intraplaque hemorrhage correlated strongly with plaque surface denudation and platelet deposition. They implied that intraplaque hemorrhage with resultant thrombus accumulation damages the overlying intimal surface and subsequently results in adherence of platelets or ulcerations or both. Thus, complicated plaque that contains hemorrhage, calcification, and lipid deposit is thought to be more frequently symptomatic and dangerous than noncomplicated fibrofatty plaque. Therefore, the identification of these types of plaque may have important clinical implications. Although this is an exciting new field of development, many authors including Wolverson et al (43), Zwiebel (41), and Thiele and Strandness (54) have warned against the diagnosis of ulceration by real-time imaging and the use of this information as a basis for clinical decisions.

At this time, the accuracy of ulcer detection is unimpressive. At some time in the future, when three-dimensional images are available for full evaluation of surface characteristics, this probably will be plausible. Until then, the designation of plaque as smooth or irregular should be the only indicator.

Transcranial Doppler Examination

An exciting new technique has been developed during the last several years for the direct evaluation of the intracranial vessels. It is now possible, by using a 2-MHz probe that allows sufficient penetration of bone, to directly examine the intracranial arteries. Three pathways of evaluation of the intracranial vessels have been used: transtemporal, transforamen magnum, and transorbital. Of particular pertinence to the evaluation of amaurosis fugax is the transorbital evaluation, which allows direct examination of the ophthalmic artery and the carotid siphon, potential sources of amaurosis fugax. This method most recently was described by Spencer and Whisler (55), who delineated the examination techniques, the methods for diagnosing intracranial arterial stenosis, and evaluation of the intracranial collaterals.

The patient is examined by placing a 2-MHz probe over the closed eyelid and directing the sound beam intracranially through the eye and the posterior orbit. Both the superior orbital fissure and the optic canal provide pathways to the parasellar and supraclinoid intracranial ICA. The entire course of the intracranial ICA can be examined through the orbit along with direct examination of the ophthalmic artery. The Doppler criteria for detecting stenosis intracranially are similar to those used extracranially. These include increased peak frequency and prominent systolic low-frequency energies with symmetrical representation above and below the baseline. Transcranial Doppler examination allows direct evaluation of siphon lesions, often a problem when tandem lesions are present in both the carotid and the siphon. Eventually, determination of the specific hemodynamic significance of each lesion and monitoring of the progression or regression of siphon stenosis may be possible by means of transcranial Doppler examinations. The transorbital approach adds to the information obtained from the extracranial duplex Doppler examination and is a promising way of evaluating ophthalmic artery occlusion, stenosis, or vasospasm. The full potential of these new transcranial approaches should be achieved in the next several years and will be specifically pertinent to the evaluation of amaurosis fugax.

Summary

With the accepted heterogenicity of the symptom amaurosis fugax, it has become clear that a variety of noninvasive techniques are necessary to evaluate this potentially serious vascular problem. Most physicians agree that true amaurosis fugax is an indication for angiography; however, the ability to separate true amaurosis fugax from other causes of transient orbital blindness is not precise. Thus, evaluation of these patients by means of noninvasive methods is appropriate.

Other than carotid stenosis, a number of entities that are known causes of amaurosis fugax can be diagnosed by using noninvasive studies. With improved duplex Doppler scanning, fibromuscular dysplasia; truncal lesions, such as in Takayasu's disease; and loops and coils in the ICA readily can be recognized. Innominate steal, an uncommon cause of amaurosis fugax, also can be identified. Moyamoya disease is now identifiable by transcranial Doppler studies, and retinal artery spasms, such as in Raynaud's disease and migraine, also can be evaluated by using transcranial methods. Even mitral valve disease as a source of emboli in amaurosis fugax can be suspected on the basis of the findings of noninvasive carotid studies. Amaurosis fugax occurs in a high percentage of patients with chronic rheumatic heart disease, and mitral valve prolapse reportedly has been associated as well. Weinberger and Goldman (56) have noted an abnormal pattern of carotid Doppler ultrasound frequency shift and an early systolic flutter in patients with normal carotid bifurcations and mitral disease. Although this method is not recommended for specific evaluation of heart disease, these findings can suggest the possibility of mitral disease, and the patient can be referred for specific tests such as echocardiography.

New developments and refinement of duplex Doppler scanning and the addition of color-coded Doppler images may further knowledge about and accuracy of flow dynamics and plaque identification in the near future.

Noninvasive Laboratory Findings in Patients with Visual Disturbances

Transient visual loss due to cerebral ocular vascular disease is a common symptom. However, because of the lack of uniform terminology regarding this heterogeneic symptom, investigation and management become difficult. Several authors have attempted systematically to clarify the terminology.

Hedges, in a report in 1984 (57), suggested that these symptoms be separated into two major headings: (1) transient blurred vision as an overall designation, and (2) TMB, which would be divided into amaurosis fugax, transient monocular blurring (more prolonged), and transient binocular blindness.

More recently, Gaul et al (58) have separated their patients with visual symptoms into 12 groups to investigate the relationship between visual disturbance and atherosclerotic plaque. They reviewed 500 consecutive records of patients with visual disturbances not related to ophthalmic pathology who were referred to the noninvasive vascular laboratory over a 3-year period. They found a strikingly high prevalence of carotid artery disease. Of the 500 patients studied, 386 (77.2%) had evidence of atherosclerotic plaque at the carotid bifurcation. They compared this to unselected autopsy series of Fisher et al (59), who reported an overall prevalence of 39.3% of disease at the carotid bifurcation, and to the findings

TABLE 15–1. Visual symptoms and carotid disease.

Classification per Gaul et al (59)	No. of patients	Total ipsilateral lesions (%)	Ipsilateral hemodynamic lesion (%)	Bilateral lesion (%)
1 Amaurosis fugax	141	75.5	33.0	69.0
2a Blurred vision, unilateral	42	59.0	29.0	56.9
2b Blurred vision, bilateral	48	62.8	25.1	52.3
3a Positive symptoms, unilateral	15	54.2	10.1	63.0
3b Positive symptoms, bilateral	9	78.1	5.0	29.9
4a Gradual visual loss, unilateral	4	68.9	9.0	49.0
4b Gradual visual loss, bilateral	0	0	0	0
5a Permanent total visual loss, unilateral	16	89.2	25.9	79.8
5b Permanent total visual loss, bilateral	1	100.0	100.0	100.0
6a Permanent partial field visual loss, unilateral	30	64.5	5.2	63.9
6b Permanent partial field visual loss, bilateral	10	75.2	4.9	43.0
7 Transient visual loss, bilateral	76	75.4	25.0	79.0
8 Ischemic retinopathy	20	18.0	9.2	73.4
9 Two visual symptoms	25	82.5	19.2	53.2
Total	437	74.3		

of Kollarits et al (17), who used carotid angiograms to evaluate patients over 60 years of age and found a prevalence of carotid atheromatas of only 24%.

By separating their cases into specific categories dependent on the patient's visual symptoms, Gaul et al (58) were able to make several important observations. They found that 114 people (22.8%) in the series had completely normal findings on noninvasive carotid studies. Therefore, a significant percentage of the population remains, especially the younger age group, in whom visual disturbance is not due to disease at the carotid bifurcation. They concluded that noninvasive carotid testing by means of B-mode imaging in conjunction with spectral analysis of the Doppler-shifted signals and OPG provides appropriate methods for evaluation of carotid artery bifurcation disease in patients with visual symptoms.

Using the classification of Gaul et al (58), we compared our results with theirs. We examined the records of 437 patients seen in the vascular laboratory between 1982 and 1986. Our results, summarized in Table 15–1, are similar to those reported by Gaul et al.

References

1. Eisenberg RL, Nemzek WR, Moore WS, et al: Relationship of transient ischemic attacks and angiographically demonstrable lesions of carotid artery. *Stroke* 1977;8:483–486.
2. Horenstein S, Hambrook G, Roat GW, et al: Arteriographic correlates of transient ischemic attacks. *Trans Am Neurol Assoc* 1972;97:132–136.
3. Janeway R, Toole JF: Vascular anatomic status of patients with transient ischemic attacks. *Trans Am Neurol Assoc* 1971;97:137–141.
4. Pessin MS, Duncan GW, Mohr JP, et al: Clinical and angiographic features of carotid transient ischemic attacks. *N Engl J Med* 1977;296:358–362.
5. Ramirez-Lassepas M, Sandok BA, Burton RC: Clinical indicators of extracranial carotid artery disease in patients with transient symptoms. *Stroke* 1973;4:537–540.
6. Barnett HJM, Stein BM, Yatsu FM, et al: *Stroke: Pathophysiology, Diagnosis and Management*. New York, Churchill Livingstone, 1986, vol 1.
7. Marshall J, Meadows S: The natural history of amaurosis fugax. *Brain* 1968;91:419–434.
8. Morax PV, Aron-Rosa D, Gautier JC: Symptoms et signes ophthalmologiques des stenoses et occlusions cartidiennes. *Bull Soc Ophthalmol Fr* 1970 suppl 1, p 169.
9. Ross Russell R: *Vascular Disease of the Cerebral Nervous System*. London, Churchill Livingstone, 1983.
10. Hunt JR: The role of the carotid arteries in the causation of vascular lesions of the brain with remarks on certain special features of the symptomatology. *Am J Med Sci* 1914;147:704–713.
11. Fisher M: Transient monocular blindness associated with hemiplegia. *Arch Ophthalmol* 1952;47:167–203.
12. Fisher CM: Occlusion of the carotid arteries. *Arch Neurol Psychiatry* 1954;72:187–204.

13. Fisher CM: Observations of the fundus oculi in transient monocular blindness. *Neurology* 1959;9:333–347.
14. Millikan CH: Siekert RG, Shick RM: Studies in cerebrovascular disease: V. The use of anticoagulant drugs in the treatment of intermittent insufficiency of the internal carotid arterial system. *Proc Mayo Clin* 1955;30:578–586.
15. Hollenhorst RW: Significance of bright plaques in the retinal arterioles. *JAMA* 1961;178:23–29.
16. Ehrenfeld WK, Hoyt WF, Wylie EJ: Embolization and transient blindness from carotid atheroma. *Arch Surg* 1966;93:787–794.
17. Kollarits CR, Lubow M, Hissong SL: Retinal strokes: I. Incidence of carotid atheromata. *JAMA* 1972;222:1273–1275.
18. Thiele BL, Young JV, Chikos PM, et al: Correlation of arteriographic findings and symptoms in cerebrovascular disease. *Neurology* 1980;30:1041–1046.
19. Futty DE, Conneally PM, Dyken ML, et al: Cooperative study of hospital frequency and character of transient ischemic attacks: V. Symptom analysis. *JAMA* 1977;238:2386–2390.
20. Zukowski AJ, Nicolaides AN, Lewis RT, et al: The correlation between carotid plaque ulceration and cerebral infarction seen on CT scan. *J Vasc Surg* 1984;1:782–786.
21. Sheng FC, Quinones-Baldrich W, Machleder HI, et al: Relationship of extracranial carotid occlusive disease and central retinal artery occlusion. *Am J Surg* 1986;152:175–178.
22. Adams HP, Putman SF, Corbett JJ, et al: Amaurosis fugax: The results of arteriography in 59 patients. *Stroke* 14:5, 1983;14:742–744.
23. Toole JF: *Cerebrovascular Disorders,* ed 3. New York, Raven Press, 1984.
24. Hershey F et al: Noninvasive diagnosis of vascular disease. Pasadena, Calif, Appleton Davies Inc, 1984.
25. Tomsak RL, Hanson M, Gutman FA: Carotid artery disease and central retinal artery occlusion. *Cleve Clin Q* 1979;46:7–11.
26. Carter JE: Chronic ocular ischemia and carotid vascular disease. *Stroke* 1985;16:721–728.
27. Brokenbrough EC: Screening for the prevention of stroke: Use of a Doppler flowmeter, product brochure. Beaverton, Ore, Parks Electronics, 1970.
28. Barnes RW, Russell HE, Bone GE, et al: Doppler cerebrovascular examination: Improved results with refinements in technique. *Stroke* 1977;8:468–471.
29. Burnbaum MD, Selhorst JB, Harbison JW, et al: Amaurosis fugax from disease of the external carotid artery. *Arch Neurol* 1977;34:532–535.
30. Gee W, Oller DW, Wylie EJ: Noninvasive diagnosis of carotid occlusion by ocular pneumoplethysmography. *Stroke* 1976;7:18–21.
31. Gee W: Ocular plethysmography, in Bernstein EF (ed): *Noninvasive Diagnostic Techniques in Vascular Disease,* ed 2. St Louis, The CV Mosby Co, 1982, pp 220–230.
32. Borozan PG, Schuler JJ, Larosa MP, et al: The natural history of isolated carotid siphon stenosis. *J Vasc Surg* 1984;1:744–749.
33. Gross WS, Verta MJ, VanBellen B, et al: Comparison of noninvasive diagnostic techniques in carotid artery occlusive disease. *Surgery* 1977;82:271–278.
34. Weinberger J, Bender AN, Yang WC: Amaurosis fugax associated with ophthalmic artery stenosis: clinical stimulation of carotid artery disease. *Stroke* 1980;11:290–293.

35. Baker JD, Barker WF, Machleder HI: Ocular pneumoplethysmography in the evaluation of carotid stenosis. *Circulation* 1980;62(suppl 1):1–3.
36. Blackshear WM Jr: Comparative review of OPG-K-M, OPG-G, and pulsed Doppler ultrasound for carotid evaluation. *Vasc Diag Ther,* November 1980, pp 43–51.
37. Eikelboom BC: Ocular pneumoplethysmography, in Bernstein EF (ed): *Noninvasive Diagnostic Techniques in Vascular Disease,* ed 3. St Louis, The CV Mosby Co, 1985, pp 330–334.
38. Barber FE, Baker DW, Nation AWC, et al: Ultrasonic duplex echo-Doppler scanner. *IEEE Trans. Biomed Eng* 1974;21:109.
39. Barber FE, Baker DW, Strandness DE Jr, et al: Duplex scanner II: For simultaneous imaging of artery tissues and flow. Ultrasonic Symposium Proceedings, IEEE Cat. — 74 CHO 896 ISU, 1974.
40. Olinger CP: Ultrasonic carotid echoarteriogrqaphy. *Am J Roentgenal Rad Ther Med* 106: 282, 1969;106:282–295.
41. Zwiebel W: Duplex carotid sonography, in *Introduction to Vascular Ultrasonography,* ed 2. Orlando, Fla, Grune & Stratton Inc, 1986, pp 139–170.
42. Spencer MP: Technique of Doppler examination, in Spencer MP, Reid JM (eds): *Cerebrovascular Evaluation with Doppler Ultrasound.* The Hague, Martinus Nijoff Publishers, 1981, pp
43. Wolverson MK, Bashiti HM, Peter GJ: Ultrasonic tissue characterization of atheromatous plaques using a high-resolution real-time scanner. *Ultrasound Med Biol* 1983;6:669–709.
44. Breslau P: Current status of ultrasonic techniques, in *Ultrasonic Duplex Scanning in the Classification of Carotid Artery Disease.* Heerlen, 1981
45. Hutchison KJ, Thiele BL, Green FM, et al: Detection of disturbed flow by computer processing of pulsed Doppler spectra, in Stevens A (ed): *Theory and Practices of Blood Flow Measurement.* 1982
46. Spencer MP, Reid JM: Quantitation of carotid stenosis with continuous-wave (CW) Doppler ultrasound. *Stroke* 1979;3:326–330.
47. Rittgers SE, Thornhill BM, Barnes RW: Quantitative analysis of carotid artery Doppler spectral waveforms: Diagnostic value of parameters. *Ultrasound Med Biol* 1983;3:225–264.
48. Blackshear WM, Phillips DJ, Chikos PM, et al: Carotid artery velocity patterns in normal and stenotic vessels. *Stroke* 1980;1:67–71.
49. Moore WS, Hall AD: Importance of emboli from carotid bifurcation in pathogenesis of cerebral ischemic attacks. *Arch Surg* 1970;101:708–716.
50. Moore WS, Boren C, Malone JM, et al: Natural history of nonstenotic asymptomatic ulcerative lesions of the carotid artery. *Arch Surg* 1978;113:1352–1359.
51. Javid H: Development of carotid plaque. *Am J Surg* 1979;138:224.
52. Javid H, Ostermiller WE, Hengesh JW, et al: Natural history of carotid bifurcation atheroma. *Surgery* 1970;67:80–86.
53. Lusby RJ, Ferrell LD, Ehrenfeld WK, et al: Carotid plaque hemorrhage. *Arch Surg* 1982;117:1479–1488.
54. Thiele BL, Strandness DE Jr: Distribution of intracranial and extracranial arterial lesions in patients with symptomatic cerebrovascular disease, in EF Bernstein (ed): *Noninvasive Diagnostic Techniques in Vascular Disease* St Louis, The CV Mosby Co, 1985, pp 316–322.
55. Spencer M, Whisler D: Transorbital Doppler diagnosis of ultracranial arterial stenosis. *Stroke* 17:5, 1986;17:916–920.

56. Weinberger J, Goldman M: Detection of mitral valve abnormalities by carotid Doppler flow study: Implications for the management of patients with cerebrovascular disease. *Stroke* 1985;16:977–980.
57. Hedges TR: The terminology of transient visual loss due to vascular insufficiency. *Stroke* 1984;15:907–908.
58. Gaul J, Marks S, Weinberger J: Visual disturbance and carotid artery disease: 500 symptomatic patients studied by noninvasive carotid artery testing including B-mode ultrasonography. *Stroke* 1986;17:393–398.
59. Fisher CM, Gore I, Okabe N, et al: Atherosclerosis of the carotid and vertebral arteries - extracranial and intracranial. *J Neuropathol Exp Neurol* 1965;24:455–476.
60. Brockenmough EC: Periorbital Doppler Velocity evaluation of Carotid Obstruction, in EF Bernstein (ed): *Noninvasive Diagnostic Techniques in Vascular Disease*. St. Louis, The CV Mosby Co, 1985, pp 335–342.

CHAPTER 16

Data from CT Scans: The Significance of Silent Cerebral Infarction and Atrophy

A.N. Nicolaides, K. Papadakis, M. Grigg, A. Al-Kutoubi, M.A. Williams, and D.F.S. Deacon

The detection of retinal emboli with the ophthalmoscope, whether shiny orange-yellow cholesterol crystals (1,2), or gray-white material consisting of platelets and fibrin (3,4), in patients with amaurosis fugax is well established. The association of this symptom with ICA stenosis and plaque ulceration (5) means that in clinical practice amaurosis fugax indicates an ulcerated atheromatous plaque of the ICA until proved otherwise (6).

Amaurosis fugax is the result of transient retinal ischemia, and, as such, it has been thought to be comparable to hemispheric TIAs. The latter are often the result of microemboli from ulcerated atheromatous carotid plaques (5,7,8), although both amaurosis fugax and hemispheric TIAs can occur as a result of hypoperfusion often precipitated by hypotension (eg, from cardiac arrhythmias in patients with severe internal carotid stenotic plaques without ulceration or in patients with carotid occlusion). Such patients have been shown by studies with radioactive xenon to have low cerebral perfusion and no reactivity to CO_2 inhalation (9), indicating the presence of maximum cerebral vascular dilatation and no reserve.

A high prevalence of "silent" cerebral infarction has been detected by CT scanning in studies performed since 1976 in patients with hemispheric TIAs (Table 16–1). These findings suggest that the new generation of high-resolution CT scanning equipment could be used to further knowledge and understanding of the pathophysiology of amaurosis fugax and TIAs, particularly their association with extracranial cerebrovascular disease. CT brain scans may provide information of equal or greater importance to that provided in the past by retinal inspection by means of the ophthalmoscope.

A search of the literature has provided little information about findings on CT scans in patients with amaurosis fugax, although the number of publications on findings in patients with TIAs and stroke is relatively large (Tables 16–1 to 16–3).

The purpose of this chapter is to present the available data from CT scans in patients with amaurosis fugax in relation to other cerebrovascular syndromes. In view of the uncertainty about the value of CT scans and the significance of silent infarcts, this is done after a review of the relevant literature.

Prevalence of Cerebral Infarction

Shortly after the introduction of CT scanning in 1973, it became obvious that this was the method of choice for detecting and localizing intracerebral hemorrhages (11,31). However, its place in the investigation of ischemic cerebrovascular disease has remained uncertain. In the early days, CT brain scans in patients with TIAs were nearly always normal (11,32), and, in general, it was not considered to be warranted as a routine investigation (33). This was aptly summarised by McDowell (6) in 1980:

> Computerised brain scanning is rarely useful in the study of patients with transient ischemic attacks. It may however, identify unsuspected intracerebral lesions, such as a tumor, intracerebral hematoma, or subdural hematoma, prior to the use of cerebral angiography. In the classic patient with transient cerebral ischemia, the CT scan should be normal, as by definition, transient cerebral ischemia should leave no detectable clinical residue. CT scan is largely useful in screening patients where the diagnosis of transient ischemia is unclear or differential diagnosis uncertain. In these instances, it can be helpful in eliminating the possibilities of other causative and treatable conditions.

Use of second-generation equipment with its higher resolution has indicated a relatively high prevalence of silent cerebral infarction in patients with TIAs, not only in the symptomatic but also in the asymptomatic hemisphere, and has led to the realization that the clinical symptomatology and the actual anatomic pathology shown on CT scans are not always correlated. The prevalence was higher in patients with reversible ischemic neurologic deficits (RINDs), partially reversible ischemic neurologic deficits (PRINDs), and stroke (Tables 16–1 to 16–3). However, even in patients with a completed stroke, the rate of detection was not 100%. It varied from 58% to 95% (ie, no infarction was found in 5% to 42%, Table 16–3). More recently, studies have indicated a high prevalence (23% to 43%) of silent cerebral infarctions on CT scans of patients with vertebrobasilar (VB) TIAs or amaurosis fugax (Table 16–2). Even in asymptomatic patients with cervical bruit or internal carotid stenosis, a prevalence as high as 21% has been reported (Table 16–2).

The finding of hypodense lesions on CT scans in patients with TIAs who had no a history of stroke and had normal findings on neurologic examinations has prompted some authors to suggest the term "cerebral infarction with transient signs" to differentiate this condition from TIAs that, in their opinion, should be diagnosed only in the absence of abnormalities on CT scans (34). Caplan (35) suggested that the terms TIA, RIND, and cerebrovascular accident (CVA) either be discarded completely or deemphasized. Recently Vollmar and his colleagues (36) proposed that

TABLE 16–1. Prevalence of cerebral infarction on CT Scans in patients with hemispheric TIAs with or without amaurosis fugax.

Study	Year	Prevalence of cerebral infarction (%)			Comments
		Patients	Symptomatic hemisphere	Asymptomatic hemisphere	
Caille et al (10)	1976	10	10	0	10 patients
Kinkel and Jacobs (11)	1976	0	0	0	30 patients
Constant et al (12)	1977	12	—	—	16 patients
Laporte et al (13)	1978	0	0	0	22 patients
Perrone et al (14)	1979	34	—	—	35 patients. ⅓ had VB TIAs and ⅔ had hemispheric TIAs.
Ladurner et al (15)	1979	18	—	—	44 patients
Allen and Preziosi (16)	1981	12	12	—	52 patients
Buell et al (17)	1981	17	17	—	95 patients. Computer-assisted radionuclide angiography revealed a hemispherical perfusion "defect" in 75% of patients.
Houser et al (18)	1982	28	14	14	—
Biller at al (19)	1982	4	2	2	45 patients with carotid TIAs
Goldenberg and Reisner (20)	1983	20	—	—	18 patients
Graber et al (21)	1984	18	—	—	79 patients
Calandre et al (22)	1984	25	—	—	88 patients with TIAs (67 hemispheric and 21 vertebrobasilar). Patients with amaurosis fugax were excluded.

Zukowski et al (5)	1984	63	—	—	36 patients with TIAs and >50% stenosis of ICA. In 26 of 36 patients, a macroscopic ulcer was present on the carotid endarterectomy specimen.
Tsementzis et al (23)	1984	70	—	—	20 patients. Emission tomography showed infarction in 95% of patients.
Ricotta et al (24)	1985	12	—	—	76 patients
Weisberg (25)	1986	18	18	—	100 patients. Scan was considered abnormal if lesion corresponded to symptoms.
Awad et al (26)	1986	32	18	13	17 patients with hemispheric and 5 patients with VB TIAs. 77% prevalence of infarction on MRI
Irvine Laboratory	1986	48	35	27	149 patients with hemispheric TIAs only (no amaurosis fugax)

CT = computed tomography; TIA = transient ischemic attack; VB-TIA = vertebrobasilar TIA; ICA = internal carotid artery; MRI = magnetic resonance imaging; dashes = no information available or not done.

TABLE 16–2. Prevalence of cerebral infarction on CT scans in patients with asymptomatic internal carotid stenosis, amaurosis fugax only (no TIAs) and VB-TIAs.

Study	Year	Prevalence %	Comments
Amaurosis fugax only (no hemispheric TIAs)			
Zukowski et al (5)	1984	23	13 patients (10 with and 3 without ulceration on carotid endarterectomy specimen)
Irvine Laboratory	1986	43	70 patients with amaurosis fugax only
Asymptomatic internal carotid stenosis			
Zukowski et al (5)	1984	8	13 patients with >50% stenosis of the ICA. Ulceration of the carotid endarterectomy specimen was present in 4 patients
Ricotta et al (24)	1985	21	24 patients
Asymptomatic cervical bruit and/or VB-TIAs			
Irvine Laboratory	1986	28	183 patients with VB-TIAs or with asymptomatic cervical bruit (no hemispheric TIAs or amaurosis fugax)
Awad et al (26)	1986	40	5 patients with VB-TIAs

CT = computed tomography; TIA = transient ischemic attack; VB-TIA = vertebrobasilar TIA; ICA = internal carotid artery.

TABLE 16–3. Prevalence of cerebral infarction on CT scans in patients with stroke (RIND, PRIND, and stroke with minimum or no recovery).

Study	Year	Prevalence %	Comments
RIND			
Perrone et al (14)	1979	60	15 patients
Goldenberg and Reisner (20)	1983	42	36 patients
Calandre et al (22)	1984	25	46 patients with RINDs (41 hemispheric and 5 vertebrobasilar)
Ricotta et al (24)	1985	55	9 patients
PRIND			
Ladurner et al (15)	1979	76	50 patients
Buell et al (17)	1981	64	59 patients (computer-assisted radionuclide angiography showed a hemispheric perfusion "defect" in 79% of patients)
Irvine Laboratory	1986	71	129 patients (major and minor strokes in the form of RIND and PRIND)
STROKE (variable or minimum recovery)			
Campbell et al (27)	1978	66	141 patients
Ladurner et al (15)	1979	95	151 patients
Buell et al (28)	1979	95	159 patients
Bradac and Oberson (29)	1980	85	200 patients (60% with major stroke and 40% with minor stroke in the form of RIND and PRIND)
Houser et al (18)	1982	78	108 patients
Oxfordshire Community Stroke Project (30)	1983	58	126 patients
Goldenberg and Reisner (20)	1983	79	119 patients
Calandre et al (22)	1984	35	79 patients
Tsementzis et al (23)	1984	81	52 patients (emission tomography showed infarction in 92%)
Ricotta et al (24)	1985	64	45 patients

CT = computed tomography; RIND = reversible ischemic neurologic deficit; PRIND = partially reversible ischemic neurologic deficit.

TABLE 16–4. Classification system for patients with cerebrovascular disease proposed by Vollmar et al (36).

Clinical findings Results of CT scan	TIA	RIND	CVA
Normal	–	–	–
Cerebral infarction	+	+	+

CT = computed tomography; TIA = transient ischemic attack; RIND = reversible ischemic neurologic deficit; CVA = cerebrovascular accident.

patients should be categorized on the basis of their clinical presentation and CT findings (Table 16–4) and that evaluation and stratification of patients in clinical trials should be based not only on the clinical presentation but also on the anatomic and pathophysiologic sequelae. The following explanation about the pathogenesis of TIAs and silent infarction has been offered: The symptoms and signs of TIAs could be from ischemia at the periphery of an infarction for which recovery is quick because of collateral blood supply. However, the explanation of silent infarcts in the absence of TIAs or in areas of the brain not corresponding to the TIA symptoms is more difficult. One possibility is that some infarcts occur in silent areas and some TIAs with infarction in appropriate areas may occur during the patient's sleep and remain unnoticed. After all, strokes do occur during sleep only to be detected on waking up.

It is now realized that many infarcts are isodense and not visible. Contrast enhancement will increase the prevalence by 5% to 10% by revealing some isodense infarcts (37,38). Other isodense lesions may be identified by computer-assisted radionuclide angiography or MRI, as indicated by studies in which both CT scanning and one of these techniques were performed in the same patients (Table 16–5). The available data now indicate that only a portion of cerebral infarcts, whether silent or not, are shown on CT scans.

Factors Affecting Prevalence

The various factors that affect the prevalence of infarction seen on CT scans are the resolution of the equipment, the time the scan is performed in relation to the onset of symptoms, whether contrast enhancement has been used, the size of the infarct, the patients' symptomatology, the presence and severity of associated atherosclerotic carotid disease, and the presence of ulceration on the carotid plaque. The effect of each one of these is summarised in the following sections.

TABLE 16–5. Prevalence of cerebral infarction in patients who had CT scans and computer-assisted radionuclide angiography or emission tomography or MRI.

Presentation	Study	Year	Cerebral infarction on CT scan (%)	Cerebral infarction on other investigations (%)	No. of patients
TIAs	Buell et al (17)	1981	17	75 (computer-assisted radionuclide angiograhy)	95
TIAs	Tsementzis et al (23)	1984	70	95 (emission tomography)	20
TIAs	Awad et al (26)	1986	32	77 (MRI)	17 with hemispheric and 5 with VB-TIAs
PRIND	Buell et al (17)	1981	64	79 (computer-assisted radionuclide angiography)	59
Stroke	Tsementzis et al (23)	1984	81	92 (emission tomography)	52

CT = computed tomography; MRI = magnetic resonance imaging; TIA = transient ischemic attack; VB-TIA = vertebrobasilar TIA; PRIND = partially reversible ischemic neurologic deficit.

Resolution of the Equipment

As mentioned before, the first generation of CT scanning equipment could detect a very small number of infarcts in patients with TIAs, but as the resolution improved, the prevalence of silent infarction increased. This occurred because the majority of infarcts in patients with TIAs are small. Current CT scanning equipment can detect infarcts 2 to 5 mm in diameter (22). Calandre et al (22) found that deep infarcts were smaller than superficial ones in all three groups of patients (TIAs, RIND, or stroke with minimum recovery), and it follows that increased resolution should be associated with a higher rate of detection of deep infarcts.

Time of Scan

Knowledge of the appearance of ischemic infarcts on CT scans and the changes that occur in time is based on serial studies of patients with clinically ischemic strokes. Initially (hours to days) the infarct is isodense and does not show on the CT scan unless an associated hemorrhage (hemorrhagic infarct) is present. This phenomenon occurs in 5% to 10% of cases. In the majority of cases, the earliest CT evidence of an infarct is a focal, poorly circumscribed, slightly hypodense zone (39,40). For this reason, infarcts visualized within the first 12 hours after the onset of symptoms are large and are the result of occlusion of major cerebral vessels. As edema increases during the third to fourth days, so does the hypodensity, making the lesion more obvious and more clearly delineated (18). After 7 to 10 days the hypodensity decreases, and a decrease in edema makes the lesion less obvious (27). Indeed, some infarcts may disappear temporarily or permanently (18). However, in the majority of the infarcts, the hypodensity continues to decrease. Within a month it may be the same as that of cerebrospinal fluid (CSF) and thus appear cystic. In patients with large infarcts, the shrinkage of infarcted brain often is associated with focal enlargement of the adjacent CSF spaces (18). If the scan is performed within three to six hours from the onset of clinical ischemic strokes, not more than 50% will be imaged (37). By the seventh day, more than 75% can be imaged, and with serial scanning the rate increases to more than 90% (18).

Use of Contrast Enhancement

Administration of IV contrast medium will result in the accumulation of iodide in the infarct or part of the infarct. Several mechanisms account for this accumulation and subsequent enhancement of the image, including hypervascularization or breakdown of the blood-brain barrier (18,21,23,38). The pattern and extent of this enhancement depend on the age of the lesion. However, the prevalence is related to both the age of the infarct and the amount of iodide injected.

Enhancement is unusual during the first three days, reaches a maximum between the second and third week, and, subsequently, decreases rapidly. It is unusual during the second month and rare after 8 weeks. Enhancement has been demonstrated in 80% of infarcts imaged during the third week by using an IV injection of 30 g of iodine (37,41). Enhancement also will occur in isodense infarcts (38), and the use of contrast medium will increase the detection rate by 5% to 10% (39,40). Some authors have advocated that scans be performed before and after administration of contrast material to optimize visualization of an infarct. However, it is thought now that enhancement is not without risk if the amount of iodine injected is greater than 42 g (41,42). For this reason, many teams do not use it routinely.

Severity of Symptoms

The size of an infarct appears to be related to the degree of clinical deficit, although exceptions to this rule exist (18). This relationship, which is partly responsible for the increased sensitivity of CT imaging, has been demonstrated by Campbell et al (27) in 108 patients with hemiparesis (Table 16–6). The association between increased rate of detection of CT infarcts and increasing severity of symptoms has been confirmed by others whose studies included patients with amaurosis fugax, TIAs, RINDs, and stroke; all studies used the same type of equipment (Table 16–7). Allen and Preziosi (16) found a prevalence of 12% in patients with focal TIAs, 45% in patients with minor stroke, and 75% in patients with major stroke.

In a series of 248 patients with ischemic episodes (44 with focal TIAs, 50 with RINDs, 151 with completed stroke and no recovery, and 13 with an intermediate type) Ladurner et al (15) considered 66 to have "dementia" according to clinical criteria or psychologic testing. Patients with dementia had an increased prevalence of hypodense lesions and atrophy (Table 16–8), and multiple bilateral lesions were significantly more common.

Presence and Severity of Internal Carotid Stenosis

The association between the detection of ischemic lesions on CT scans and the presence of stenotic disease on angiography was pointed out by

TABLE 16–6. Grade of hemiparesis and prevalence of supratentorial infarction detected on CT scans in 108 patients.

Grade of weakness	No. of patients	Prevalence of infarction on CT scan (%)
1	27	63
2	30	73
3	15	80
4	36	92

CT = computed tomography.
[From Campbell JK, Houser W, Stevens JC, et al, 1978 (27).]

TABLE 16–7. Association between rate of CT detection of infarcts and increasing severi of symptoms.

Study	Year	Asymptomatic carotid stenosis (%)	Amaurosis fugax	TIAs (%)	RIND (%)	PRIND (%)	Stro (%
Ladurner et al (15)	1979	—	—	18	—	76	95
Buell et al (17)	1981	—	—	17	—	—	64
Allen and Preziosi (16)	1981	—	—	12	—	—	53
Houser et al (18)	1982	—	—	28	—	—	78
Goldenberg and Reisner (20)	1983	—	—	20	42	—	73
Tsementzis et al (23)	1984	—	—	70	—	—	80
Zukowski et al (5)	1984	8	23	63*	—	—	—
Ricotta et al (24)	1985	21	—	12	55	—	64
Irvine Laboratory	1986	28†	43	48	—	—	7

*All patients had >50% internal carotid stenosis. Prevalence varied, depending on the presence or abse of carotid plaque ulceration.
†Some patients had vertebrobasilar TIAs.
All studies used the same kind (models) of equipment.
CT = computed tomography; TIA = transient ischemic attack; RIND = reversible ischemic neurolo deficit; PRIND = partially reversible ischemic neurologic deficit
dashes = no information available.

Perrone et al (14) in 1979 in a series of 35 patients with TIAs and 15 patients with RINDs. The prevalence of infarcts on CT scans was increased in the patients who had angiographic evidence of internal carotid stenosis (Table 16–9).

Subsequently, in 1983, Goldenberg and Reisner (20) found a highly significant correlation beween the size of the infarct visualized with CT and the reduction in luminar diameter shown by angiography in a series of patients with TIAs, RINDs, and stroke.

In our series of 70 patients with amaurosis fugax only (no TIAs), 104 with hemispheric TIAs (no amaurosis fugax), 185 with VB-TIAs and/or asymptomatic cervical bruit, and 129 with stroke who made a moderate

TABLE 16–8. Prevalence of hypodense lesions and atrophy on CT scans in relation to dementia in 248 patients with ischemic episodes.

Ischemic episode	n	No. with hypodense lesion (%)	No. with atrophy (%)
With dementia	66	58 (88)*	57 (86)†
Without dementia	182	131 (72)	115 (63)

*$X^2 = 6.75$; $p < .01$.
†$X^2 = 12.24$; $p < .001$.
CT = computed tomography.
[From Ladurner G, Sager WD, Hiff LD, et al, 1979 (15).]

TABLE 16–9. Prevalence of hypodense lesions on CT scans in relation to angiographic evidence of internal carotid stenosis.

Findings on angiography	Hypodense lesions present (%)	Hypodense lesions absent	Total
Internal carotid stenosis	13 (59)	9	22
No evidence of internal carotid stenosis	1 (13)	7	8

35 patients had transient ischemic attacks, and 15 had reversible ischemic neurologic deficits. By Fisher's exact test, $p = .027$. [From Perrone P, Candelise L, Scott G, et al, 1979 (14).]

to full recovery, the prevalence of infarcts seen on CT scans increased as the degree of carotid stenosis increased. Determination of this correlation was possible because all patients had been studied by means of duplex Doppler scanning (Fig. 16–1).

In an earlier study (5), specimens obtained by carotid endarterectomy were examined for macroscopic ulceration, and the findings were correlated with the prevalence of cerebral infarction on the CT scan in 65

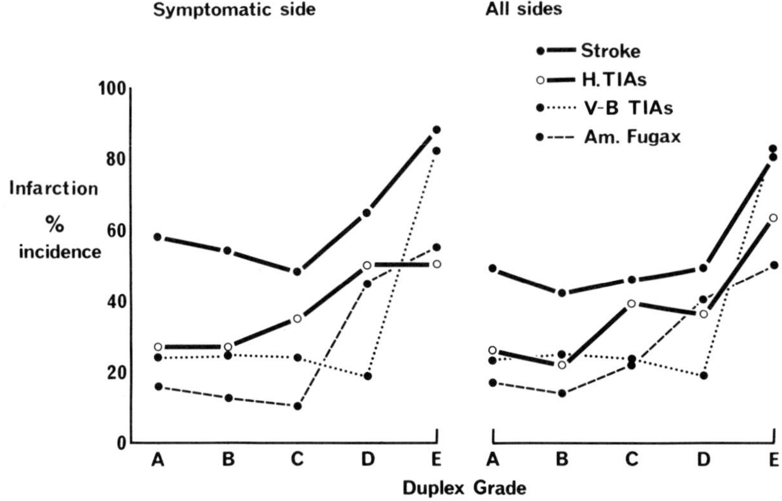

FIGURE 16–1. Prevalence of infarction seen on CT scans in relation to internal carotid stenosis in 70 patients with amaurosis fugax only (no TIAs), 104 with hemispheric TIAs (no amaurosis fugax), 185 with vertebrobasilar (VB) TIAs and/ or asymptomatic cervical bruit, and 129 with stroke who made a moderate to full recovery. Grading of internal carotid stenosis by duplex Doppler scan: A = no evidence of stenosis, B = 1%–15% stenosis, C = 16%–49% stenosis, D = 50%–99% stenosis, E = occlusion.

patients. Thirty-six had carotid TIAs, 13 had amaurosis fugax, 13 were asymptomatic but had severe internal carotid stenosis requiring aorto-coronary bypass, and six had stroke and a good recovery. A macroscopic ulcer was found in 42 specimens (three bilateral operations). Twenty-six (62%) of the patients with ulceration had one or more ipsilateral infarcts. Only two (8%) of the 26 patients without ulcer had infarcts. In the 36 patients who had carotid TIAs, ipsilateral silent infarcts were detected in 26. Ulceration was present in 23 (88%) of these 26. This data showed a strong association between internal carotid plaque ulceration and silent infarction detected on CT scans.

Significance of Silent Cerebral Infarction

No studies are available on the natural history of patients with or without silent cerebral infarction. However, some information is available from studies of patients undergoing carotid endarterectomy. In one retrospective review (21) of 79 patients with no history of stroke who had a CT scan before endarterectomy, the prevalence of a postoperative permanent neurologic deficit was 14%, compared with 1.5% in patients who had a normal scan. The prevalence of transient neurologic deficit was 14%, compared with 3%.

Other teams (36,43,44) have suggested that the prevalence of intraoperative ischemia requiring shunting is increased in patients who have evidence of infarcts on CT scans.

Further studies are needed on the natural history of patients with amaurosis fugax and carotid TIAs in relation to silent infarcts seen on CT scans.

Prevalence of Atrophy

Table 16–10 shows the prevalence of atrophy seen on CT scans in several studies. Kinkel and Jacobs (11) in 1976 were the first to observe cortical atrophy excessive for the patient's age in two (6%) of 30 patients with carotid TIAs who were scanned during the period of January 1974 to May 1975. Ventricular asymmetry and/or unilateral focal atrophy were found in 20% of 50 patients (35 with TIAs and 15 with RINDs) by Perrone et al (14) in 1979 who noted a strong association with internal carotid stenosis. At the same time, Ladurner et al (15) in 1979 reported atrophy in 43% of patients with focal TIAs, in 68% of patients with PRIND, and in 82% of patients with completed stroke. In addition, they found a higher prevalence of atrophy in patients with dementia (Table 16–8) and a strong association with multiple infarcts. In our series, the prevalence of atrophy (age was not taken into consideration) was 15% in patients with amaurosis fugax and no focal TIAs, 22% in patients with focal TIAs and no amaurosis fugax, 25% in patients with asymptomatic cervical bruit and/or VB-TIAs, and 36% in patients with a stroke and a moderate-to-full recovery (RIND or PRIND).

TABLE 16–10. Prevalence of atrophy seen on CT scans.

Study	Year	Prevalence (%)	Comments
Patients with TIAs with or without amaurosis fugax			
Kinkel and Jacobs (11)	1976	6	30 patients with carotid TIAs
Perrone et al (14)	1979	20	35 patients with TIAs and 15 with RIND
Ladurner et al (15)	1979	43	44 patients (homolateral atrophy, 11%; general atrophy, 32%)
Biller et al (19)	1982	20	45 patients with carotid TIAs
Irvine Laboratory	1986	22	104 patients with carotid TIAs (no amaurosis fugax)
Patients with amaurosis fugax			
Irvine Laboratory	1986	15	70 patients with amaurosis fugax (no carotid TIAs)
Patients with asymptomatic cervical bruit and/or vertebrobasilar TIAs			
Irvine Laboratory	1986	25	183 patients
Patients with PRIND			
Ladurner et al (15)	1979	68	50 patients (homolateral atrophy, 16%; general atrophy, 56%)
Irvine Laboratory	1986	36	129 patients with moderate to full recovery
Patients with stroke			
Ladurner et al (15)	1979	82	141 patients with "completed stroke" (homolateral atrophy, 18%)

CT = computed tomography; TIA = transient ischemic attack; RIND = reversible ischemic, neurologic deficit; PRIND = partially reversible neurologic deficit.

Factors Affecting Prevalence

Three factors are associated with the finding of cerebral atrophy on CT scan: age, cerebral infarction, and atherosclerotic cerebrovascular disease.

Age

The prevalence of atrophy increases with age, so many neuroradiologists do not consider it abnormal and do not report it unless it is excessive for the patient's age. Unfortunately, atrophy, as indicated by increased CSF spaces, is difficult to define, and its detection is subjective, especially in borderline cases. Other factors, such as atherosclerotic cerebrovascular disease, silent infarcts, and hypertensive changes, are frequent findings in an aging population. At the moment, it is not possible to say whether age per se is a factor in atrophy or whether atrophy found in older people is the result of other coincidental factors.

Cerebral Infarction

The association of atrophy with cerebral infarction detected on CT scan has been noted (18). After the edema subsides, many infarcts become cystic and, presumably because of loss of brain tissue, most large infarcts are associated with local dilatation of the adjacent CSF spaces. Sometimes enlargement of these spaces is the only evidence of an infarct that is isodense and therefore not visualized or subsequently has become isodense. It is not surprising that multiple infarcts are associated with a higher prevalence of atrophy (15).

The increased prevalence of atrophy in association with the presence of silent infarctions, particularly bilateral or multiple lesions, also was found in our patients who had amaurosis fugax and focal TIAs. The prevalence was 12% in the absence of hypodense lesions, 14% in the presence of a single unilateral infarct, 33% in the presence of single bilateral infarcts, and 70% in the presence of multiple infarcts (Table 16–11). In our patients with stroke (RIND and PRIND), the prevalence of atrophy was 43% in the absence of hypodense lesions, 23% in the presence of a single unilateral infarct, 38% in the presence of single bilateral infarcts, and 64% in the presence of multiple infarcts (Table 16–12).

At this point, it should be remembered that CT scans detect only a fraction of infarcts (30% to 60%) shown by other methods such as MRI (Table 16–5). It is not surprising that atrophy was found in 12% of patients with amaurosis fugax and focal TIAs and in 43% with stroke and no evidence of infarction on CT scans. A likely explanation is that isodense undetected infarcts were present, particularly in the patients with stroke. Further evidence of the association of atrophy with silent cerebral infarction is being presented in the following sections.

TABLE 16–11. Prevalence of atrophy in patients with amaurosis fugax and hemispheric TIAs in relation to the number of infarctions seen on CT scans.

Infarction on CT scan	No atrophy	Atrophy (%)	Total
None	66	9 (12)	75
Single, unilateral	43	7 (14)	50
Single, bilateral	10	5 (33)	15
Multiple	3	7 (70)	10

TIA = transient ischemic attack; CT = computed tomography.

Internal Carotid Stenosis

The association of cerebral atrophy with internal carotid stenosis observed by Perrone et al (14) in 1979 has been confirmed by us in patients with amaurosis fugax and in patients with VB-TIAs and/or asymptomatic cervical bruit (Fig. 16–2). However, further analysis of the data in relation to both internal carotid stenosis and silent cerebral infarction indicated that it was not the internal carotid disease per se that was related to the atrophy but the cerebral infarction. Patients without silent cerebral infarction, even with high grades of internal carotid stenosis, have a very low prevalence of atrophy.

Findings from the Irvine Laboratory

For the purpose of this study, from the records of the Irvine Laboratory, we identified 70 patients with amaurosis fugax only (no focal TIAs), 104 with hemispheric TIAs only (no amaurosis fugax), 129 with stroke who had moderate-to-full recovery, and 185 with VB-TIAs and/or asymptomatic cervical bruit. All these patients had both CT scanning and duplex Doppler

TABLE 16–12. Prevalence of atrophy in patients with stroke in relation to the number of infarctions on CT scans.

Infarction on CT scan	No atrophy	Atrophy (%)	Total
None	25	19 (43)	44
Single, unilateral	41	12 (23)	53
Single, bilateral	15	9 (38)	24
Multiple	4	7 (64)	11

CT = computed tomography.

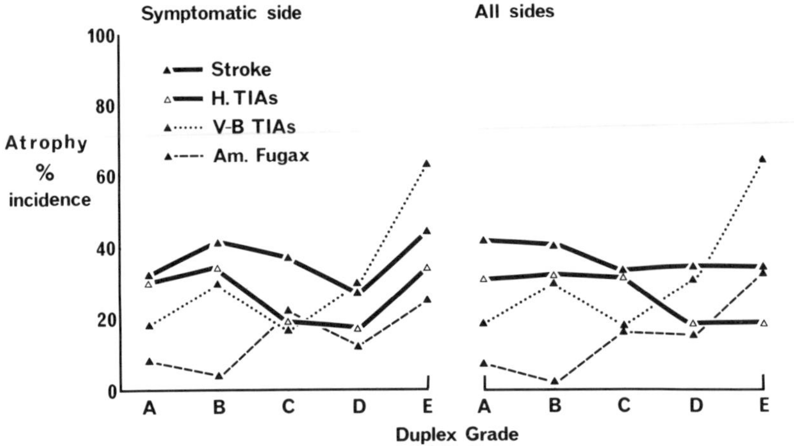

FIGURE 16–2. Prevalence of atrophy seen on CT scans in relation to internal carotid stenosis in the same patients as in FIGURE 16–1.

scanning (ATL Model 500) as part of the routine investigative procedures used at the Irvine Laboratory since 1982. The relationship between the duplex Doppler gradings A to E and the degree of internal carotid stenosis (diameter) is as follows: A, no evidence of stenosis; B, 1% to 15%; C, 16% to 49%; D, 50% to 99%; and E, occlusion. The accuracy of duplex Doppler scanning, in our hands, has been validated in a series of more

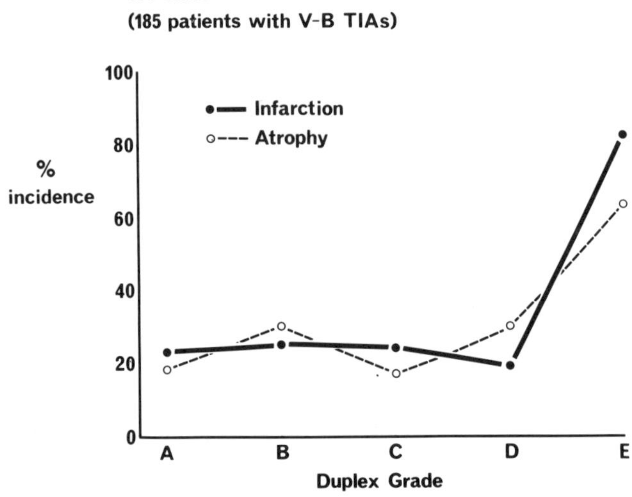

FIGURE 16–3. Prevalence of infarction and atrophy seen on CT scans in relation to internal carotid stenosi in 370 sides of 185 patients with VB-TIAs and/or asymptomatic cervical bruit. (Reproduced from J Vasc Surg by kind permission of the editor: Grigg et al, in press)

than 300 patients who had angiography (*kappa* = .8). Patients who had both TIAs and AF have been excluded.

In the 185 patients with VB-TIAs and/or asymptomatic cervical bruit, the overall prevalence of infarction seen on CT scans was 28% and of atrophy, 25%. The relationship between the prevalence of infarction and atrophy and the degree of carotid stenosis is shown in Fig. 16–3. The prevalence of both infarction and atrophy seen on CT scans was increased for grade E. However, the increased prevalence of atrophy was the result of more frequent atrophy in patients with CT infarction (Fig. 16–4).

In the 70 patients with amaurosis fugax, the overall prevalence of infarction seen on CT scans was 43% and of atrophy, 25%. The prevalences of both infarction and atrophy increased as the prevalence of internal carotid stenosis increased (Fig. 16–5). This was found in both the symptomatic and the asymptomatic side. It was more obvious when both sides were considered together (Fig. 16–6). The increased prevalence of atrophy shown in Figs. 16–5 and 16–6 in grades D and E was the result of atrophy in patients with silent infarction (Fig. 16–7).

In the 104 patients with hemispheric TIAs, the overall prevalences were 48% for cerebral infarction and 22% for atrophy. The prevalence of infarction on both the symptomatic and asymptomatic sides seen on CT scans increased as the prevalence of internal carotid stenosis increased (Fig. 16–8). Unlike the findings in the previous groups, this was not accompanied by an increased prevalence of atrophy. Indeed, if anything, the prevalence of atrophy decreased in grades D and E. This was more

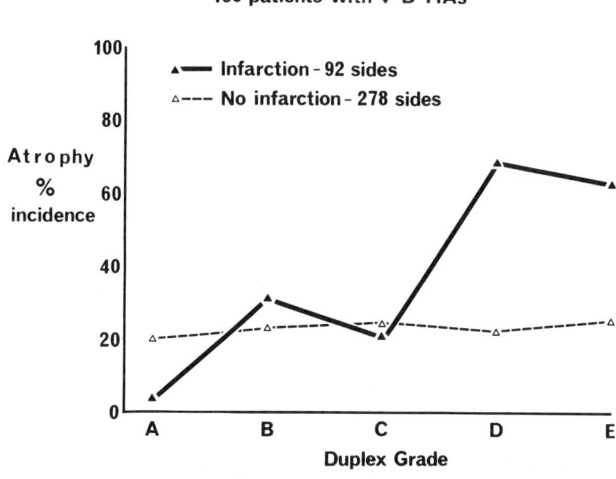

FIGURE 16–4. Prevalence of atrophy seen on CT in 287 sides without and 92 sides with infarction in relation to internal carotid stenosis in 185 patients with VB-TIAs and/or asymptomatic cervical bruit. (Reproduced from J Vasc Surg by kind permission of the editor: Grigg et al, in press)

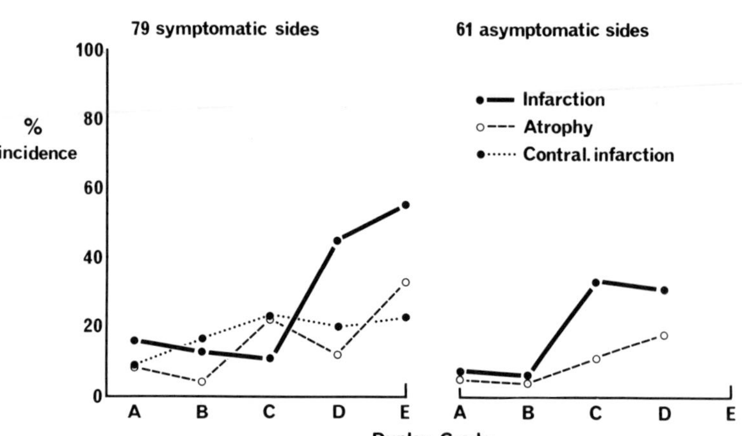

FIGURE 16–5. Prevalence of infarction and atrophy seen on CT scans in relation to internal carotid stenosis in 70 patients with amaurosis fugax. (Reproduced from J Vasc Surg by kind permission of the editor: Grigg et al, in press)

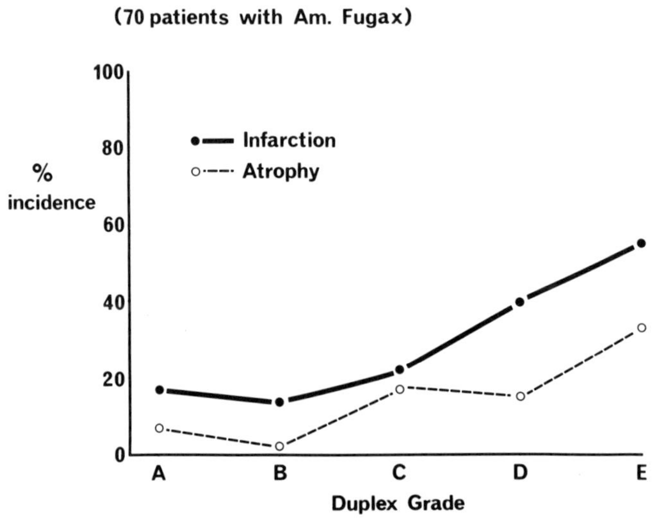

FIGURE 16–6.—Prevalence of infarction and atrophy seen on CT scans in relation to internal carotid stenosis in 140 sides of 70 patients with amaurosis fugax. (Reproduced from J Vasc Surg by kind permission of the editor: Grigg et al, in press)

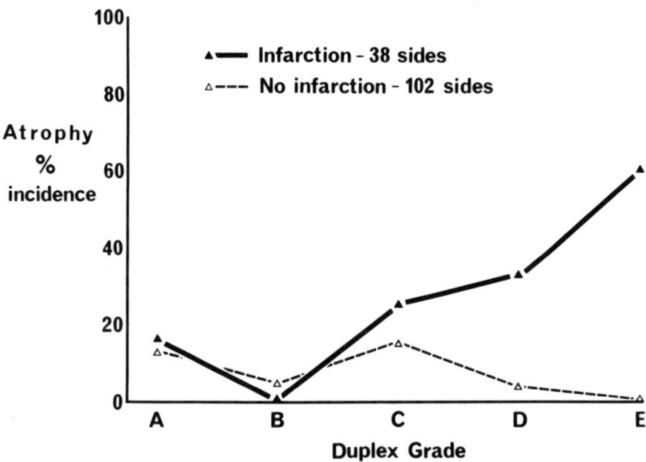

FIGURE 16–7. Prevalence of atrophy seen on CT scans in 102 sides without and 38 sides with infarction in relation to internal carotid stenosis in 70 patients with amaurosis fugax. (Reproduced from J Vasc Surg by kind permission of the editor: Grigg et al, in press)

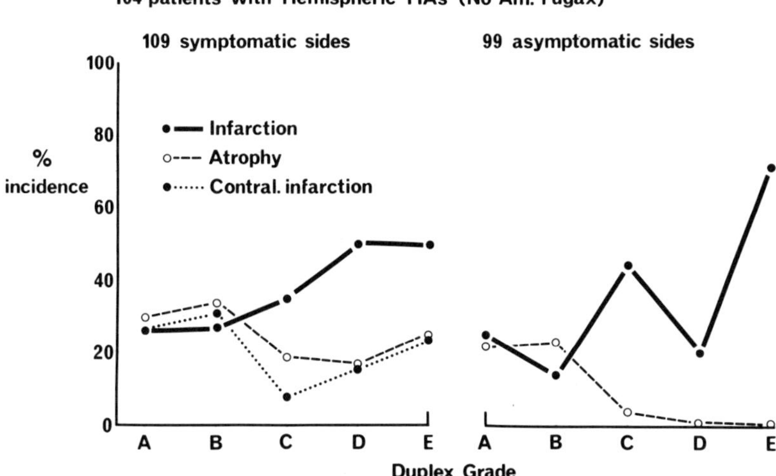

FIGURE 16–8. Prevalence of infarction and atrophy seen on CT scans in relation to internal carotid stenosis in 104 patients with hemispheric TIAs. (Reproduced from J Vasc Surg by kind permission of the editor: Grigg et al, in press)

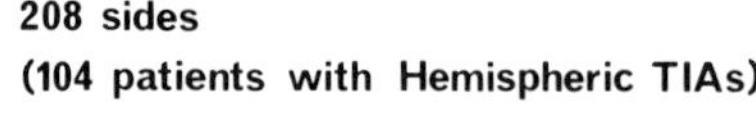

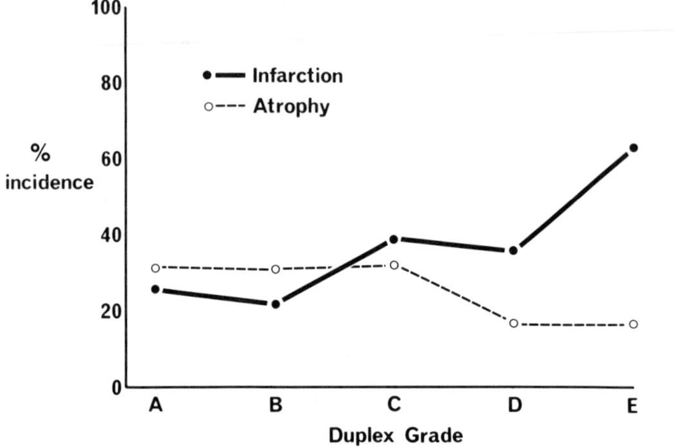

FIGURE 16–9. Prevalence of infarction and atrophy seen on CT scans in relation to internal carotid stenosis in 208 sides of 104 patients with hemispheric TIAs. (Reproduced from J Vasc Surg by kind permission of the editor: Grigg et al, in press)

104 patients with Hemispheric TIAs

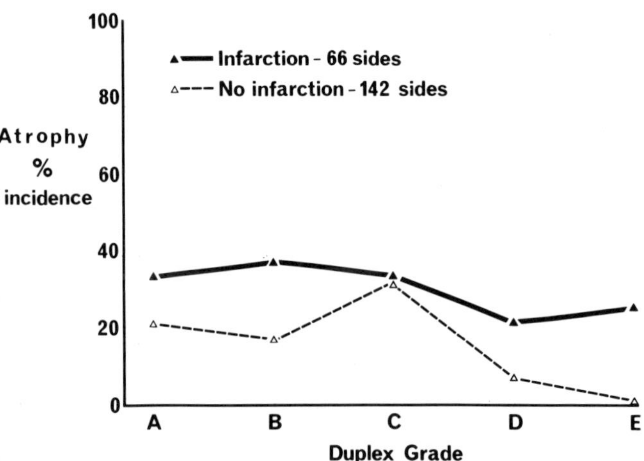

FIGURE 16–10. Prevalence of atrophy seen on CT scans in 142 sides without and 66 sides with infarction in relation to internal carotid stenosis in 104 patients with hemispheric TIAs. (Reproduced from J Vasc Surg by kind permission of the editor: Grigg et al, in press)

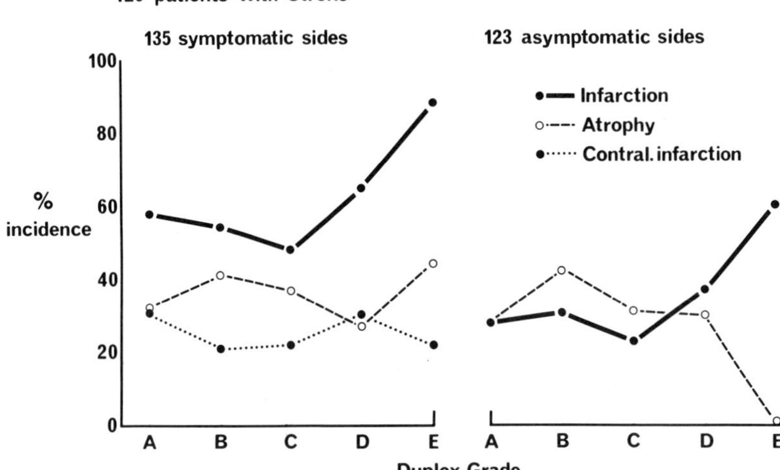

FIGURE 16–11. Prevalence of infarction and atrophy seen on CT scans in relation to internal carotid stenosis in 129 patients with stroke. (Reproduced from J Vasc Surg by kind permission of the editor: Grigg et al, in press)

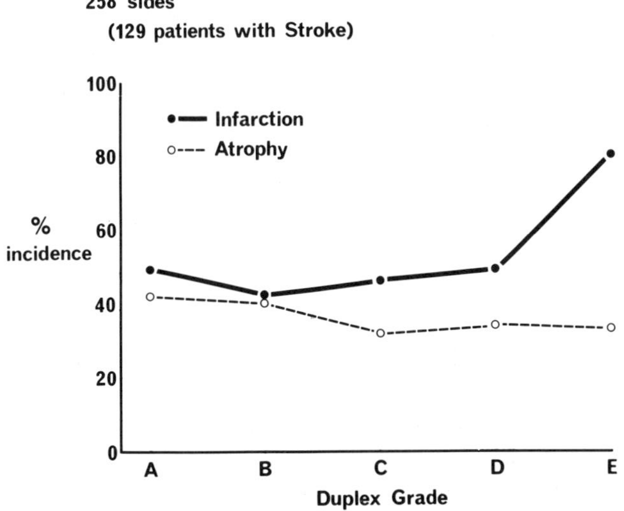

FIGURE 16–12. Prevalence of infarction and atrophy seen on CT scans in relation to internal carotid stenosis in 258 sides of 129 patients with stroke. (Reproduced from J Vasc Surg by kind permission of the editor: Grigg et al, in press)

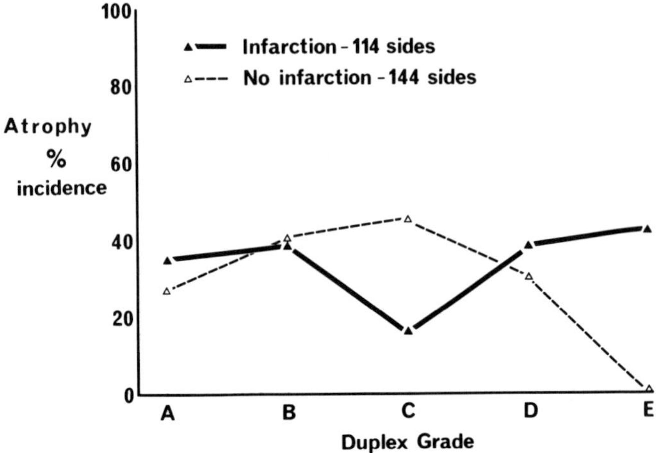

FIGURE 16–13. Prevalence of atrophy seen on CT scans in 144 sides without and 114 sides with infarction in 129 patients with stroke. (Reproduced from J Vasc Surg by kind permission of the editor: Grigg et al, in press)

obvious when both sides were considered together (Fig. 16–9). Nevertheless, the prevalence of atrophy in Groups D and E was the result of atrophy mainly in the patients with infarction (Fig. 16–10).

In the 129 patients with stroke (RIND and PRIND), the overall prevalences were 71% for cerebral infarction and 36% for atrophy. The prevalences of cerebral infarction and atrophy in relation to the severity of internal carotid stenosis showed a similar trend to that found in the patients with hemispheric TIAs. The prevalence of infarction associated with grades D and E was increased in both the symptomatic and the asymptomatic sides (Figs. 16–11 and 16–12). This increased prevalence was not accompanied by an increased prevalence of atrophy. Indeed, atrophy was absent in the asymptomatic side with internal carotid occlusion (Fig. 16–11). In the sides with occluded ICAs, the increased prevalence of atrophy was the result of atrophy in the patients with infarction (Fig. 16–13).

General Discussion and Conclusions

It is now evident that patients with asymptomatic internal carotid stenosis, amaurosis fugax, and TIAs have a high prevalence of small, silent cerebral infarcts seen on CT scans. These infarcts occur not only on the symptomatic but also, to a lesser extent, on the asymptomatic side and are only a fraction of the total, as indicated by MRI. Many infarcts are not detected by CT scans because they are isodense.

The prevalence of silent infarction increases as the prevalence of carotid stenosis increases, but is also appreciable in patients with normal carotids

(17% in patients with amaurosis fugax and 31% in patients with hemispheric TIAs). Presumably, the infarcts in these patients are the result of either intracranial disease or emboli from areas more central than the carotid bifurcation.

Cerebral atrophy, sometimes ipsilateral, but more often general, also is associated with an increased prevalence of carotid stenosis and is very likely the result of infarction. This is supported by the higher prevalence of atrophy in patients with bilateral or multiple infarcts (Table 16–11). In addition, in patients without any carotid stenosis, a close association exists between the prevalences of infarction and atrophy in all the groups (ie, patients with VB-TIAs, amaurosis fugax, hemispheric TIAs, and stroke). (See Figs. 16–3, 16–5, 16–6, 16–8, 16–9, 16–11, and 16–12.)

In patients with amaurosis fugax, the increased prevalence of atrophy found in the presence of severe internal carotid disease is the result of atrophy in the patients with silent infarcts (Fig. 11–7). In view of the fact that these infarcts are small and many are not even detectable by CT scan (though they may be visible with MRI), it can be hypothesized that showers of small emboli occur (platelet aggregates or cholesterol crystals) that, because of their size, do not produce symptoms unless they enter the retinal artery. Nevertheless, they produce small silent infarcts and atrophy.

In patients with amaurosis fugax and ipsilateral ICA occlusion or very severe ICA stenosis (some patients with grade D and patients with grade E), the presence of infarction (often small and multiple) could be the result of hemodynamic rather than embolic ischemia. This also could be the case in patients with VB-TIAs and/or asymptomatic cervical bruit in whom the prevalence of infarction is increased only in the presence of an occluded carotid artery (Fig. 16–3) and in whom the increased prevalence of atrophy is found mainly in the presence of carotid occlusion (Fig. 16–4).

Further support of the aforementioned hypothesis is provided by the fact that in patients with amaurosis fugax, atrophy is not found in the presence of carotid occlusion and absence of cerebral infarction (grade E, Fig. 16–7). It can be postulated that the occluded carotid artery protects the brain from emboli and the good collateral circulation protects it from infarcts (the collateral circulation should be good if no CT evidence of infarction is found in the presence of an occluded carotid). Amaurosis fugax in the presence of ipsilateral ICA occlusion is well documented (34).

The different pattern of prevalence of atrophy in relation to the grade of internal carotid stenosis (ie, the lack of increased prevalence of atrophy in association with the increased prevalence of infarction) found in patients with hemispheric TIAs (Figs. 16–8 and 16–9) and stroke (Figs. 16–11 and 16–12) does not contradict the aforementioned hypothesis. Larger emboli may occur in these patients (or more severe hemodynamic ischemic events in patients with ICA occlusion), producing larger infarcts. Because of the relatively larger area of cerebral damage by caused ischemia, these patients have hemispheric TIAs, RINDs, PRINDs, or stroke with minimal recovery. These conditions usually are investigated before any additional ischemic events of this magnitude or smaller (producing silent multiple infarction with subsequent atrophy) can occur. This can explain the relatively low prevalence of atrophy found in patients with grades D and, particularly, grade E who have hemispheric TIAs and stroke (Figs. 16–8 to 16–13). The atrophy found in these patients is the result of the relatively large volume of the infarcts producing the symptoms rather than the silent small lesions detectable on CT or MRI.

In conclusion, the retina is a small but very sensitive part of the nervous system that can detect (in the form of amaurosis fugax) very small emboli or ischemic episodes of hemodynamic origin that normally do not produce an otherwise clinically detectable effect in the brain although they produce small silent infarcts and, eventually, atrophy. This concept argues against the belief that amaurosis fugax is produced by emboli entering the retinal artery only because of selective streaming of blood flow in the ICA.

This hypothesis is an oversimplification because it does not include the effect of other factors, such as hypertension, raised hematocrit, cardiac arrhythmias seen on the CT scan, and the size of the infarcts. Finally, it is essential that patients with cerebrovascular symptoms who have normal or abnormal CT scans be followed up so that the clinician can learn more of their natural history and the prognostic significance of the CT scan.

References

1. Fisher CM: Observations of the fundus oculi in transient monocular blindness. *Neurology* 1959;9:333–347.
2. Hollenhorst RW: The ocular manifestations of internal carotid arterial thrombosis. *Med Clin North Am* 1960;44:897–908.
3. McBrien OJ, Bradley RD, Ashton N: The nature of retinal emboli in stenosis of the internal carotid artery. *Lancet* 1963;1:697–699.
4. Ross Russell RW: The source of retinal emboli. *Lancet* 1968;2:789–792.
5. Zukowski AJ, Nicolaides AN, Lewis RT, et al: The correlation between carotid plaque ulceration and cerebral infarction. *J Vasc Surg* 1984;1:782–786.
6. McDowell FH: Transient cerebral ischaemia: Diagnostic considerations. *Prog Cardiovasc Dis* 1980;22:309–324.
7. Imparato AM, Riles TS, Gorstein F: The carotid bifurcation plaque: Pathologic findings associated with cerebral ischemia. *Stroke* 1979;10:238–245.
8. Lusby RJ, Ferrell LD, Ehrenfeld WK, et al: Carotid plaque hemorrhage: Its role in the production of cerebral ischemia. *Arch Surg* 1982;117:1479–1488.
9. Nicolaides AN, Salmasi A-M, Sonecha TN: How should we investigate the arteriopath for coexisting lesions. *J Cardiovasc Surg* 1986;27:515–533.
10. Caillé JM, Constant P, Dop A, et al: Aspects and evolution of cerebrovascular accidents. *J Neuroradiol* 1976;3:297–312.
11. Kinkel WR, Jacobs L: Computerised axial transverse tomography in cerebrovascular disease. *Neurology* 1976;26:924–930.
12. Constant P, Renou AM, Caillé JM, et al: Follow up study of cerebral ischaemia with computer tomography. *Acta Neurol Scand* 1977;56(suppl 64):164–165.

13. Laporte A, Renou AM, Mazeaux JM, et al: Comparative results of ^{99m}Tc-pertechnate scintigraphy and computerised tomography after contrast injection in cerebral pathology. *Neuroradiology* 1978;16:173–177.
14. Perrone P, Candelise L, Scott G, et al: CT evaluation in patients with transient ischemic attacks: Correlation between clinical and angiographic findings. *Eur Neurol* 1979;18:217–221.
15. Ladurner G, Sager WD, Hiff LD, et al: A correlation of clinical findings and CT in ischaemic cerebrovascular disease. *Eur Neurol* 1979;18:281–288.
16. Allen GS, Preziosi TJ: Carotid endarterectomy: A prospective study of its efficacy and safety. *Medicine* 1981;60:298–309.
17. Buell U, Scheid KF, Lanksh W, et al: Sensitivity of computer-assisted radionuclide angiography in transient ischemic attack and prolonged reversible ischemic neurological defect. *Stroke* 1981;12:829–834.
18. Houser OW, Campbell JK, Baker HL Jr, et al: Radiologic evaluation of ischemic cerebrovascular syndromes with emphasis on computed tomography. *Radiol Clin North Am* 1982;20:123–142.
19. Biller J, Laster DW, Howard G, et al: Cranial computerised tomography in carotid artery transient ischemic attacks. *Eur Neurol* 1982;21:98–101.
20. Goldenberg G, Reisner TH: Angiographic findings in relation to clinical course and results of computed tomography in cerebrovascular disease. *Eur Neurol* 1983;22:124–130.
21. Graber JN, Vollmar RW, Johnson WC, et al: Stroke after carotid endarterectomy: Risk as predicted by preoperative computerised tomography. *Am J Surg* 1984;147:492–497.
22. Calandre L, Gomara S, Bermejo F, et al: Clinical CT correlations in TIA, RIND and strokes with minimum residum. *Stroke* 1984;15:663–666.
23. Tsementzis SA, Hitchcock ER, Woolley JL: Emission and transmission tomography of the brain in cerebrovascular disease. *Surg Neurol* 1984;21:385–390.
24. Ricotta JJ, Ouriel K, Green R, et al: Use of computerised cerebral tomography in selection of patients for elective and urgent carotid endarterectomy. *Ann Surg* 1985;202:783–787.
25. Weisberg LA: Computerised tomographic abnormalities in patients with hemispheric transient ischemic attacks. *South Med J* 1986;79:804–807.
26. Awad I, Modic M, Little J, et al: Focal parenchymal lesion in transient ischemic attacks: Correlation of computed tomography and magnetic resonance imaging. *Stroke* 1986;17:399–403.
27. Campbell JK, Houser W, Stevens JC, et al: Computed tomography and radionuclide imaging in the evaluation of ischemic stroke. *Radiology* 1978;126:695–702.
28. Buell U, Kazner E, Rath M, et al: Sensitivity of computed tomography and serial scintigraphy in cerebrovascular disease. *Radiology* 1979;131:393–398.
29. Bradac GB, Oberson R: CT and angiography in cases with occlusive disease of supravententorial cerebral vessels. *Neuroradiology* 1980;19:193–200.
30. Oxfordshire Community Stroke Project: Incidence of stroke in Oxfordshire: First year's experience of a community stroke register. *Br Med J* 1983;287:713–717.
31. Scott WR, New PFJ, Davis KR, et al: Computerised axial tomography of intracerebral and intraventricular hemorrhage. *Radiology* 1974;112:73–80.

32. Brahme FJ: CT diagnosis of cerebrovascular disorders: A review. *Comput Tomogr* 1978;2:173–181.
33. Bentson JR: CT in the diagnosis of cerebral vascular disease. *Bull Los Angeles Neurol Soc* 1980;45:21–25.
34. Bogousslawaky J, Regli F: Cerebral infarction with transient signs (CITS): Do TIAs correspond to small deep infarcts in internal carotid artery occlusion? *Stroke* 1984;15:536–539.
35. Caplan LR: Are terms such as completed stroke or RIND of continued usefulness? *Stroke* 1983;14:431–433.
36. Vollmar RW, Eldrup-Jorgensen J, Hoffman MA: The role of cranial computed tomography in carotid surgery. *Surg Clin North Am* 1986;66:255–268.
37. Inoue Y, Takemoto K, Miyamoto T, et al: Sequential computed tomography scans in acute cerebral infarction. *Radiology* 1980;135:655–662.
38. Wing SD, Normal D, Pollock JA, et al: Contrast enhancement of cerebral infarcts in computed tomography. *Radiology* 1976;121:89–92.
39. Clasen RA, Huckman MS, Von Roenn KA, et al: Time course of cerebral swelling in stroke: A correlative autopsy and CT study, in Cervos-Navarro J, Ferszt R: *Advances in Neurology: Brain Edema*. New York, Raven Press, 1980, vol 28, pp
40. Lukin RR, Chambers AA, Thornsick TA: Cerebrovascular lesions: Infarction, hemorrhage, aneurysm and arteriovenous malformation. *Semin Roentgenol* 1977;12:75–87.
41. Pullicine P, Kendall BE: Contrast enhancement in ischaemic lesions: 1. Relationship to prognosis. *Neuroradiology* 1980;19:235–239.
42. Hayman LA, Evans RA, Bastion FO, et al: Delayed high dose contrast CT: Identifying patients at risk of massive hemorrhagic infarction. *Am J Neuroradiol* 1981;2:139–147.
43. Rosenthal D, Stanton PE, Lamis PA: Carotid endarterectomy: The unreliability of intraoperative monitoring in patients having had stroke or reversible neurologic deficit. *Arch Surg* 1981;116:1569–1575.
44. Whittemore AD, Ruby ST, Couch NP, et al: Early carotid endarterectomy in patients with small fixed neurologic deficits. *J Vasc Surg* 1984;1:795–799.

CHAPTER 17

Angiography in Amaurosis Fugax

Michael J.G. Harrison

The idea that embolism to the eye or brain may arise from the heart or from the carotid artery is of course an ancient one (1,2), though intensive investigation of patients for such sources has been pursued only in the last 20 years or so.

Despite increasing sophistication in noninvasive methods of assessment and imaging of the carotid artery, angiography remains the gold standard for the identification of atheromatous changes that might be relevant to the production of symptoms in the ipsilateral retina or cerebral hemisphere. It must be accepted, however, that angiography underestimates the extent of minor plaques that do not encroach on the lumen, and it is not accurate in the recognition of ulceration of more complicated plaques (3). Nor does it identify mural thrombi in the lumen of a diseased carotid bifurcation more than rarely, despite their presence in surgical specimens (4). The concentration on the carotid bifurcation as a responsible lesion for ocular ischemia has meant that few studies have provided detailed information on the carotid siphon or the ophthalmic artery.

This chapter considers the results of angiography in the investigation of patients with amaurosis fugax. It compares the findings with those in patients with cerebral tumours (who represent the only control cases available) in an attempt to define the significance of the vascular pathology detected. It then compares and contrasts the angiographic findings in patients with amaurosis fugax with those with cerebral TIAs and with patients with retinal strokes (CRA occlusion and branch occlusions with persistent field defects).

The literature quoted concerns more than 1,000 cases investigated by angiography, and the results refer to the findings in the ipsilateral ICA. Some studies characterize the findings on angiograms as normal or as showing irregularity due to plaque formation, stenosis (meaning plaque encroachment on the lumen), or occlusion. Others additionally report miscellaneous findings, such as fibromuscular dysplasia, kinks or loops, or isolated intracranial changes, as "other" abnormalities. The reports with such categorization of the findings are listed in Table 17–1. The results

TABLE 17–1. Angiographic findings in amaurosis fugax.

Study	No. of cases	Angiographic findings				
		Normal	Wall irregularity	Stenosis	Occlusion	Other
Harrison, Marshall (5)	19	6	6	4	3	0
Hooshmand et al (6)	34	2	18	12	2	0
Pessin et al (7)	33	8	5	15	5	0
Wilson, Ross Russell (8)*	67	32	8	16	7	4
Eisenberg, Mani (9)	40	5	7	19	9	0
Thiele et al (10)	28	2	10	16	0	0
Parkin et al (11)*	38	1	12	20	4	1
Adams et al (12)*	59	20	8	15	10	6
Total	318	76	74	117	40	11
Percent		24	23	37	13	3

*Includes amaurosis fugax and transient ischemic attacks.

appear fairly homogeneous. In 318 cases, 24% of the angiograms were normal, 23% showed irregularity of the walls only, 37% showed stenosis, 13% showed occlusions, and 3% showed other abnormalities.

In three of these studies (8,11,12), patients were included who had cerebral TIAs as well as amaurosis fugax. As a subgroup they showed little difference from those patients who apparently had amaurosis fugax as their only clinical manifestation.

To these figures can be added those from studies that separated atheroma from occlusion or normality of the ICA even though they did not distinguish between plaque formation and stenosis of the lumen (Table 17-2).

Most of these studies included patients who had both amaurosis fugax and TIAs. The overall figures remain as before. Twenty-five percent had normal angiograms, 59% had atheromatous changes of the carotid short of occlusion, and 14% had occlusions.

To these data can be added those from studies that referred only to the findings of extracranial disease (atheroma) without reporting separately irregularity, stenosis, or occlusion. These and the combined figures from Tables 17–1 and 17–2 are shown in Table 17–3. The total number of cases of amaurosis fugax was 1027, of whom about half (575) may have had

TABLE 17–2. Angiographic findings in amaurosis fugax.

Study	No. of cases	Angiographic findings			
		Normal	Wall irregularity or stenosis	Occlusion	Oth
Table 17–1	318	76	191	40	1
Marshall, Meadows (13)	21	10	7	4	[illegible]
Ramirez-Lassepas et al (14)*	27	1	20	6	[illegible]
Sandok et al (15)*	43	1	30	12	[illegible]
Lemak, Fields (16)*	234	51	150	33	[illegible]
Poole, Ross Russell (17)*	60	35	15	6	[illegible]
Total	703	174	413	101	1
Percent		25	59	14	[illegible]

*Includes amaurosis fugax and transient ischemic attacks.

TABLE 17–3. Angiographic findings in amaurosis fugax.

Study	No. of cases	Angiographic findings		
		Normal	ISO	Other
Table 17–2	703	174	514	15
Mungas, Baker (18)*	107	12	95	0
Hurwitz et al (19)	90	22	68	0
Harrison, Marshall (20)	55	8	39	8
Bogousslavsky et al (21)	55	21	34	0
Hedges et al (DSA) (22)	17	6	11	0
Total	1027	243	761	23
Percent		24	74	2

*Includes amaurosis fugax and transient ischemic attacks. ISO = wall irregularities, stenoses, and occlusions combined; DSA = digital subtraction angiography.

cerebral ischaemic attacks also. Seventy-four percent had visible changes attributable to local atheromas. A small minority (2%) had other abnormalities, but this group was probably under reported.

Comparison with Control Cases

This very high prevalence of atheromatous disease in the ipsilateral ICA is evidence in favour of the belief that small friable emboli that cause fleeting visual loss commonly originate at the carotid bifurcation. This inference clearly would be strengthened by a comparison with a control population. No study has collected such data prospectively, nor could it in view of the invasive procedures that would be required. Data are available, however, on the appearance of the carotid bifurcation in patients having angiography for cerebral tumours. A series from The National Hospital, Queen Square, showed the following results (Table 17–4). No patient with a proven tumour as a reason for angiography had a carotid occlusion. Only 2% had a stenotic lesion, but 24% (the same as the prevalence in cases of amaurosis fugax) had minor atheromatous irregularity. In 74% of the cases, no evidence of arterial disease was seen. The contrast shows, therefore, that stenotic occlusive disease of the ICA can be associated with the symptoms of amaurosis fugax but that the relevance of minor atheromatous change is by no means certain.

The ages of the tumor population and of the patients with amaurosis fugax may differ a little, but this cannot account for the striking differences

'ABLE 17–4. Angiographic findings in amaurosis fugax and in tumors.

	No. of cases	Angiographic findings (%)			
		Normal	Wall irregularity	Stenosis	Occlusion
.maurosis fugax (Table 17–1)	318	23	22	35	8
umors (personal data)	211	74	24	2	0

TABLE 17–5. Prevalence of angiographic abnormalities.

Appearance of carotid bifurcation	Tumor	Infarct	Transient ischemic attack
No. of patients	66	44	40
Normal findings (%)	86	57*	45*
Irregular wall (%)	11	15	10
Stenosis, all grades (%)	3	14†	40*
Occlusion (%)	0	14†	5

*$p < .001$
†$p < .01$
(From Harrison MJG, Marshall J, 1976 [23].)

seen ($\chi^2 = 173, p < 10^{-10}$). When a group of men 50 to 59 years old who had TIAs (including amaurosis fugax) were compared with a group of patients who had tumors (23), the difference in findings was similar (Table 17–5).

Another clue to the etiologic relevance of carotid stenosis in amaurosis fugax is available from a comparison of the symptomatic and asymptomatic sides in patients in whom bilateral angiography has been reported. The results of two such studies (15,24) are shown in Table 17–6. The side of the attacks of amaurosis fugax had a significantly more severe spectrum of atheromatous disease ($\chi^2 = 25, p < .0001$).

Cerebral Transient Ischemic Attacks

Do the findings in patients with amaurosis fugax differ from those in patients with hemispheric TIAs also in the carotid territory?

Clinical differences suggest that the nature of the embolic material or the ischemic process may be somewhat different. For example, attacks of amaurosis fugax are often much briefer than cerebral TIAs. Although this might reflect different tissue sensitivity to embolic obstruction of nutrient vessels, it is also possible that the sources of embolism might differ. To explore this further, it is necessary to compare angiographic findings in the two conditions (Table 17–7).

TABLE 17–6. Angiographic findings in amaurosis fugax: ipsilateral versus contralateral carotid artery.

	No. of cases		Angiographic findings					
			Normal (%)		Stenosis (%)		Occlusion (%)	
Study	IPS	CON	IPS	CON	IPS	CON	IPS	CON
Kollarits et al (24)	19	19	0	32	35	8	21	10
Sandok et al (15)	43	47	2	35	70	60	28	5
Combined data (15, 24)			2	34	72	59	26	7

IPS = ipsilateral; CON = contralateral.

TABLE 17–7. Angiographic findings in amaurosis fugax and cerebral transient ischemic attacks.

Study	Amaurosis fugax			Cerebral transient ischemic attacks		
	Normal	ISO	Other	Normal	ISO	Other
Pessin et al (7)	8	30	0	9	40	3
Eisenberg, Mani (9)	5	35	0	7	40	0
Harrison, Marshall (20)	8	39	8	32	33	27
Hurwitz et al (19)	22	68	0	73	103	0
Total	43	167	8	121	216	0
Percent	20	77	3	33	59	8

ISO = Wall irregularities, stenosis, and occlusions combined.

Disease of the carotid artery is more common in patients with amaurosis fugax, suggesting that episodic retinal ischemia usually is associated with such changes ($\chi^2 = 19.4$, $p < .0002$). By contrast, the pathogenesis of cerebral TIAs may be more heterogeneous, and embolism from the heart or aorta may account for a bigger proportion of cases. Patients who have both amaurosis fugax and hemispheric TIAs are particularly likely to have angiographic evidence of carotid disease (5) (Table 17–8). If these attacks are synchronous, carotid occlusion or hemodynamically tight stenosis prevails (25).

Retinal Infarction

Carotid stenosis is found more commonly in patients with TIAs than in patients with completed strokes (23). A comparable difference occurs between patients with transient retinal ischemia (amaurosis fugax) and those with completed retinal strokes with retinal infarction and persistent visual loss and field defects. An inspection of the findings of two studies of cases

TABLE 17–8. Angiographic findings according to clinical findings in 211 patients.

Angiographic finding	Retinal ischemia		Retinal and hemispheric ischemia		Hemispheric ischemia only — Ipsilateral bruit: With		Hemispheric ischemia only — Ipsilateral bruit: Without		Total	
	No.	%	No.	%	No.	%	No.	%	No.	%
Normal	6	32	8	27	6	21	71	53	91	43
Stenosis	4	21	10	33	17	61	17	13	48	23
Atheroma	6	32	4	13	4	14	34	25	48	23
Occlusion	3	16	8	27	1	4	6	5	18	9
Branch occlusion							6	5	6	3
Total	19	100	30	100	28	100	134	100	211	100

[From Harrison MJG, Marshall J, 1975 (5).]

TABLE 17–9. Angiographic findings in amaurosis fugax and retinal stroke.

	Angiographic findings				
	Normal	Wall irregularity	Stenosis	Occlusion	Other
Amaurosis fugax (5–12)					
No. of cases	76	74	117	40	11
Percentage	24	23	37	13	3
Retinal stroke (26, 27)					
No. of cases	36	15	28	9	1
Percentage	40	17	32	10	1

of CRA occlusion and branch occlusion (26,27) shows that normal angiograms are more likely with the completed lesions in parallel with stroke data. ($\chi^2 = 10.4$, $p < .03$). This has been thought to reflect a greater relevance of cardiac embolism in retinal stroke (26) (Table 17–9).

Intracranial Arterial Disease

As mentioned before, the published series have made little mention of the role of intracranial stenoses and occlusions in the pathogenesis of amaurosis fugax. Anecdotal reports have attested to the occasional association of amaurosis fugax with disease of both the carotid siphon and the ophthalmic artery (28,29). Data on 37 cases of isolated amaurosis fugax with no hemispheric symptoms are shown in Table 17–10. Extracranial occlusive disease clearly is the preponderant finding. When tandem lesions are found, it is difficult to decide which is the responsible abnormality.

TABLE 17–10. Extracranial and intracranial angiographic findings in amaurosis fugax.

Finding	No. of cases
Occlusion of cervical carotid artery	3
Stenosis of cervical carotid artery	19
Irregularity of cervical carotid artery	4
Total extracranial abnormalities	26
Occlusion of carotid siphon	0
Stenosis of carotid siphon	0
Irregularity of carotid siphon	1
Irregularity of cervical carotid artery and carotid siphon	2
Irregularity of cervical carotid artery and stenosis of carotid siphon	1
Abnormality of intracranial branches	1
Total intracranial plus extracranial abnormalities	5
Other changes (loops, kinks, dysplasia)	2
Normal angiograms	4
Total	37

Some observers have suggested that the siphon narrowing seen in some cases of tight carotid stenosis is an artifact due to flow conditions because the appearance of the intracranial vessel may revert to normal after successful endarterectomy at the bifurcation.

Thus, only two patients showed isolated intracranial abnormalities. In one of these, the irregularity of branches from the middle cerebral artery was of no relevance to the presenting symptoms. This small series suggests that intracranial disease is rarely the cause of amaurosis fugax.

Digital Subtraction Angiography

The safety of IV digital subtraction angiography (DSA) makes it attractive for the outpatient investigation of patients with amaurosis fugax. However, its safety advantage over arterial angiography must be set against the problem that an adequate study is not always obtained. Hedges et al (22) reported a series of 122 patients studied ophthalmologically who were referred for IV DSA. In 22, the studies failed to provide films of diagnostic quality. The adequacy of visualization in the carotid siphon and ophthalmic artery was not mentioned. Intravenous DSA is accepted in most centers as an appropriate screening test to be followed by intra-arterial studies (perhaps DSA) if a potentially operable lesion is seen or if the IV study is inadequate and the patient is a surgical candidate. Because stenoses of the siphon and the ophthalmic artery are not amenable to surgery, the use of arterial studies to identify such lesions when less invasive techniques have failed to reveal a carotid stenosis at the bifurcation probably is not justified.

Discussion and Conclusions

Angiographic studies of patients with amaurosis fugax, particularly those who are more than 50 years of age, have shown that atheromatous disease of the ipsilateral ICA is present in 75% of cases. This exceeds the prevalence seen in angiography of the carotid bifurcation in patients with cerebral hemispheric TIAs, strokes, or retinal strokes, and in a control group (tumour patients). The implication must be that the size and type of emboli that play a causative role in the genesis of amaurosis fugax most likely arise at the carotid bifurcation. The cause of hemispheric TIAs and strokes is more heterogeneous and more frequently involves cardiac embolism.

Disease of the carotid syphon and the ophthalmic artery may be responsible for comparable attacks but must be rare. Improved methods still are needed for detection of plaque rupture and the presence of mural thrombi in the carotid artery. Although the limits of angiography have not been reached, and computer-assisted three-dimensional reconstruction imaging looks promising, CT or MRI may be required for resolution of these problems.

References

1. Van Graefe A: Ueber Embolie der Arteria Centralis Retinae als Ursacht plötzhcher Erblindung. *Albrecht von Graefes Arch Klin Exp Ophthalmol* 1859;5:136–157.
2. Chiari H: Ueber des Verhalten des Terlurgswinbels der Carotis communis bei der endarteritis chronica deformans *Verh Dtsch Ges Pathol* 1905;9:326–330.
3. Croft RJ, Ellam LD, Harrison MJG: Accuracy of carotid angiography in the assessment of atheroma of the internal carotid artery. *Lancet* 1980;1:997–1000.
4. Harrison MJG, Marshall J: The finding of thrombus at carotid endarterectomy and its relationship to the timing of surgery. *Br J Surg* 1977;64:511–512.
5. Harrison MGJ, Marshall J: Indicators for angiography and surgery in carotid artery disease. *Br Med J* 1975;1:616–617.
6. Hooshmand H, Vines FS, Lee HM, et al: Amaurosis fugax: Diagnostic and therapeutic aspects. *Stroke* 1974;5:643–647.
7. Pessin MS, Duncan GW, Mohr JP, et al: Clinical and angiographic features of carotid transient ischemic attacks. *N Engl J Med* 1977;296:358–362.
8. Wilson LA, Ross Russell RW: Amaurosis fugax and carotid artery disease: Indications for angiography. *Br Med J* 1977;2:435–437.
9. Eisenberg RL, Mani RL: Clinical and arteriographic comparison of amaurosis fugax with hemispheric transient ischemic attacks. *Stroke* 1978;9:254–255.
10. Thiele BL, Young JV, Chikos PM, et al: Correlation of angiographic findings and symptoms in cerebrovascular disease. *Neurology* 1980;30:1041–1046.
11. Parkin PJ, Kendall BE, Marshall J, et al: Amaurosis fugax: Some aspects of management. *J Neurol Neurosurg Psychiatry* 1982;45:1–6.
12. Adams HP, Putman SF, Corbett JJ, et al: Amaurosis fugax: The results of arteriography in 59 patients. *Stroke* 1983;14:742–744.
13. Marshall J, Meadows SM: The natural history of amaurosis fugax. *Brain* 1986;91:419–433.
14. Ramirez-Lassepas M, Sandok BA, Burton RC: Clinical indicators of extracranial carotid artery disease in patients with transient symptoms. *Stroke* 1973;4:537–540.
15. Sandok BA, Trautmann JC, Ramirez-Lassepas M, et al: Clinical angiographic correlations in amaurosis fugax. *Am J Ophthalmol* 1974;79:137–142.
16. Lemak NA, Fields WS: The reliability of clinical prediction of extracranial artery disease. *Stroke* 1976;7:377–379.
17. Poole CMJ, Ross Russell RW: Mortality and stroke after amaurosis fugax. *J Neurol Neurosurg Psychiatry* 1985;48:902–905.
18. Mungas JE, Baker WH: Amaurosis fugax. *Stroke* 1977;8:232–235.
19. Hurwitz BJ, Heyman A, Wilkinson WE, et al: Comparison of amaurosis fugax and transient cerebral ischemia: A prospective clinical and arteriographic study. *Ann Neurol* 1985;18:698–704.
20. Harrison MJG, Marshall J: Arteriographic comparison of amaurosis fugax and hemispheric transient ischaemic attacks. *Stroke* 1985;16:795–797.
21. Bogousslavsky J, Hachinski VC, Barnett HJM: Causes cardiaques et artérielles de cécite monoculaire transitoire. *Rev Neurol* 1985;141:774–779.
22. Hedges TR, Giliberti OL, Margargal LE: Intravenous digital subtraction angiography and its role in ocular vascular disease. *Arch Ophthalmol* 1985;103:666–669.

23. Harrison MJG, Marshall J: Angiographic appearance of carotid bifurcation in patients with completed stroke, transient ischaemic attacks and cerebral tumour. *Br Med J* 1976;1:205–207.
24. Kollaritis CR, Lubow M, Hissong SM: Retinal stroke incidence of carotid Atheroma. *JAMA* 1972;222:1273–1275.
25. Harrison MJG: Pathogenesis, *in* Transient Ischaemic Attacks, Warlow CP, Mortis P (eds): New York, Marcel Dekker Inc, 1984, pp
26. Wilson LA, Warlow CP, Ross Russell RW: Cardiovascular disease in patients with retinal artery occlusion. *Lancet* 1979;1:292–294.
27. Sham HG, Brown GC, Goldberg RE: Digital subtraction carotid angiography and retinal arterial obstruction. *Ophthalmology* 1985;92:68–72.
28. Weinberger J, Bender AN, Yang WS: Amaurosis fugax associated with ophthalmic artery stenosis: Clinical simulation of carotid artery disease. *Stroke* 1980;11:290–293.
29. Kadir S, Roberson GH: Bracheocephalic atherosclerosis: A cause of amaurosis fugax. *Radiology* 1979;130:171–173.

CHAPTER 18

Aspirin Trials in the United States

William S. Fields and Noreen A. Lemak

By the late 1960s, information about the platelet and its role in thrombosis was emerging. By that time it already had been established that thromboembolism was an important pathogenetic mechanism in cerebrovascular disease. Therefore, a controlled clinical trial of antiplatelet therapy for cerebral ischemia was considered appropriate. A small conference was convened in Houston, Texas, in 1970, to discuss the scientific background for the implementation of such a trial. Participants included neurologists, hematologists, radiologists, vascular surgeons, clinical pharmacologists, and epidemiologists. The outcome of the conference was a book, *Aspirin, Platelets and Stroke: Background for a Clinical Trial* (1), published in 1970. Subsequently, with support from the National Heart, Lung, and Blood Institute, the Aspirin in Transient Ischemic Attacks (AITIA) Study was launched in 1972 and reported in 1977 (2) and 1978 (3). In the United States, this has been the only major clinical trial evaluating the effectiveness of aspirin versus placebo in patients with TIAs, either hemispheric or monocular.

It was logical that early investigations into platelet-active drugs focused on aspirin, a simple, relatively harmless, over-the-counter compound used by millions of people worldwide. Weiss, in 1971 (4), stated, "I think it is interesting to note that aspirin, which has been used extensively for treating minor headaches, is now being considered as prophylaxis against headaches of a more serious nature (strokes)." Clinicians were very surprised to learn at that time that they would have to apply to the US Food and Drug Administration for an investigational new drug number before they could conduct a controlled study of the use of their old friend aspirin for the prevention of stroke.

Although some anecdotal information had been available before, two reports of limited experience with aspirin for TIAs appeared in 1971. Harrison and colleagues (5) related that aspirin, at a dosage of 600 mg daily, had stopped frequent attacks of amaurosis fugax in two patients. Mundall et al (6) reported the disappearance of episodes of TMB in a patient who was treated with aspirin at a dosage of 600 mg four times daily. This patient also had thrombocytosis, and her platelets aggregated spontaneously in vitro. On aspirin therapy, aggregation returned to normal.

These reports stimulated the obvious need for a prospective, controlled trial that not only would be double-blind, with patients randomly allocated to either aspirin or placebo, but also would have well-defined criteria for eligibility, would control concomitant medications, monitor adherence and comorbidity, and include a sufficient number of cases to test the hypothesis adequately.

The AITIA Study

Organization

The AITIA study was described by a professor of biomathematics at Oxford as "a model example of careful organization and protocol design" (7). Nevertheless, partway through the study, the participants ran into formidable difficulties when the long-term financial support originally approved for the study was lost. This resulted in curtailment of admissions and a relatively short period of follow-up. According to statisticians, these two drawbacks forestalled the possibility of attaining a statistically significant differential in favor of aspirin for stroke because of the large numbers of patients and follow-up years required for detection of a substantial reduction in the frequency of stroke. However, the study did provide significance in favor of aspirin when death, cerebral or retinal infarction, and the occurrence of TIAs were considered together as end points.

The objective of the AITIA study was to determine whether oral administration of aspirin would protect against TIAs, cerebral or retinal infarcts, or stroke-related mortality. Ten institutions throughout the United States plus a Central Registry–Drug Distribution Center (see Appendix) participated, and patients were allocated randomly to aspirin (650 mg twice daily) or an identically appearing placebo. All tablets were film-coated so they would not dissolve in the mouth, and a bitter-tasting vegetable material (quassin) was added to disguise the familiar aspirin taste.

The study consisted of two simultaneous clinical trials for persons having carotid territory TIAs: one trial evaluated aspirin for medical management; the second evaluated aspirin as an adjunct to surgical reconstruction of the carotid artery. All patients had four-vessel arteriography before admission. If a patient had an accessible, appropriate carotid lesion, a clinical decision was made by the patient's physician to either enter the patient in the medical trial or advise surgical intervention before randomization.

The medical component consisted of 178 patients; 51% of these had appropriate lesions that caused greater than 50% narrowing of the artery or were ulcerated or both (occlusions not included). The surgical component consisted of 125 patients who had reconstructive operations and, five days after surgery, were allocated randomly to an aspirin or placebo regimen. Aspirin was not started before surgery for two reasons: (1) the surgeons believed it would interfere with hemostasis during the perioperative period, and (2) they also believed that the double-blind aspect of the study would be broken as they were confident they could recognize at surgery those persons on aspirin. Both of these objections have been proven false, and, by waiting until five days after surgery to admit and randomize patients, those individuals who had strokes or other complications during or after surgery were automatically excluded from consideration for admission.

Analyses of the data covered three major areas: baseline characteristics of the study population at the time of randomization; life-table analysis of stroke, stroke-related mortality and total mortality; and occurrence of TIAs within 6 months after treatment assignment.

Results

Baseline Comparisons

Twenty-one baseline characteristics of the medical and surgical groups are presented in Tables 18–1 and 18–2. In general, the randomization process produced homogeneous groups for the comparison of aspirin and placebo treatments.

Life-Table Analysis

The 24-month life table for the group treated medically is shown in Table 18–3. The end points are death from any cause, cerebral infarction, or retinal infarction. The differences in the cumulative event rates provide one measure of the efficacy of aspirin therapy.

In the medical group, 32 events (13 aspirin, 19 placebo) were reported. Three deaths (one intracerebral hemorrhage, two myocardial infarctions) occurred in the aspirin group, whereas eight deaths (one cancer, one cerebral infarct, two brainstem infarcts, four cardiovascular events) occurred in the placebo group.

Although the relative risk of an event was consistently greater than 1 throughout the 24-month period (Table 18–3); the results of the log-rank test for differences between the aspirin and placebo groups were not significant at the 5% level. Restriction of end-point events to fatal or nonfatal cerebral or retinal infarctions yielded a similar comparison. However, the data were consistent with a ⅓ reduction in risk of a fatal or nonfatal cerebral or retinal infarction by the use of aspirin.

The life-table analysis for the surgical group is shown in Table 18–4. Sixteen events were reported (eight aspirin, eight placebo). All eight of the end points among the placebo patients were brain infarcts; six of these occurred within 10 months after randomization. Among the aspirin-treated patients, six of the eight end points were cardiovascular deaths; four of these occurred after 11 months of follow-up.

TABLE 18–1. Medical group—number and percentage of patients with selected baseline findings, by treatment.

Demographic and historical data on admission	Treatment			
	Aspirin (n = 88)		Placebo (n = 90)	
	number	%	number	%
1. Age (years) at entry				
≥75	7	8.0	8	8.8
≥65	25	28.4	34	37.8
≥55	62	70.4	63	70.0
≥45	80	90.9	86	95.6
2. Sex - male	60	68.2	58	64.4
3. Race - nonwhite	22	25.0	22	24.4
4. Months from first TIA to entry				
≥24	17	19.3	6	6.7
≥12	21	23.9	9	10.0
5. Weeks from last TIA to entry				
≥8	7	8.0	6	6.7
≥4	21	23.9	27	30.0
6. TIA symptoms				
Single	26	29.5	36	40.0
Multiple	62	70.5	54	60.0
7. Patients reporting hemispheric events during month before randomization	68	77.3	67	74.4
8. History of amaurosis fugax and hemispheric events	13	14.8	3	3.3
9. History of hypertension	39	44.3	45	50.0
10. History of myocardial infarction	17	19.3	16	17.8
11. History of angina pectoris	13	14.8	12	13.3
12. History of peripheral vascular disease	12	13.6	4	4.4
13. History of diabetes	13	14.8	12	13.3
14. History of peptic ulcer	6	6.8	11	12.2
15. History of malignancy	4	4.5	2	2.2
16. History of renal disease	3	3.4	6	6.7
17. No history of the above (9–16) diseases	20	22.7	29	32.2
18. Cigarette smoking	48	54.5	45	50.0
19. Lesions appropriate to presenting symptoms	63	71.6	66	73.3
20. Deficit on admission	21	23.9	29	32.2
21. Previous platelet antiaggregate therapy	6	6.8	14	15.5

TIA = transient ischemic attack.
[From Fields et al, 1977 (2). Reproduced with permission of the publisher.]

Life-table analysis of end points for the surgical group did not reveal a statistically significant difference between the aspirin and placebo treatments over the 24-month period, but when nonstroke-related events were eliminated, there was a significant difference in favor of aspirin. However, too few patients were studied, and the follow-up was too short to infer that aspirin prevents stroke.

TABLE 18–2. Surgical group—number and percentage of patients with selected baseline findings, by treatment.

Demographic and historical data on admission	Treatment			
	Aspirin (*n* = 65)		Placebo (*n* = 60)	
	number	%	number	%
1. Age (years) at entry				
≥75	3	4.6	3	5.0
≥65	18	27.7	22	36.7
≥55	48	78.8	44	73.3
≥45	64	98.5	57	95.0
2. Sex - male	50	76.9	43	71.7
3. Race - nonwhite	5	7.7	3	5.0
4. Months from first TIA to entry				
≥24	2	3.1	4	6.7
≥12	9	13.8	10	16.7
5. Weeks from last TIA to entry				
≥8	7	10.8	7	11.7
≥4	28	43.1	24	40.0
6. TIA symptoms				
Single	17	26.2	17	28.3
Multiple	48	73.8	43	71.7
7. Hemispheric events during month before randomization	42	64.6	40	66.7
8. Amaurosis fugax plus hemispheric events	12	18.5	11	18.3
9. Hypertension	27	41.5	32	53.3
10. Myocardial infarction	9	13.8	13	21.7
11. Angina pectoris	11	16.9	7	11.7
12. Peripheral vascular disease	15	23.1	6	10.0
13. Diabetes	9	13.8	9	15.0
14. Peptic ulcer	5	7.7	5	8.3
15. Malignancy	5	7.7	1	1.7
16. Renal disease	3	4.6	3	5.0
17. No history of above (9–16) diseases	19	29.2	17	28.3
18. Cigarette smoking	34	52.3	28	46.7
19. Neurologic deficit on admission	23	35.4	21	35.0
20. Previous platelet antiaggregate therapy	6	9.2	9	15.0
21. Days from surgery to randomization				
≤7	39	60.0	42	70.0
≤13	57	87.7	54	90.0

TIA = transient ischemic attack.
[From Fields et al, 1978 (3). Reproduced with permission of the publisher.]

Occurrence of Transient Ischemic Attacks

The occurrence of TIAs was included in the evaluation of treatments as this was also part of the major objective. An outcome was considered unfavorable if the patient suffered a hard end point (death or cerebral or retinal infarction) during the first 6 months of follow-up, or if the number of TIAs during that period was greater than or equal to the number of

TABLE 18–3. Medical group—total mortality, nonfatal cerebral and retinal infarction for 178 patients by treatment modality summarized in an actuarial life table.

Months after randomization	Alive at start of interval		Events during interval		Withdrawals during interval		Proportion having event during interval		Cumulative proportion surviving event-free		Standard error	
	Aspirin	Placebo	Aspirin	Placebo	Aspirin	Placebo	Aspirin	Placebo	Aspirin	Placebo	Aspirin	Placebo
0–1	88	90	3	6	3	3	0.035	0.068	0.965	0.932	0.020	0.027
1–2	82	81	2	0	3	4	0.025	0.000	0.941	0.932	0.026	0.027
2–3	77	77	0	1	2	5	0.000	0.013	0.941	0.920	0.026	0.029
3–4	75	71	1	2	3	1	0.014	0.028	0.929	0.894	0.028	0.034
4–5	71	68	1	4	0	2	0.014	0.060	0.915	0.840	0.031	0.041
5–6	70	62	0	1	2	1	0.000	0.016	0.915	0.827	0.031	0.042
6–7	68	60	1	0	2	1	0.015	0.000	0.902	0.827	0.033	0.042
7–8	65	59	0	1	0	2	0.000	0.017	0.902	0.812	0.033	0.044
8–9	65	56	2	0	2	4	0.031	0.000	0.874	0.812	0.038	0.044
9–10	61	52	0	1	5	2	0.000	0.020	0.874	0.796	0.038	0.046
10–11	56	49	0	1	1	1	0.000	0.021	0.874	0.780	0.038	0.048
11–12	55	47	0	0	5	6	0.000	0.000	0.874	0.780	0.038	0.048
12–13	50	41	0	0	3	4	0.000	0.000	0.874	0.780	0.038	0.048
13–14	47	37	1	0	1	2	0.022	0.000	0.855	0.780	0.041	0.048
14–15	45	35	0	1	2	3	0.000	0.030	0.855	0.757	0.041	0.052
15–16	43	31	0	0	3	3	0.000	0.000	0.855	0.757	0.041	0.052
16–17	40	28	0	1	2	2	0.000	0.037	0.855	0.729	0.041	0.057
17–18	38	25	1	0	1	0	0.027	0.000	0.832	0.729	0.046	0.057
18–19	36	25	0	0	2	2	0.000	0.000	0.832	0.729	0.046	0.057
19–20	34	23	1	0	5	3	0.032	0.000	0.806	0.729	0.052	0.057
20–21	28	20	0	0	1	3	0.000	0.000	0.806	0.729	0.052	0.057
21–22	27	17	0	0	0	0	0.000	0.000	0.806	0.729	0.052	0.057
22–23	27	17	0	0	3	2	0.000	0.000	0.806	0.729	0.052	0.057
23–24	24	15	0	0	6	3	0.000	0.000	0.806	0.729	0.052	0.057
Total			13	19								

[From Fields et al, 1977 (2). Reproduced with permission of the publisher.]

TABLE 18–4. Surgical group—total mortality, nonfatal cerebral and retinal infarction for 125 patients by treatment modality summarized in an actuarial life table.

Months after randomization	Alive at start of interval		Events during interval		Withdrawals during interval		Proportion having event during interval		Cumulative proportion surviving event-free		Standard error	
	Aspirin	Placebo	Aspirin	Placebo	Aspirin	Placebo	Aspirin	Placebo	Aspirin	Placebo	Aspirin	Placebo
0–1	65	60	1	1	2	2	0.016	0.017	0.984	0.983	0.016	0.017
1–2	62	57	0	0	5	4	0.000	0.000	0.984	0.983	0.016	0.017
2–3	57	53	1	2	4	2	0.018	0.038	0.966	0.945	0.023	0.031
3–4	52	49	0	0	2	2	0.000	0.000	0.966	0.945	0.023	0.031
4–5	50	47	0	1	0	4	0.000	0.022	0.966	0.924	0.023	0.037
5–6	50	42	0	0	2	1	0.000	0.000	0.966	0.924	0.023	0.037
6–7	48	41	1	1	1	0	0.021	0.024	0.946	0.902	0.031	0.042
7–8	46	40	0	0	0	1	0.000	0.000	0.946	0.902	0.031	0.042
8–9	46	39	0	0	1	2	0.000	0.000	0.946	0.902	0.031	0.042
9–10	45	37	0	1	1	1	0.000	0.027	0.946	0.877	0.031	0.048
10–11	44	35	0	0	1	1	0.000	0.000	0.946	0.877	0.031	0.048
11–12	43	34	1	0	1	2	0.024	0.000	0.924	0.877	0.037	0.048
12–13	41	32	0	0	2	2	0.000	0.000	0.924	0.877	0.037	0.048
13–14	39	30	0	1	1	1	0.000	0.034	0.924	0.847	0.037	0.055
14–15	38	28	0	0	0	1	0.000	0.000	0.924	0.847	0.037	0.055
15–16	38	27	0	1	4	2	0.000	0.038	0.924	0.815	0.037	0.061
16–17	34	24	0	0	0	0	0.000	0.000	0.924	0.815	0.037	0.061
17–18	34	24	0	0	3	2	0.000	0.000	0.924	0.815	0.037	0.061
18–19	31	22	1	0	1	1	0.033	0.000	0.862	0.815	0.047	0.061
19–20	29	21	1	0	2	1	0.036	0.000	0.862	0.815	0.055	0.061
20–21	26	20	0	0	3	3	0.000	0.000	0.862	0.815	0.055	0.061
21–22	23	17	1	0	3	3	0.047	0.000	0.822	0.815	0.065	0.061
22–23	19	14	1	0	1	1	0.054	0.000	0.777	0.815	0.075	0.061
23–24	17	13	0	0	5	4	0.000	0.000	0.777	0.815	0.075	0.061
Total			8	8								

[From Fields et al, 1978 (3). Reproduced with permission of the publisher.]

TABLE 18–5. Medical group—clinical outcome 6 months after randomization by treatment group.

Outcome	Aspirin	Placebo
Unfavorable		
Death - cerebral infarction	0	2
Death - cardiovascular	1	4
Death - intracerebral hemorrhage	1	0
Nonfatal cerebral infarction	4	8
Retinal infarction	1	0
Excessive ratio of transient ischemic attacks	8	20
Favorable	63	43
Less than 6 months follow-up	10	13
Total	88	90

[From Fields et al, 1977 (2). Reprinted with permission of the publisher.]

TIAs reported for the 3 months before randomization. An approximate 50% reduction in reported TIAs during the 6-month period was required for a treatment to be judged as successful. All the remaining patients who completed 6 months of follow-up were classified as having favorable outcomes.

The results for the medical group are shown in Table 18–5. Substantially more cases (20 *v* 8) were classified as unfavorable by the criterion of excessive ratios of TIAs in the placebo compared with the aspirin group. Fifteen patients in the aspirin group and 34 in the placebo group had unfavorable outcomes, a statistically significant difference ($p < .01$).

The percentage of unfavorable cases also was analyzed by a treatment group for those variables in Table 18–1 that were distributed unequally at baseline. When all of these variables were considered simultaneously, the difference between the aspirin and placebo groups remained significant.

The results for the surgical group are shown in Table 18-6. Six patients

TABLE 18–6. Surgical group—clinical outcome 6 months after randomization by treatment group.

Outcome	Aspirin	Placebo
Unfavorable		
Death - cerebral infarction	0	1
Death - cardiovascular	1	0
Nonfatal cerebral infarction	1	3
Excessive ratio of transient ischemic attacks	4	8
Favorable	46	37
Less than 6 months follow-up	13	11
Total	65	60

[From Fields et al, 1978 (3). Reprinted with permission of the publisher.]

in the aspirin group and 12 in the placebo group had unfavorable outcomes. Although not significant at the 5% level, the result was consistent with the finding for the medical cohort. In general, surgical patients had a more favorable prognosis overall than the medical group.

Significance in favor of aspirin treatment was found mainly in patients with a history of multiple TIAs and, in the medical group, was most evident in those who had carotid lesions anatomically appropriate to the TIA symptoms.

Addendum

Because large multicenter trials are expensive, and because we think it is important to obtain as much information as possible from them, we recently reviewed the AITIA data and published an article providing information on several topics not previously reported (8). Among these was an analysis to determine whether patients with amaurosis fugax reponded differently to aspirin than patients with hemispheric TIAs did. Briefly, the effectiveness of aspirin was not significantly different between the two groups, and this finding was consistent in both the medical and surgical cohorts.

Comparison of AITIA Study with Other Major Trials of Aspirin for Cerebrovascular Disease

The three other clinical trials to be compared are the Canadian (9), the French (Accidents, Ischemiques Cerebraux Lies a l'Atherosclerose or AICLA) (10), and the Danish (11) trials. The Hospital Frequency Study (12) is not a clinical trial, but it is the largest American prospective follow-up of patients with TIAs (969 patients).

The Canadian, American, and French trials were different in terms of both the design and methods and the type of patients admitted, but their findings were similar. The Canadian Cooperative Study Group (CCSG) admitted patients over a period of 56 months; the AICLA, 38 months; and the AITIA, 31 months. Patients having vertebrobasilar TIAs only were not admitted to the AITIA trial but were accepted by the CCSG and the AICLA. Cerebral angiography was mandatory in the AITIA study but optional in the Canadian and French trials.

The Canadians had a study sample of 585 patients *v* 178 in the AITIA medical group and 125 in the AITIA surgical group. In the CCSG trial, patients were randomized to one of four regimens: sulfinpyrazone, 200 mg four times daily; aspirin, 325 mg four times daily; both drugs; or placebo. Because no synergistic interaction between aspirin and sulfinpyrazone was found and sulfinpyrazone was proven to be ineffective, it could be considered as a placebo. Consequently, for purposes of analysis, all patients were essentially on aspirin or placebo, and this more than doubled the number of patients available for analysis in the two groups. (Some clinicians were confused by this design because the aspirin-only takers experienced 26 strokes and deaths against 27.2 expected; the second number was generated by the log-rank life-table method of Peto et al (13) on the assumption that all four regimens are equally efficacious.)

Both the CCSG and AITIA trials supported the conclusion that aspirin is of benefit to patients with threatened stroke, although the benefit in the Canadian study was confined to men. In the AITIA trials, the difference in favor of aspirin was mainly in patients with an appropriate carotid lesion and in those with a history of multiple TIAs, but this finding was not apparent in the Canadian trial.

The AITIA published results did not contain separate analyses for men and women. However, in light of the conclusion reached by the CCSG, this data subsequently was analyzed separately for men and women. Overall, women had a greater proportion of favorable outcomes than men did, and the effect of aspirin did not differ according to sex.

The French trial also found that aspirin was beneficial to men and women equally. This double-blind, randomized clinical trial assigned 604 patients with atherothrombotic cerebral ischemic events to aspirin (1 g/day), placebo, or aspirin plus dipyridamole. It was concluded that aspirin had a significantly beneficial effect (in the prevention of cerebral infarction) that was not enhanced by the addition of dipyridamole; no sex difference in the response to aspirin was seen; and the incidence of myocardial infarction was reduced in the two treated groups.

There is no satisfactory explanation why aspirin would benefit men only—no known biochemical basis for a less impressive action in women. Aspirin blocks production of thromboxane A_2 and increases bleeding time equally in men and in women. Platelets from healthy men and women produce comparable amounts of thromboxane and aggregate comparably to a variety of agents, provided adjustments are made for sex differences in hemoglobin concentration, which create differences in plasma concentration of anticoagulants in vitro (14).

Data from the AITIA, CCSG, and Hospital Frequency Study tend to show that the natural history of cerebrovascular disease may be more benign for women than for men (15). Among patients taking placebo, the incidence of subsequent death or stroke was for men and women, respectively, 14% and 5% per year in the AITIA medical group and 12% and 6% per year in the Canadian study. In the Hospital Frequency Study, among patients not taking aspirin or anticoagulants, the prevalence of TIA, stroke, or death was 10% in men and only 3% in women. These figures suggest that TIAs do not present such a dire warning in women as in men, whatever the reason, and this possibility will present problems for trial designs in the future (15). Also, a study (16) from Evans County, Georgia, has shown that asymptomatic cervical arterial bruits are a significant risk factor for stroke and coronary death in men, but not in women. It seems possible, then, that the Canadian stroke study could have missed a benefit of aspirin in women because of the relatively few women in the trial and a relatively benign natural history of TIAs in women—a type II error (14).

Since 1974, six major controlled trials of aspirin therapy in patients who had had a myocardial infarction (17–22) have shown trends toward a decreased prevalence of death or recurrent infarction, but none have achieved statistical significance. A recent Veterans Administration Cooperative Study (23) selected unstable angina as the subject of a controlled trial because it is associated with transient, potentially reversible, limitations in coronary blood flow. In published results from that trial, it was concluded that the prevalence of death or acute myocardial infarction was 51% lower in the aspirin group than in the placebo group.

On the other hand, when cerebrovascular disease is considered, most of the major trials have shown a positive effect for aspirin. In addition to the results cited previously for the AITIA study, the Canadian Cooperative Study observed that men had a 48% reduction in stroke or death ($p < .005$). The French study showed a significant reduction ($p < .05$) of cerebral infarction (fatal or nonfatal) in the aspirin group compared with the placebo group. The Hospital Frequency Study, which was an analysis of risk factors in patients having TIAs, reported mortality rates at 1 year of 3% and 7% in the aspirin and control groups, respectively.

The only large study of cerebrovascular disease not showing fewer end points among aspirin takers was the Danish randomized trial. This study included 101 patients on aspirin and 102 on placebo. Many of these persons discontinued study medications before an end point occurred, leaving only 77 on aspirin and 71 on placebo. These numbers are too small for a satisfactory analysis of stroke end points, and a difference between aspirin and placebo treatments may have been missed (type II error). Also, the Danish report stated that patients referred for carotid surgery were excluded from the trial. This may have eliminated many persons with appropriate ulcerated lesions, a group for whom the AITIA trial found the benefit of aspirin most evident.

Although the AITIA study was the only one that listed retinal infarction as a hard end point and the only one known to investigate the group with amaurosis fugax separately, all of the major aspirin trials included patients who were having retinal as well as cerebral ischemic events.

Low-Dose Aspirin

Aspirin acetylates and inactivates cyclooxygenase and thus blocks the formation of thromboxane A_2 in platelets and the formation of prostacyclin (PGI_2) in vessel walls. Thromboxane A_2 is a potent vasoconstrictor and also causes aggregation of platelets, whereas prostacyclin antagonizes these actions. Many studies are underway to find the dose of aspirin that would inhibit synthesis of thromboxane A_2 without affecting prostacyclin production—a dose that may vary among patients. Also, it may be impossible to find a dose of aspirin low enough to have no effect on prostacyclin production; it has been reported that a single 20-mg dose of aspirin inhibits PGI_2 synthesis (24). Clinical trials have shown efficacy for both low and high doses of aspirin, and the exact dose may not be important (14), although lower doses would have fewer side effects and would achieve improved compliance from patients placed on a daily regimen. The problem of the correct dose is further complicated. Within 4 hours after oral low dose aspirin, enough new nonacetylated platelets circulate to make possible full platelet aggregation; only 10% of nonacetylated platelets restore the potential for normal function to the entire platelet population (25).

Salicylate has a half-life in plasma of two to three hours when taken in low doses, but aspirin has a half-life of only 15 minutes (26). Recent work (27) has shown that after four to seven days of 80 mg of slow-release aspirin daily, platelet cyclooxygenase activity is inhibited 91% to 96%; consequently, production of thromboxane A_2 is inhibited almost completely. It has been advised that until slow-release, low-dose aspirin is readily available, 20 mg of aspirin taken orally every four to six hours throughout the day (eg, quartered pediatric aspirin tablets) would give much more effective aspirin coverage than one standard aspirin tablet daily, without any risk of gastrointestinal disturbance (28).

Most aspirin trials in cerebrovascular disease have used dosages from 325 mg to 1,300 mg daily. If tolerable to the patient, it might be wise for physicians to continue advising such dosages until smaller amounts have been proven successful in large clinical trials. To our knowledge, no large trials using very low-dose aspirin in cerebrovascular disease are underway at the present time. Even the long-awaited United Kingdom TIA Study (2,400 patients), which was designed to help settle the low-dose question, used 300 mg/day.

Persantine-Aspirin Trial in Cerebral Ischemia

The clinical trials on the use of aspirin for medical management of patients with a history of transient cerebral ischemia made it apparent that many patients did not benefit from aspirin therapy. Physicians throughout the world had been using aspirin together with dipyridamole empirically, but no controlled trial in patients with stroke symptoms had tested whether that combination of drugs was more effective than aspirin alone.

The Persantine-Aspirin Trial, started in 1978, was designed to answer that question. Fifteen centers in the United States and Canada participated, and 890 individuals were admitted and allocated randomly to either aspirin (325 mg) plus placebo or aspirin plus Persantine (75 mg) four times daily. The results were reported in 1985 (29), and the conclusion was that dipyridamole contributed no additional benefit when prescribed with aspirin.

Although several factors may contribute to the occurrence of a hemispheric attack, amaurosis fugax episodes are thought to be caused almost exclusively by emboli. In the Persantine-Aspirin Trial, 74 subjects had had only amaurosis incidents before admission. It was of interest to determine whether the combination of aspirin and Persantine was more effective than aspirin alone in this small subgroup of persons. Analysis revealed a relative risk of 1.64 ($\chi^2 = 0.49$, $p = .52$), indicating that patients assigned to aspirin only were observed to have a 64% greater risk of having an end point than those taking aspirin plus Persantine. Because the associated *p*-value is relatively high, it cannot be concluded that this observed difference was due to the effect of Persantine rather than variation in the data.

Appendix

Participants in the AITIA Study

University of Texas Health Science Center at Houston—Central Registry	William S. Fields, MD, Coordinator
Institution	*Principal Investigator*
Bowman-Gray School of Medicine Winston-Salem, NC	Lawrence A. Pearce, MD
Indiana University Medical Center Indianapolis, IN	Mark L. Dyken, MD
New York University School of Medicine New York, NY	William K. Hass, MD
San Francisco General Hospital San Francisco, CA	Frank M. Yatsu, MD Barbara D. Barnes, MD
University of Alabama School of Medicine Birmingham, AL	James H. Halsey, MD
University of Cincinnati Medical School Cincinnati, OH	Charles P. Olinger, MD
University of Rochester School of Medicine Rochester, NY	Richard Satran, MD
University of Virginia School of Medicine Charlottesville, VA	George R. Hanna, MD
Veterans Administration Hospital San Francisco, CA	Wesley S. Moore, MD
Wayne State University School of Medicine Detroit, MI	Raymond B. Bauer, MD

Central Registry Staff

Noreen A. Lemak, MD
R. Denise Keating, MS
Paul W. Callen, BS
Mary M. Preslock, BS

Statistical Consultants

Ralph F. Frankowski, PhD
Robert J. Hardy, PhD
University of Texas
School of Public Health

References

1. Fields WS, Hass WK: *Aspirin, Platelets and Stroke: Background for a Clinical Trial*. St Louis, Warren H Green Inc, 1970.
2. Fields WS, Lemak NA, Frankowski RF, et al: Controlled trial of aspirin in cerebral ischemia. *Stroke* 1977;8:301–316.
3. Fields WS, Lemak NA, Frankowski RF, et al: Controlled trial of aspirin in cerebral ischemia: Part II. Surgical group. *Stroke* 1978;9:309–319.
4. Schindler PE Jr: *Aspirin Therapy*. New York, Walker & Co, 1978.
5. Harrison MJG, Marshall J, Meadows JC, et al: Effect of aspirin in amaurosis fugax. *Lancet* 1971;2:743–744.
6. Mundall J, Quintero P, von Kaulla K, et al: Transient monocular blindness and increased platelet aggregability treated with aspirin: A case report. *Neurology* 1971;21:402.
7. Armitage P: The statistician's comments on the AITIA study, in *The Challenge of Clinical Trials in Thrombosis*. New York, Schattauer Verlag, 1978.
8. Lemak NA, Fields WS, Gary HE Jr: Controlled trial of aspirin in cerebral ischemia: An addendum. *Neurology* 1986;36:705–712.
9. Canadian Cooperative Study Group: A randomized trial of aspirin and sulfinpyrazone in threatened stroke. *N Engl J Med* 1978;299:53–59.
10. Bousser MG, Eschwege E, Haguenau M, et al: "AICLA" controlled trial of aspirin and dipyridamole in the secondary prevention of atherothrombotic cerebral ischemia. *Stroke* 1983;14:5–14.
11. Sørensen PS, Pedersen H, Marquardsen J, et al: Acetyl-salicylic acid in the prevention of stroke in patients with reversible cerebral ischemic attacks: A Danish study. *Stroke* 1983;14:15–22.
12. Conneally PM, Dyken ML, Futty DE, et al: Cooperative study of hospital frequency and character of transient ischemic attacks: VIII. Risk factors. *JAMA* 1978;240:742–746.
13. Peto R, Pike MC, Armitage P, et al: Design and analysis of randomized clinical trials requiring prolonged observation of each patient: II. Analysis and examples. *Br J Cancer* 1977;35:1–39.
14. Eichner ER: Platelets, carotids and coronaries: Critique on antithrombotic role of antiplatelet agents, exercise, and certain diets. *Am J Med* 1984;77:513–523.
15. Sherry S: Clinical aspects of antiplatelet therapy. *Semin Hematol* 1985;22:125–134.
16. Heyman A, Wilkinson WE, Heyden S, et al: Risk of stroke in asymptomatic persons with cervical arterial bruits: A population study in Evans County, Georgia. *N Engl J Med* 1980;302:838–841.

17. Elwood PC, Cochrane AL, Burr ML, et al: A randomized controlled trial of acetyl salicylic acid in the secondary prevention of mortality from myocardial infarction. *Br Med J* 1974;1:436–440.
18. Coronary Drug Project Research Group: Aspirin in coronary heart disease. *J Chronic Dis* 1976;29:625–642.
19. Breddin K, Loew D, Lechner K, et al: Secondary prevention of myocardial infarction: Comparison of acetylsalicylic acid, phenprocoumon and placebo: A multicenter two-year prospective study. *Thromb Haemost* 1979;41:225–236.
20. Elwood PC, Sweetnam PM: Aspirin and secondary mortality after myocardial infarction. *Lancet* 1979;2:1313–1315.
21. Aspirin Myocardial Infarction Study Research Group: A randomized, controlled trial of aspirin in persons recovered from myocardial infarction. *JAMA* 1980;243:661–669.
22. Persantine-Aspirin Reinfarction Study Research Group: Persantine and aspirin in coronary heart disease. *Circulation* 1980;62:449–461.
23. Lewis HD Jr, Davis JW, Archibald DG, et al: Protective effects of aspirin against acute myocardial infarction and death in men with unstable angina: Results of a Veterans Administration cooperative study. *New Engl J Med* 1983;309:396–403.
24. Davi G, Custro N, Novo S, et al: The effect of two low doses of aspirin on whole blood thromboxane and prostacyclin generation in healthy subjects. *Thromb Haemost* 1982;50:669–670.
25. Cerskus AL, Ali M, Davies BJ, et al: Possible significance of functional platelets in a population of aspirin-treated platelets *in vitro* and *in vivo*. *Thromb Res* 1980;18:389–397.
26. Goodman LS, Gilman AG, Gilman A: *The Pharmacological Basis of Therapeutics*, ed 6. London, Baillière Tindall, 1980, p 694.
27. Jakubowski JA, Stampfer MJ, Vaillancourt R, et al: Cumulative antiplatelet effect of low-dose enteric coated aspirin. *Br J Haematol* 1985;60:635–642.
28. Eastham RD: The low dose aspirin controversy solved at last? *Br Med J* 1985;291:738–739.
29. American-Canadian Co-operative Study Group: Persantine aspirin trial in cerebral ischemia: Part II. Endpoint results. *Stroke* 1985;16:406–415.

CHAPTER 19

Antithrombotic Therapy in Patients with Transient Ischemic Attacks or Amaurosis Fugax

Laurence A. Harker

The indications for the clinical use of antithrombotic agents are established for a few cerebral vascular disorders. However, for many cerebral ischemic settings, the use of these agents is not entirely clear despite extensive, basic, experimental animal and clinical studies. This uncertainty is, in part, explained by the lack of knowledge of the precise pathogenesis of many cerebral vascular syndromes, by the lack of suitable pharmacologic agents for definitive clinical testing, and by the inconclusive results obtained in some of the clinical studies (1,2).

The evaluation of antithrombotic therapy in cerebrovascular ischemia is difficult because of limited availability of suitable patients and the low frequency of the two clinically important outcome events: stroke and death. Therefore, large-scale multicenter trials with long-term follow-up are necessary. Basic principles and issues considered to be of fundamental importance in the evaluation of clinical trials include specific inclusion-exclusion criteria, randomization, stratification for important prognostic factors, double-blind administration of therapy, assessment of drug compliance and contamination, appropriate and well-defined outcome events, assessment of adverse effects, and the use of sound statistical methods (1–4).

Kinetic studies (5) using radioactively labeled platelets and fibrinogen have indicated that arterial thrombosis is characterized by selective platelet consumption that can be interrupted by inhibitors of platelet function but not by heparin, whereas venous thrombosis produces combined and equivalent consumption of both platelets and fibrinogen that is blocked by anticoagulant therapy but not by drugs that modify platelet function. Some thrombotic disorders, such as those associated with prosthetic heart valves, may require a combination of platelet-active agents and anticoagulant drugs to achieve complete antithrombotic efficacy.

Antithrombotic therapy has been evaluated in several cerebral vascular thrombotic disorders, from TIAs to completed strokes. Because both platelets and the coagulation mechanisms are involved in the genesis of arterial thrombi, both platelet-inhibitory drugs and conventional anticoagulants have been evaluated for prevention and treatment.

Pathogenesis

Considerable evidence has indicated that platelet thromboemboli may be implicated in transient cerebral ischemia, including amaurosis fugax and TIAs. Fisher (6) and others (7,8) have reported that white bodies may pass through the retinal arterial circulation in patients during episodes of amaurosis fugax. Gunning et al (9) observed platelet-fibrin thromboemboli in the cerebral and retinal blood vessels at autopsy in a series of patients with cerebral and retinal ischemia associated with atherosclerotic lesions. In addition, platelet-containing material often has been observed in the ulcerative lesions of extracranial vessels at the time of surgery.

In addition to platelet-fibrin emboli, emboli of atheromatous debris may cause cerebral ischemia. Bright plaques in the retinal circulation in patients with carotid disease and stroke have been described (10,11). However, a complete understanding of how these emboli are formed and what conditions are essential for their formation still is lacking. Experimental models have provided support for the concept that the endothelium must be damaged to be thrombogenic. Traumatic lesions in the proximal middle cerebral artery of rats have produced platelet-fibrin emboli that lodged in small peripheral branch arteries (12).

The prostaglandin system and its metabolic products may contribute to the ischemia produced by platelet-fibrin emboli (13, 14). Most cells are able to produce prostaglandins. All cells oxidize arachnidonic acid via a cyclooxygenase to an intermediate cyclic endoperoxide. In platelets, thromboxane A_2 is produced from the endoperoxides by thromboxane synthetase. Thromboxane A_2 is the most potent naturally occurring vasoconstrictor and platelet aggregator known. It has a half-life of approximately 32 seconds at 37°C. Thromboxane A_2 rapidly is converted to thromboxane B_2, an inactive metobolite. In endothelial cells, the cyclic endoperoxides are converted to prostacyclin. Prostacyclin is the most potent vasodilator and inhibitor of platelet aggregation known. Prostacyclin is unstable in aqueous solution, with a half-life of two minutes. It is metabolized rapidly to 6-keto-$PGF_{1\alpha}$.

As originally suggested by Moncada and Vane (15), vascular patency may be maintained, in part, by a balance between the proaggregatory and vasconstrictor forces of thromboxane on the one hand and the antiaggregatory and vasdilatory action of prostacyclin on the other. A disruption of this balance in favor of thromboxane could lead to an increased thrombotic tendency and vasoconstriction. At a site of stenosis, plaque disruption and ulceration may produce vascular narrowing by both formation and embolization of thrombus together with thromboxane A_2-mediated vasoconstriction.

Approximately 25% to 40% of patients with TIA will develop cerebral infarction within 5 years of the initial event (16–19). The period of greatest risk is the first year after the onset of TIA. Recurrent TIAs carry a particularly poor prognosis for the development of cerebral infarction. After the first year, the rate of stroke occurrence is approximately 5% per year, which is at least five times as great as the stroke rate in the general population of similar age. Most patients who have TIAs die of vascular causes, one third of them with stroke and two thirds with other vascular diseases, primarily myocardial infarction.

Whether the ulcerative nonstenotic plaque is a nidus for embolus formation is uncertain. A review of the pathology of carotid plaques from the side appropriate to focal cerbral symptoms revealed no instances of isolated plaque. Rather, all symptomatic plaques were associated with either intramural plaque disruptions, greater than 70% stenosis of the vessel lumen, or both. Furthermore, when previously asymptomatic plaques became symptomatic, it was always in the presence of progression of the plaque (16,17).

It is now established that atherosclerotic lesions of arteries supplying the brain give rise to microthromboemboli that produce amaurosis fugax, TIAs, and stroke (16,17). Two thirds of the angiographically demonstrable atherosclerotic lesions are extracranial and therefore surgically accessible, and most of these are located at the carotid bifurcation. Present evidence suggests that carotid endarterectomy reduces the risk of TIAs and stroke, although no controlled data are available to prove this claim. Nevertheless, carotid endarterectomy is recommended for selected patients with symptoms of cerebral ischemia and angiographic abnormalities of the extracranial arterial supply to the brain. Because the endarterectomy procedure involves surgical removal of the arteriosclerotic intimal lesion, platelets are deposited rapidly on the nonendothelial subintimal carotid surface. Although acute occlusion with thrombus is rare after carotid endarterectomy, platelet-dependent intimal thickening predictably occurs because of proliferation smooth muscle cells, probably mediated through the chemotactic and mitogenic properties of platelet-derived growth factor (20). Consequently, in about 20% of patients undergoing carotid endarterectomy, clinically detectable restenosis may develop during the year after surgery, thereby compromising the surgery and sometimes requiring reoperation. Some strategy to reduce the process of restenosis would be beneficial to patients who have had endarterectomies.

Drug Actions

Aspirin

Aspirin, a nonsteroidal antiinflammatory agent, potently and irreversibly inactivates platelet cyclooxygenase by acetylation (15,21). Although all of aspirin's antithrombotic effects have been attributed to this blockade of formation of thromboxane A_2 by platelets, evidence exists of antithrombotic effects independent of aspirin's inactivation of cyclooxygenase (22).

At present, interest in aspirin therapy for vascular disease is intense.

Aspirin has been shown in well-designed clinical trials to be beneficial in at least five and possibly six clinical settings relevant to cardiovascular disease:

1. Reduction of thromboembolic complications associated with artificial heart valves (23,24)
2. Prevention of stroke and death in patients with TIAs (18,19)
3. Decrease in thrombotic occlusion of arteriovenous Silastic cannula in uremic patients undergoing hemodialysis (25)
4. Reduction in acute myocardial infarction (AMI) and cardiac death in patients with unstable angina (26,27)
5. Possibly, a decrease in the secondary prevention of AMI (28)
6. In one study (which requires confirmation), increase in the patency of saphenous vein coronary bypass grafts (29)

These reported benefits of aspirin require some comment. First, the antithrombotic effects of aspirin in patients with prosthetic mitral valves is evident in association with oral anticoagulant therapy, and this combination is associated with an unacceptably high frequency of gastrointestinal bleeding (30). Second, the capacity of low doses of aspirin to reduce the thrombotic complications of arteriovenous cannulas was shown in patients undergoing long-term hemodialysis, who thus had associated significant platelet dysfunction (25). It cannot be assumed that a similar dose would be antithrombotic in the absence of associated platelet dysfunction. Third, the pathogenetic mechanisms of TIA and unstable angina may not be thrombotic but vasospastic. Thus, the benefits of aspirin in those clinical settings may reflect blockade of thromboxane A_2-mediated vasospasm rather than inhibition of platelet-dependent thrombus formation.

Sulfinpyrazone

Sulfinpyrazone is a urocosuric agent with weak antiinflammatory properties. Its mechanism of antithrombotic action remains to be defined (22,31), although a protective effect of reducing endothelial injury has been postulated (32). The combination of aspirin and sulfinpyrazone may have a synergistic antithrombotic effect (22).

Sulfinpyrazone reduces occlusion of arteriovenous cannulas (33) and early occlusion of coronary artery saphenous vein grafts (34). Because the claimed benefit in reducing mortality in the secondary prevention of AMI remains controversial (35,36), no recommendations can be made about that possible indication.

Dipyridamole

Dipyridamole, a coronary vasodilator with weak inhibitory effects on phosphodiesterase activity (1–4,22) appears to increase inhibitory cyclic adenosine monophosphate (cAMP) levels in platelets by elevating blood adenosine levels via the blockade of adenosine uptake by red cells and vascular wall cells (37,38). Aspirin potentiates the antithrombotic effects of dipyridamole in the baboon by mechanisms independent of platelet inactivation of platelet cyclooxygenase (22).

Dipyridamole decreases thromboembolism in patients with artificial heart valves (in combination with anticoagulants) (39). Dipyridamole in association with aspirin appears to be more effective than aspirin alone in reducing the progression of peripheral vascular disease (40). When used in combination with aspirin, it has been shown to decrease coronary mortality and nonfatal myocardial infarction in patients who previously have sustained an AMI (41), to reduce both early and late occlusion of coronary artery saphenous vein grafts (42, 43), and to preserve renal function in patients with membranoproliferative glomerulonephritis (44). The benefit of adding dipyridamole to aspirin in these latter settings remains to be established.

Ticlopidine

Of the antiplatelet drugs currently available for clinical investigation, ticlopidine is one of the most potent and has several important theoretical advantages over existing drugs (45). Ticlopidine is unrelated chemically to other antiplatelet drugs and appears to have a unique, albeit unknown, mechanism of action. It is neither a prostaglandin synthesis inhibitor nor a cAMP-phosphodiesterase inhibitor. Several reports have indicated that ticlopidine may act on the platelet membrane to alter its reactivity to activating stimuli. The broad spectrum of antiplatelet activity of ticlopidine, the prolonged duration of suppressed platelet function, and the apparently novel mechanism of action set ticlopidine apart from currently available antiplatelet agents. The fact that ticlopidine does not inhibit PGI_2 synthesis in the arterial wall but can still inhibit aggregation induced by thromboxane A_2 and prostaglandin endoperoxide gives it a theoretical advantage over aspirin. A number of important, well-designed multicenter trials are in progress (46,47).

Suloctidil

Suloctidil, a peripheral vasodilator without a well-defined antithrombotic mechanism (48), normalizes platelet survival in patients with prosthetic heart valves. In a well-designed clinical trial, suloctidil has shown no benefit in reducing stroke and death in patients with a recent thromboembolic stroke (49).

Heparin

Heparin is a family of mucopolysaccharides with molecular weights between 6×10^3 and 14×10^3 daltons and a plasma half-life of 30 to 60 minutes when administered IV. Its anticoagulant activity is mediated through binding to antithrombin III (AT III), thereby facilitating the inactivation of thrombin; factors VIIIa, IXa, Xa, and XIa; and plasmin (50). Significantly, AT III deficiency can be associated with venous thrombosis, arterial thrombotic occlusions, or intracerebral arterial thrombosis (51). Heparin therapy is monitored by means of the activated partial thromboplastin time.

Oral Anticoagulants

Vitamin K antagonists act as competitive inhibitors of vitamin K, blocking the final carboxylation step in the synthesis of the vitamin K–dependent (extrinsic pathway) clotting factors II, VII, IX, and X and proteins C and S (52,53). Coumarin therapy is monitored by means of the prothrombin time. Approximately 1 week or more of coumarin administration is required to achieve a therapeutically significant reduction of the vitamin K factors.

Coumarins have been used in long-term (3 to 6 months) treatment of thromboemboli with presumed cardiac sources. Their usefulness in high-grade stenosis of the extracranial and intracranial arteries supplying the brain has not been established by controlled trials (54,55).

Trials with Antiplatelet Agents in Patients with Transient Ischemic Attacks or Amaurosis Fugax

Evans (56) carried out a double-blind crossover study in which each of 20 patients with amaurosis fugax received either sulfinpyrazone or an identical-appearing placebo and then after 6 weeks was crossed over to the alternative therapy for a further 6 weeks. A clinically important improvement for individual patients was defined as a 50% reduction in the number of attacks as compared with the 6-week period immediately before the trial. Whereas five patients showed improvement on both treatments, and two did not improve on either, the remaining 13 patients all showed significant improvement on sulfinpyrazone therapy, but none on placebo. The difference was statistically highly significant. The study was limited because it did not include the more important long-term end points of stroke and death. In addition, in current long-term, multicenter trials of transient cerebral ischemia, no single center has produced 20 cases of amaurosis fugax in 4 years of study. This shortcoming therefore raises some questions about the accuracy of the diagnosis in Evans's study.

A study by Fields et al (18) was designed to test, in a double-blind manner, the effectiveness of aspirin in the prophylaxis of cerebrovascular ischemic events. Only patients with carotid system TIAs were admitted to the study, and they were allocated randomly to receive either 650 mg aspirin twice a day or an identical-appearing placebo. The primary outcome was defined as stroke-free survival with reduced TIAs during the first 6 months of follow-up. Among the 178 patients studied, favorable outcomes were reported in 81% of the aspirin-treated group, compared with 56% in the placebo control group ($p < .01$). When only stroke or death was considered as the composite outcome event, the beneficial effect of aspirin was confined to men (47% risk reduction *v* 0% risk reduction for women). When TIAs were included as part of the outcome, and results were classified as favorable or unfavorable, no significant sex difference was seen in the observed response.

Fields et al (57) carried out a second study to assess the effect of aspirin in 125 patients who had had operations of the carotid artery after episodes of TIA. These patients were assigned randomly to aspirin, 300 mg four times daily, or a placebo. Favorable outcomes, defined as stroke-free survival with reduced TIAs during the first 6 months, occurred in 89% of the aspirin-treated group and in 76% of the placebo-treated group. Aspirin had no significant effect either on overall mortality rate or on the frequency of cerebral or retinal infarctions. When deaths that were not stroke-related were eliminated from this analysis, an appreciable observed reduction in the frequency of fatal or nonfatal cerebral and retinal infarctions occurred in the aspirin-treated group compared with the placebo-treated group. However, because of the small number of patients and the short period of follow-up, these results by themselves did not establish convincingly that aspirin was effective in preventing cerebral infarction.

The Canadian Cooperative Study Group (19) carried out a double-blind, randomized, multicenter study to assess the relative efficacy of aspirin and sulfinpyrazone, singly and in combination, in the reduction of continuing TIAs, stroke, or death. Five hundred and eighty-five patients (70% of them men) who had had one or more cerebral or retinal ischemic attacks within 3 months before entry were followed for an average of 26 months. The four treatment regimens were placebo, aspirin (325 mg four times daily), sulfinpyrazone (200 mg four times daily), and aspirin plus sulfinpyrazone at the same dosage. For the entire group, aspirin reduced the risk of continued TIA, stroke, or death by 19% ($p < .05$). If only stroke or death was considered, aspirin reduced the risk by 31% ($p < .05$). No statistically significant reduction in these events attributable to sulfinpyrazone was found. A striking difference was found between men and women in their therapeutic response to aspirin ($p = .003$). In terms of stroke or death, men had a 48% reduction of risk, whereas women had no observable benefit.

Guiraud-Chaumeil et al (58) randomly allocated 440 patients with TIAs to one of three treatment groups, all of which received dihydroergocornine (4.5 g daily). One group received nothing else, one group received aspirin also (300 mg three times daily), and the the third group received aspirin (300 mg three times daily) plus dipyridamole (50 mg three times daily). The investigators in this single-center, unblinded trial concluded that differences in outcomes were not statistically significant. However, although the actuarial curves for the outcomes of stroke or death were very similar for the aspirin and aspirin-plus-dipyridamole groups, they were both appreciably better than for the group who received dihydroergocornine alone.

Sorensen et al (59) recently published the results of a trial involving 203 patients, 148 men and 55 women, who during the last month before admission had experienced at least one reversible cerebral ischemic attack of less than 72 hours' duration. The patients were assigned randomly to treatment with either aspirin (two 500-mg tablets once daily) or a placebo and followed for an average of 25 months. The frequency of stroke or death was 21% in the aspirin group and 17% in the placebo group. Moreover, the occurrence of TIAs during the treatment period also was not reduced by aspirin treatment. Fewer myocardial infarctions were observed in the aspirin group (5.9%) than in the placebo group (13.7%); this difference, however, also was not statistically significant ($p = .10$). This study was not of sufficient size to exclude the possibility that aspirin treatment could be truly effective.

Bousser et al (60) carried out a controlled cooperative trial in France to evaluate the effect of aspirin given singly or in combintion with dipyridamole in the secondary prevention of cerebral ischemic accidents. A total of 604 patients with atherothrombotic cerebral ischemic events (transient, 16%, or minor stroke, 84%) referrable either to the carotid or to the vertebrobasilar circulation were entered into the double-blind, randomized clinical trial to compare the effects of aspirin (325 mg three times daily) or aspirin (325 mg three times daily) in combination with dipyridamole (75 mg three times daily) and were followed up for 3 years. Randomization produced comparable treatment groups; adherence to the protocol and drug compliance were good. However, side effects, particularly symptoms of peptic ulcer and hemorrhagic events, were significantly more frequent ($p < .03$) in the two treatment groups who received aspirin. At the end of the study, the number of fatal and nonfatal cerebral infarctions was 31 in the placebo group, 17 in the aspirin group, and 18 in the combination aspirin-dipyridamole group, corresponding to cumulative rates of 18% in the placebo group and 10.5% in each of the two active treatment groups. A statistically significant difference at the 6% level was present between placebo and combination aspirin-dipyridamole and between placebo and aspirin. Clearly, no difference between aspirin and aspirin plus dipyridamole was observed. Among other diseases occurring during the trial, the only significant difference concerned myocardial infarction, which was less frequent in the two treated groups ($p < .05$). Interestingly, subgroup analysis failed to show a significant sex difference in the efficacy of aspirin.

Recently, the American-Canadian Cooperative Study Group (61) has completed a multicenter, randomized trial to determine if the combination of aspirin (325 mg four times daily) plus dipyridamole (75 mg four times daily) offered any benefit over aspirin (325 mg four times daily) alone. A total of 890 patients with a history of recent carotid territory TIAs were followed up for an average of 25 months, and the outcomes in the two groups were almost identical.

In a recently completed study of TIA patients in the United Kingdom (62), the effect of different aspirin doses was compared. In this study, 2,449 patients with TIAs were allocated randomly to a placebo, 300 mg aspirin daily, or 300 mg aspirin four times daily. The preliminary results showed that stroke and death were reduced by aspirin therapy, without evidence for a differential effect of dose on the outcome. The full report has not been published yet.

The Ticlopidine-Aspirin Stroke Study (47) is an ongoing, multicenter study to evaluate the efficacy of ticlopidine *v* aspirin in the prevention of ischemic stroke. Study patients have histories of one or more attacks of reversible ischemic neurologic disease or of a minor stroke followed by a greater than 80% functional recovery within 3 months before trial entry (currently 82% have transient cerebral or retinal ischemia as the qualifying event). It is planned to enter 3,000 patients over a 3-year recruitment period with a 2- to 5-year follow-up. Results are expected to be reported in 1988.

Anticoagulant Therapy in Patients with Transient Ischemic Attacks or Amaurosis Fugax

The role of anticoagulation in TIAs or amaurosis fugax is poorly defined. Ten clinical trials have evaluated the effect of anticoagulants on cerebral TIAs. Four of these trials were randomized, and six were nonrandomized. The four prospective, randomized trials involved a small number of patients and short duration of follow-up (63–66). Only one of the studies was double-blind. The results of the studies indicated that anticoagulants have no effect on the prevalence of stroke or death. However, in two of the studies, the frequency of recurrent TIA was reduced.

The results of the nonrandomized studies showed that mortality was not reduced in the anticoagulant treatment group, although a decrease in the frequency of stoke in the treated group was reported.

Thus, the evidence is unconvincing that anticoagulant therapy is beneficial in patients with TIAs. The evidence that anticoagulants are beneficial in reducing the frequency of recurrent TIAs is equivocal (67). Furthermore, the morbidity and mortality associated with the long-term use of anticoagulants should be considered when assessing the value of this form of treatment in the long term.

Conclusions

Aspirin has been shown convincingly to reduce stroke or death in men with TIAs and possibly may be beneficial to women also. A single aspirin once a day appears to be as efficacious as 1.0 to 1.5 g of aspirin a day.

Because the gastrointestinal side effects are related directly to dose, the lower dose is recommended. No additional benefit has been shown by combining aspirin with dipyridamole and probably not with sulfinpyrazone. No benefit has been found for using sulfinpyrazone, dipyridamole, or suloctidil alone in the prevention of stroke or death in patients with cerebrovascular disease. Results with ticlopidine are pending. No convincing evidence indicates that anticoagulants are beneficial in reducing stroke, death, or transient events in these patients. The results of the trials with aspirin do not discriminate between platelet thrombi or vasospasm as the underlying mechanism of TIA because aspirin-inactivated cyclooxygenase would block thromboxane-mediated vasoconstriction also.

Acknowledgment. This work was supported in part by research grants (HL 31950 and RR00833) from the National Institutes of Health. Manuscript No. 4721-BCR from the Research Institute of Scripps Clinic and Research Foundation, La Jolla, California.

References

1. Genton E, Gent M, Hirsh J, et al: Platelet-inhibiting drugs in the prevention of clinical thrombotic disease. *N Engl J Med* 1975;293:1174–1178.
2. Harker LA: Antiplatelet drugs in the management of patients with thrombotic disorders. *Sem Thromb Hemost* 1986;12:134–155.
3. Braunwald E, Friedewald WT, Furberg CD (eds): Proceedings of the workshop on platelet-active drugs in the secondary prevention of cardiovascular events. *Circulation* 1980;62(supplV):1–135.
4. Weiss HJ: *Platelets: Pathophysiology and Antiplatelet Drug Therapy*. New York: Alan R. Liss Inc, 1982, p 1.
5. Harker LA, Slichter SJ: Platelet and fibrinogen consumption in man. *N Engl J Med* 1972;287:999–1005.
6. Fisher CM: Observations of the fundus oculi in transient monocular blindness. *Neurology* 1959;9:333–347.
7. Ross Russell RW: Observations on the retinal blood vessels in monocular blindness. *Lancet* 1961;2:1422–1428.
8. Ashby M, Oakley N, Lorentz I, et al: Recurrent transient monocular blindness. *Br Med J* 1963;2:894–897.
9. Gunning AJ, Pickering GW, Robb-Smith AHT, et al: Mural thrombosis of the internal carotid artery and subsequent embolism. *Q J Med* 1964;33:155–195.
10. Hollenhorst RW: Significance of bright plaques in the retinal arterioles. *JAMA* 1961;178:23–29.
11. Beal MF, Williams RS, Richardson EP, et al: Cholesterol embolism as a cause of transient ischemic attacks and cerebral infarction. *Neurology* 1981;31:860–865.
12. Denny-Brown D: Recurrent cerebrovascular episodes. *Arch Neurol* 1960;2:194–210.
13. Hamberg M, Svensson J, Samuelsson B: Thromboxanes: A new group of biologically active compounds derived from prostaglandin endoperoxides. *Proc Natl Acad Sci USA* 1975;72:2994–2998.

14. Moncada S, Gryglewski R, Bunting S, et al: An enzyme isolated from arteries transforms prostaglandin endoperoxides to an unstable substance that inhibits platelet aggregation. *Nature* 1976;263:663–665.
15. Moncada S, Vane JR: Arachidonic acid metabolites and the interactions between platelets and blood-vessel walls. *N Engl J Med* 1979;300:1142–1147.
16. Turpie AG, Hirsh J: Thromboembolic cerebral vascular diseases, in Kwaan HC, Bowie EJW (eds): *Thrombosis*. Philadelphia: WB Saunders Co, 1982, pp 154–167.
17. Whisnant JP, Matsumoto N, Elveback LR: Transient cerebral ischemic attacks in a community: Rochester, MN, 1955 through 1969. *Mayo Clin Proc* 1973;48:194–198.
18. Fields WS, Lemak NA, Frankowski RF, et al: Controlled trial of aspirin in cerebral ischemia. *Stroke* 1977;8:301–316.
19. The Canadian Cooperative Study Group: A randomized trial of aspirin and sulfinpyrazone in threatened stroke. *N Engl J Med* 1978;299:53–59.
20. Friedman RJ, Stemerman MB, Wenz B, et al: The effect of thrombocytopenia on experimental arteriosclerotic lesion formation in rabbits: Smooth muscle cell proliferation and re-endothelialization. *J Clin Invest* 1977;60:1191–1201.
21. Majerus PW (1983) Arachidonate metabolism in vascular disorders. *J Clin Invest* 1983;72:1521–1525.
22. Hanson SR, Harker LA, Bjornsson TD: Effects of platelet-modifying drugs on arterial thromboembolism in baboons: Aspirin potentiates the antithrombotic actions of dipyridamole and sulfinpyrazone by mechanism(s) independent of platelet cyclooxygenase inhibition. *J Clin Invest* 1985;75:1591–1599.
23. Dale J, Myhre E, Storstein O, et al: Prevention of arterial thromboembolism with acetylsalicylic acid: A controlled clinical study in patients with aortic ball valves. *Am Heart J* 1977;94:101–111.
24. Altman R, Boullon F, Rouvier J, et al: Aspirin and prophylaxis of thromboembolic complications in patients with substitute heart valves. *J Thorac Cardiovasc Surg* 1976;72:127–129.
25. Harter HR, Burch JW, Majerus PW, et al: Prevention of thrombosis in patients on hemodialysis by low-dose aspirin. *N Engl J Med* 1979;301:577–579.
26. Lewis HD, Davis JW, Archibald DG, et al: Protective effects of aspirin against acute myocardial infarction and death in men with unstable angina. *N Engl J Med* 1983;309:396–403.
27. Cairns JA, Gent M, Singer J, et al: Aspirin, sulfinpyrazone or both in unstable angina: results of a Canadian multicenter trial. *N Engl J Med* 1985;313:1369–1375.
28. Aspirin after myoicardial infarction, editorial. *Lancet* 1980;1:1172.
29. Lorenz RL, Weber M, Kotzur J, et al: Improved aorto-coronary bypass patency by low-dose aspirin (100 mg daily): Effects on platelet aggregation and thromboxane formation. *Lancet* 1984;1:1261–1264.
30. Chesebro JH, Fuster V: Thromboembolism in heart valve replacement, in Kwaan HC, Bowie EJW (eds): *Thrombosis*. Philadelphia, WB Saunders Co, 1982, pp 146–153.
31. McGregor M, Mustard JF, Oliver MF, et al (eds): *Cardiovascular Action of Sulfinpyrazone: Basic and Clinical Research*. Miami, Symposium Specialists Medical Books, 1980.
32. Harker LA, Harlan JM, Ross R: Effect of sulfinpyrazone on homocysteine-induced endothelial injury and arteriosclerosis in baboons. *Circ Res* 1983;53:731–739.

33. Kaegi A, Pineo GF, Shimizu A, et al: Arteriovenous-shunt thrombosis: Prevention by sulfinpyrazone. *N Engl J Med* 1974;290:304–306.
34. Baur HR, Van Tassel RA, Pierach CA, et al: Effects of sulfinpyrazone on early graft closure after myocardial revascularization. *Am J Cardiol* 1982;49:420–424.
35. The Anturane Reinfarction Trial Research Group: Sulfinpyrazone in the prevention of sudden death after myocardial infarction. *N Engl J Med* 1980;302:250–256.
36. Temple R, Pledger GW: The FDA's critique of the Anturane Reinfarction Trial. *N Engl J Med* 1980;303:1488–1492.
37. Sollevi A, Ostergren J, Hiemdahl P, et al: The effect of dipyridamole on plasma adenosine levels and skin microcirculation in man. *J Clin Chem Clin Biochem* 1982;20:420–421.
38. Crutchley DJ, Ryan US, Ryan JW: Effects of aspirin and dipyridamole on the degradation of adenosine diphosphate by cultured cells derived from bovine pulmonary artery. *J Clin Invest* 1980;66:29–35.
39. Sullivan JM, Harken DE, Gorlin R: Pharmacologic control of thromboembolic complications of cardiac-valve replacement. *N Engl J Med* 1971;284:1391–1394.
40. Hess H, Mietaschk A, Deichsel G: Drug-induced inhibition of platelet function delays progression of peripheral occlusive arterial disease: A prospective double-blind arteriographically controlled trial. *Lancet* 1985;1:415–418.
41. Klimt CR, Knatterud GL, Stamler J: Persantine-Aspirin Reinfarction Study: Part II. Secondary coronary prevention with persantine and aspirin. *J Am Coll Cardiol* 1986;7:251–269.
42. Chesebro JH, Clements IP, Fuster V, et al: A platelet inhibitor-drug trial in coronary-artery bypass operations: Benefit of perioperative dipyridamole and aspirin therapy on early postoperative vein-graft patency. *N Engl J Med* 1982;307:73–78.
43. Chesebro JH, Fuster V, Elveback LR, et al: Effect of dipyridamole and aspirin on late vein-graft patency after coronary bypass operations. *N Engl J Med* 1984;310:209–214.
44. Donadio JV Jr, Anderson CF, Mitchell JC III, et al: Membranoproliferative glomerulonephritis: A prospective clinical trial of platelet-inhibitor therapy. *N Engl J Med* 1984;310:1421–1426.
45. O'Brien JR: Ticlopidine. *Haemostasis* 1983;13(suppl 1):1–53.
46. Gent M, Ellis D: Canadian American Ticlopidine Study (CATS) in thromboembolic stroke. *Agents Actions* 1984;15(suppl):283–296.
47. Hass WK, Kamm B: The North American Ticlopidine Aspirin Stroke Study: Structure, stratification variables, and patient characteristics. *Agents Actions* 1984;15(suppl):273–278.
48. Roba J, Defreyn G, Biagi G: Antithrombotic activity of suloctidil. *Thromb Res* 1985 suppl IV, pp 53–58.
49. Gent M, Blakely JA, Hachinski V, et al: A secondary prevention, randomized trial of suloctidil in patients with a recent history of thromboembolic stroke. *Stroke* 1985;16:416–424.
50. Rosenberg RD: Actions and interactions of antithrombin and heparin. *N Engl J Med* 1976;292:146–151.
51. Thaler E, Lechner K: Antithrombin III deficiency and thromboembolism. *Clin Haematol* 1981;10:369–390.

52. O'Reilly RA: Vitamin K and other oral anticoagulant drugs. *Annu Rev Med* 1976;27:249–261.
53. Loeliger EA: The optimal therapeutic range in oral anticoagulation: History and proposal. *Thromb Haemost* 1979;42:1141–1152.
54. Furlan AJ, Cavalier SJ, Hobbs RE, et al: Hemorrhage and anticoagulation after nonseptic embolic brain infarction. *Neurology* 1982;32:280–282.
55. Cerebral Embolism Study Group: Immediate anticoagulation of embolic stroke: Brain hemmorrhage and management options. *Stroke* 1984;15:779–789.
56. Evans G: Effect of drugs that suppress platelet surface interaction on incidence of amaurosis fugax and transient cerebral ischemia. *Surg Forum* 1972;23:239–241.
57. Fields WS, Lemak NA, Frankowski RF, et al: Controlled trial of aspirin in cerebral ischemia: Part II: Surgical group. *Stroke* 1978;9:309–319.
58. Guiraud-Chaumeil B, Rascol A, David J, et al: Prevention des recidives des accidents vasculaires cerebraux ischemiques par les antiagregants plaquettaires. *Rev Neurol (Paris)* 1982;138:367–385.
59. Sorensen PS, Pedersen H, Marquardsen J, et al: Acetylsalicylic acid in the prevention of stroke in patients with reversible cerebral ischemic attacks: A Danish cooperative study. *Stroke* 1983;14:15–22.
60. Bousser MG, Eschwege E, Haguenau M, et al: "AICLA" controlled trial of aspirin and dipyridamole in the secondary prevention of athero-thrombotic cerebral ischemia. *Stroke* 1983;14:5–14.
61. The American-Canadian Co-operative Study Group: Persantine aspirin trial in cerebral ischemia: Part II. Endpoint results. *Stroke* 1985;16:406–415.
62. The UK-TIA Study Group: Design and protocol of the UK-TIA aspirin study, in Tognoni G, Garattini S (eds): *Drug Treatment and Prevention in Cerebrovascular Disorders: Clinical Pharmacology and Drug Epidemiology*. Amsterdam, Elsevier, 1979, vol 2, pp 387–394.
63. Veterans Administration Co-operative Study of Atherosclerosis, Neurology Section: An evaluation of anticoagulant therapy in the treatment of cerebrovascular disease. *Neurology* 1961;11(4, part 2):132–138.
64. Fisher CM: The use of anticoagulants in cerebral thrombosis. *Neurology* 1958;8:311–332.
65. Baker RN, Schwartz WS, Rose AS: Transient ischemic strokes. *Neurology* 1966;16:841–847.
66. Baker RN, Broward JA, Fang HC, et al: Anticoagulant therapy in cerebral infarction: Report on cooperative study. *Neurology* 1962;12:823–835.
67. Brust JCM: Transient ischemic attacks: Natural history and anticoagulations. *Neurology* 1977;27:701–707.

CHAPTER 20

The Safety of Carotid Endarterectomy for Amaurosis Fugax

Nicolee C. Fode and Thoralf M. Sundt

This chapter is based on a survey of 46 institutions and 3,328 carotid endarterectomies performed in the year 1981. It was a retrospective study sponsored by the American Association of Neurological Surgeons. The purpose of this audit was to determine the relative safety of carotid endarterectomy in institutions of various sizes and academic affiliations. The study was incomplete in that the number of contributing institutions was disappointingly low. The survey fell far short of the goal of 10,000 cases from 100 institutions. Nevertheless, some information was gathered that might be useful for a judgment about the profile of carotid endarterectomy in the United States today. The results of this study have been published previously in the 1986 May/June issue of *Stroke* (1).

The aim of this chapter is to place in perspective the relative safety of carotid endarterectomy. In the audit, it appeared that patients who underwent carotid endarterectomy for amaurosis fugax fared better than patients who underwent surgery for hemispheric TIAs or for a minor stroke. However, it is necessary to further analyze these figures before leaping to any conclusions about the merit of carotid endarterectomy for a particular disease process divorced from considerations about the type of surgery performed, the presence or absence of monitoring during the operation, and the experience of the operative team.

This audit was conducted by the American Association of Neurological Surgeons and therefore could have a built-in bias in favor of neurosurgeons. Those neurosurgeons who had good results were eager to report their experience, and in institutions in which neurosurgeons did not perform the surgery, and results were poor, a similar eagerness might be present to share this information. Thus, although the audit did show favorable results for neurosurgeons compared to other surgeons, this material is of questionable validity and has not been analyzed.

Case Material

Overall, the risk of transient neurological dysfunction after surgery was 2.5% and the risk of stroke or death was 6%. Those institutions with more than 700 beds had a statistically lower prevalence of stroke or death than did other institutions (Table 20–1). The prevalence of stroke or death postoperatively was significantly lower for patients who were operated on for amaurosis fugax or for unspecified reasons (Table 20–2). Prevalence of postoperative stroke or death was related to the type of arterial repair; vein patch grafting was statistically better than both fabric patch grafting and primary closure (Table 20–3). Patients who were monitored with EEG during surgery fared better than those without monitoring (Table 20–4). The prevalence of stroke or death in patients undergoing combined coronary artery bypass surgery and carotid endarterectomy was 13.3% (Table 20–5).

The highest risk group for complications among patients undergoing surgery in the various institutions during the period of the retrospective audit was the group of patients who were neurologically unstable (ie, patients with progressing strokes). Although there is some controversy about the indications for surgery in this group, it must be remembered that this group has the highest risk for a major stroke if they do not have surgery, and surgical intervention in these patients can have dramatic beneficial results.

The risk of carotid endarterectomy at the participating institutions varied tremendously, and, curiously enough, the risks reported in the audit varied according to the obvious attention given to the audit forms by the participating neurologist or neurosurgeon. The highest complication rate, for

ABLE 20–1. Size of institution versus major morbidity and mortality.

Size of stitution	Total # of cases	Minor stroke able to work	Major stroke-unable to work: Able to care for self	Major stroke-unable to work: Unable to care for self	Death: Stroke	Death: MI	Total death & stroke
0–199	12	0	0	0	0	0	0
0–299	150	4 (2.7%)	2 (1.3%)	1 (0.7%)	1 (0.7%)	5 (3%)	13 (8.7%)
0–399	104	0	1 (1%)	6 (5.8%)	1 (1%)	1 (1%)	9 (8.7%)
0–499	446	4 (1%)	7 (1.6%)	10 (2.2%)	9 (2%)	4 (1%)	34 (7.6%)
0–599	588	10 (1.7%)	8 (1.4%)	8 (1.4%)	6 (1%)	4 (0.7%)	36 (6.1%)
0–699	327	8 (2.4%)	6 (1.8%)	6 (1.8%)	8 (2.4%)	6 (1.8%)	34 (10.4%)
0–799	255	1 (0.4%)	2 (0.8%)	1 (0.4%)	4 (1.6%)	0	8 (3%)
0–899	199	3 (1.5%)	3 (1.5%)	7 (3.5%)	1 (0.5%)	0	14 (7%)
ver 900	1242	14 (1.1%)	16 (1.3%)	12 (1%)	10 (0.8%)	6 (0.5%)	58 (4.7%)

I = myocardial infarction.
rom Fode NC et al, 1986 (1). Reproduced by permission of the publisher.]

TABLE 20–2. Indication for surgery versus major morbidity and mortality.

Indication for surgery	Total # of cases	Minor stroke able to work	Major stroke-unable to work: Able to care for self	Major stroke-unable to work: Unable to care for self	Death: Stroke	Death: MI	Total stroke & death
Amaurosis fugax	461	0	5 (1.1%)	6 (1.3%)	0	3 (0.7%)	14 (3%)
Asymptomatic bruit	396	3 (0.8%)	3 (0.8%)	4 (1%)	7 (1.8%)	4 (1%)	21 (5.3%)
TIA	1283	25 (1.9%)	16 (1.2%)	20 (1.6%)	10 (0.8%)	11 (0.9%)	82 (6.4%)
Dizziness, vertigo, syncope	336	5 (1.5%)	5 (1.5%)	6 (1.8%)	7 (2%)	1 (0.3%)	24 (7%)
Minor stroke	388	4 (1%)	9 (2.3%)	7 (1.8%)	8 (2.1%)	2 (0.5%)	30 (7.7%)
Major stroke	51	0	0	0	4 (7.8%)	1 (2%)	5 (9.8%)
Progressing stroke	38	2 (5.3%)	2 (5.3%)	2 (5.3%)	2 (5.3%)	0	8 (21.1%)
Prelude to surgery elsewhere	176	4 (2.3%)	3 (1.7%)	3 (1.7%)	1 (0.6%)	3 (1.7%)	14 (8%)
Other or unspecified	195	1 (0.5%)	2 (1%)	3 (1.5%)	1 (0.5%)	1 (0.5%)	8 (4%)

MI = myocardial infarction; TIA = transient ischemic attack.

[From Fode NC et al, 1986 (1). Reproduced by permission of the publisher.]

TABLE 20–3. Type of procedure versus major morbidity and mortality.

Type of procedure	Total # of cases	Minor stroke able to work	Major stroke unable to work		Death		Total death & stroke
			Able to care for self	Unable to care for self	Stroke	MI	
Primary closure	2714	37 (1.4%)	41 (1.5%)	44 (1.6%)	35 (1.3%)	22 (0.8%)	179 (6.6%)
Vein patch graft	266	3 (1.1%)	0	2 (0.8%)	0	1 (0.4%)	6 (2.3%)
Fabric patch graft	257	3 (1.2%)	4 (1.6%)	5 (1.9%)	5 (1.9%)	1 (0.4%)	18 (7.0%)
Unknown	84	1 (1.2%)	0	0	0	1 (1.2%)	2 (2.4%)

MI = myocardial infarction.
[From Fode NC et al, 1986 (1). Reproduced by permission of the publisher.]

TABLE 20–4. Cerebral protection versus major morbidity and mortality.

Cerebral protection	Total # of cases	Minor stroke able to work	Major stroke unable to work		Death		Total death & stroke
			Able to care for self	Unable to care for self	Stroke	MI	
No monitor							
Shunt	953	19 (2.0%)	19 (2.0%)	10 (1.0%)	20 (2.1%)	13 (1.4%)	81 (8.5%)
No shunt	955	6 (0.6%)	9 (0.9%)	23 (2.4%)	10 (1.0%)	5 (0.5%)	53 (5.5%)
EEG							
Shunt	462	2 (0.4%)	0	2 (0.4%)	2 (0.4%)	2 (0.4%)	8 (1.7%)
No shunt	511	7 (1.4%)	8 (1.6%)	5 (1.0%)	3 (0.6%)	3 (0.6%)	26 (5%)
Stump pressure							
Shunt	41	2 (4.9%)	0	0	1 (2.4%)	0	3 (7.3%)
No shunt	135	0	2 (1.5%)	3 (2.2%)	0	0	5 (3.7%)
Other/unknown	262	8 (3.0%)	7 (2.7%)	7 (2.7%)	4 (1.5%)	3 (1.1%)	29 (11%)

MI = myocardial infarction; EEG = electroencephalograph.
[From Fode NC et al, 1986 (1). Reproduced by permission of the publisher.]

TABLE 20–5. Classification of operation versus major morbidity and mortality.

Classification of operation	Total # of cases	Minor stroke able to work	Major stroke unable to work: Able to care for self	Major stroke unable to work: Unable to care for self	Death: Stroke	Death: MI	Total stroke & death
Single stage unilateral endarterectomy	2535	31 (1.2%)	38 (1.5%)	39 (1.5%)	32 (1.3%)	12 (0.5%)	152 (6%)
Simultaneous bilateral endarterectomy	27	0	0	1 (3.7%)	2 (7.4%)	1 (3.7%)	4 (15%)
Staged bilateral one week or more apart	623	8 (1.3%)	6 (1.0%)	5 (0.8%)	6 (1.0%)	8 (1.3%)	33 (5.3%)
Combined with peripheral vascular procedure	39	2 (5.0%)	0	1 (2.6%)	0	1 (2.6%)	4 (10.3%)
Combined with coronary bypass	98	3 (3.1%)	1 (1.0%)	5 (5.1%)	0	4 (4.1%)	13 (13.3%)

MI = myocardial infarction.

[From Fode NC et al, 1986 (1). Reproduced by permission of the publisher.]

example, was reported by a neurologist who was obviously quite disturbed about the results of endarterectomies performed in his hospital. He reported a 21% complication rate of major proportions in patients undergoing surgery at his hospital that was unrelated to the specialty of the surgeon involved—neurosurgeon, vascular surgeon, general surgeon—all were equally bad.

In the overall audit, patients who had EEG monitoring during surgery fared better than patients who did not have monitoring ($p < .005$). In nonmonitored patients, cases in which a shunt was not used during surgery did significantly better than those in which a shunt was used ($p < .005$). Thus, if no monitoring was used, it appeared to be safer to operate on the patient without a shunt than with a shunt.

Patients who had the vessel repaired with a vein patch graft did statistically better ($p < .01$) than those who had fabric patch grafting, and both did better than patients in whom the vessel was closed primarily. This data could be skewed, as one large center with a low morbidity rate used a vein patch graft routinely.

Results of Surgery for Amaurosis Fugax

Thirty-four percent of patients operated upon for amaurosis fugax had EEG monitoring *v* 29% for the group as a whole. This was statistically significant ($p < .05$). Twenty-five percent of patients with amaurosis fugax had the vessel repaired with a saphenous vein patch graft or dacron patch graft *v* 16% of the group as a whole. This was statistically also significant ($p < .0005$). No patients having surgery for amaurosis fugax had a minor complication. All irreversible complications were major complications that led to hemiplegia or death.

Institutions with a high complication rate for patients undergoing surgery for amaurosis fugax also had high complication rates in general. For example, one institution had a major morbidity and mortality of 14% overall in 63 patients and a 33% major complication rate for patients with amaurosis fugax (there were only three cases). Another institution with a 15% overall complication rate for 42 patients undergoing surgery during 1981 had a 29% complication rate among seven patients undergoing surgery for amaurosis fugax (major complications). Another institution with a 21% overall complication rate (78 cases undergoing surgery) had a 17% major complication rate among 12 patients undergoing surgery for amaurosis fugax. A fourth institution had a 14% overall complication rate for 63 patients undergoing carotid endarterectomy and a 25% complication rate among eight patients undergoing endarterectomy for amaurosis fugax. A fifth institution had an overall 13% complication rate among 107 patients undergoing surgery and a 10% complication rate (major stroke and death) among 19 patients undergoing surgery for amaurosis fugax.

The audit of these institutions included a category called "other complications," which included minor (wound hematomas, transient cranial nerve deficits) to major (nonfatal MI, death from pulmonary problems) complications. This category was not included in the statistical analysis. However, the overall prevalence of "other" complications was 9%. In patients with amaurosis fugax, these other complications included pulmonary emboli, blindness, nonfatal MI, and a central cord syndrome possibly related to positioning of a patient with severe cervical spondylosis (there was some question about this being related to "emboli from the heart"—unlikely in our judgment).

In conclusion, if it is safe to do an endarterectomy at Institution A in general, it is safe to do an endarterectomy for amaurosis fugax at Institution A. On the other hand, if it is dangerous to do an endarterectomy at Institution B, it is dangerous to do the operation for amaurosis fugax or any other indication at Institution B.

Conclusion

It is our bias that meticulous attention to detail in both the neurologic monitoring of the patient and the technique of arterial reconstruction are far more important than the indication for the operative procedure in terms of the safety of the operation. No margin for error is available for these individuals, and the penalty for a complication can be devastating. No room exists for a cavalier attitude, and the results of this analysis indicate that the situation in some institutions at the present time is indeed grim.

It seems advisable at this point to identify the best technique for vascular reconstruction. It seems that it would be appropriate for major and minor institutions to pool their data and find out exactly what is going on with this operation.

The following recommendations might be considered:

1. All patients having a carotid endarterectomy should undergo a detailed postoperative neurologic examination by a qualified neurologist.
2. All patients should undergo postoperative DSA. Digital subtraction angiograms are not useful in many patients who have thick atherosclerotic plaques before surgery but are ideal for postoperative studies. We have reported our results in patients undergoing this procedure with saphenous vein patch grafting (2) and Little et al (3) from the Cleveland Clinic have compared primary closure with patch graft closures as well (6% *v* 0% postoperative occlusion rates, respectively). A recent paper from Italy also has supported this contention (4). To our knowledge, no such study has been reported of patients in whom the vessel has been closed primarily, yet most institutions still maintain that primary arterial closure has results equal to those obtained with patch grafting.

This belief cannot be substantiated by the data currently available, and it should be established positively or negatively. Noninvasive testing suggests a restenosis or occlusion rate as high as 35% (5) to 49% (6) in patients in whom the artery was repaired primarily. This type of postoperative and follow-up evaluation falls short of a DSA.

3. Participating institutions should provide detailed records of the preoperative neurologic state of the patient and sufficient details of the operative procedures to make such an analysis meaningful.

Unfortunately, one of the major problems with this retrospective audit was the reluctance of surgeons in participating institutions to have their patients reviewed. If the results of carotid endarterectomy are as spectacular as claimed by the surgical community, established surgeons should not be reluctant to have their patients examined and audited. This seems far preferable to a randomized trial, which, in our judgment, has major ethical problems.

References

1. Fode NC, Sundt TM Jr, Robertson JT, et al: Multicenter retrospective review of results and complications of carotid endarterectomy in 1981. *Stroke* 1986;17(3):370–376.
2. Sundt TM Jr, Houser OW, Whisnant JP, et al: Correlation of postoperative and two-year follow-up angiography with neurological function in 99 carotid endarterectomies in 86 consecutive patients. *Ann Surg* 1986;203(1):90–100.
3. Little JR, Bryerton BS, Furlan AJ: Saphenous vein patch grafts in carotid endarterectomy. *J Neurosurg* 1984;61:743–747.
4. Deriu GP, Ballotta E, Bonavina L, et al: The rationale for patch-graft angioplasty after carotid endarterectomy: Early and long-term follow-up. *Stroke* 1984;15(6):972–979.
5. Norvving B, Nilsson B, Olsson JE: Progression of carotid disease after endarterectomy: A Doppler ultrasound study. *Ann Neurol* 1982;12:548–552.
6. Bodily DC, Zierler RE, Marinelli MR, et al: Flow disturbances following carotid endarterectomy. *Surg Gynecol Obstet* 1980;151:77–80.

CHAPTER 21

Long-Term Results of Surgical Therapy for Amaurosis Fugax

Daniel P. Connelly, Steven Okuhn,
and William K. Ehrenfeld

The relationship between amaurosis fugax and ipsilateral extracranial cerebrovascular disease and subsequent stroke was not adequately appreciated until 1952 when Fisher (1) described seven patients with monocular loss of vision and contralateral hemiplegia. It has become clear that amaurosis fugax can be a marker for surgically correctable extracranial arterial lesions, and these lesions are repaired with the view toward prevention of retinal or cerebral stroke. Many surgical series that evaluate cerebrovascular reconstruction have been reported (2–9). These studies have indicated that perioperative and long-term results vary with the preoperative indication for surgery. Patients who are operated on for amaurosis fugax and retinal stroke have a longer stroke-free survival than patients operated on for other TIAs or cerebral stroke (9,10). What has not been shown, however, is to what extent cerebrovascular reconstruction prevents subsequent ipsilateral amaurosis fugax, ipsilateral retinal stroke, or ipsilateral cerebral stroke.

This investigation was undertaken to evaluate the perioperative and long-term results of extracranial cerebrovascular reconstruction performed for amaurosis fugax and retinal stroke. Special attention was directed towards determining the postoperative occurrence of ipsilateral ocular and ipsilateral cerebral ischemic events.

Methods and Clinical Material

The patients selected for this study underwent cerebrovascular reconstruction between 1974 and 1985 at the University of California, San Francisco (UCSF) and fell into two groups. Group I patients were operated on between 1974 and 1977 and were selected from the operative registry to provide a population for long-term follow-up. Group II consisted of patients operated upon between 1983 and 1985 who were selected similarly and already had been entered into a vascular database. They were included to increase the power of subsequent statistical analysis. Retrospective chart review was used in both groups to determine the indication for operation, angiographic findings, the operation performed, and perioperative results. Long-term follow-up was obtained by review of recent office records or telephone interviews with the patient, a family member, or the patient's private physician. If current contact could not be made, then the date and clinical status of the patient at the last office visit were used as the most recent follow-up. For patients who died, neurologic status before death was ascertained, and the date of death was used as the date of last contact.

The data were analyzed by using Cox regression and life-table survival analyses. The SAS software system running on an IBM 4381 computer was used to perform these statistical procedures.

Surgical Experience

Group I

From 1974 to 1977, 400 patients underwent cerebrovascular reconstruction at UCSF, and the records of 375 of these patients were available for review. The records indicated that 66 patients underwent 72 operations in which amaurosis fugax (64) or retinal stroke (seven) was the primary or secondary indication for operation (Tables 21–1, 21–2). One operation was performed for a nonspecific visual disturbance and a Hollenhorst plaque noted on funduscopic examination. Six patients underwent a second operation for amaurosis fugax (four for ipsilateral recurrent amaurosis fugax and two for contralateral amaurosis fugax). A TIA (10 patients) or a completed stroke (five patients) was an associated indication for operation. One patient with a stroke in evolution and amaurosis fugax underwent a contralateral carotid bifurcation thromboendarterectomy for contralateral high-grade stenosis and ipsilateral carotid artery occlusion. Angiography showed that five additional patients had ipsilateral ICA occlusion, and 10 patients had contralateral ICA occlusion.

The majority of operative procedures (67 of 72), were directed towards reconstruction of the carotid artery bifurcation, 56 primary and six reoperative bifurcation thromboendarterectomies (Table 21–3). Two patients underwent interposition grafting for recurrent disease. Another patient underwent bifurcation thromboendarterectomy and common carotid endarterectomy for an occlusion of the common carotid artery. Two additional

TABLE 21–1. Surgical experience for amaurosis fugax.

Group	No. of operations	No. of patients
I (1974–1977)	72	66
II (1983–1985)	61	56
Total	133	122

TABLE 21–2. Indication for operation.

	Group I		Group II	
	No.	%	No.	%
Indication				
Amaurosis fugax	64	89	52	85
Retinal stroke	7	10	9	15
Nonspecific visual problem + Hollenhorst plaque	1	1.4		
Associated Preoperative Findings				
Stroke in evolution	1	1.4	1	1.6
Completed stroke	5	7	3	4.9
Transient ischemic attack (hemispheric, nonocular)	10	14	20	33

patients had contralateral carotid bifurcation thromboendarterectomy because of an ipsilateral ICA occlusion that was associated with a significant stenosis of the contralateral carotid bifurcation. One of these 67 patients had ligation of the ICA after a failed bifurcation thromboendarterectomy.

Of the remaining five patients, three underwent external carotid thromboendarterectomy for an ipsilateral ICA occlusion and external carotid artery disease associated with amaurosis fugax. Another patient had an innominate artery thromoboendarterectomy for an ulcerated stenosis. The final patient had his operation limited to exploration only when the carotid bifurcation was found to be thrombosed.

Group II

From July 1983 to December 1985, 364 patients underwent cerebrovascular reconstruction. Within this group were 56 patients who underwent 61 operations for which amaurosis fugax (52) or retinal stroke (nine) was the primary or secondary indication (Tables 21–1, 21–2). Five patients underwent a second operation for amaurosis fugax (one for ipsilateral recurrent

TABLE 21–3. Surgical procedures.

	Group I (72 operations)		Group II (61 operations)	
	No.	%	No.	%
Carotid bifurcation procedure	67	93	49	80
External carotid thromboendarterectomy	3	4	5	8
Carotid dilatation	0		4	7
Innominate artery thromboendarterectomy	1	1.3	3	5
Exploration only (vessels occluded)	1	1.3	0	

amaurosis fugax and four for contralateral amaurosis fugax). A TIA (20 patients) or a completed stroke (three patients) was an associated indication for operation. One patient with a stroke in evolution and amaurosis fugax had an ipsilateral high-grade stenosis of the ICA and underwent emergency carotid bifurcation thromboendarterectomy. Review of angiographic findings showed ipsilateral ICA occlusion in five patients and contralateral ICA occlusion in four.

Of the operative procedures performed, 49 (80%) involved a carotid bifurcation procedure. Forty-four patients underwent primary carotid bifurcation thromboendarterectomy, and three patients had a reoperative carotid bifurcation thromboendarterectomy (Table 21–3). One patient had a reversed saphenous vein interposition graft from the proximal common carotid artery to the bifurcation, and another patient in this group had a bifurcation thromboendarterectomy with resection and reanastomosis of a redundant ICA.

Of the remaining 12 operations, five were ipsilateral external carotid thromboendarterectomies (all in patients with associated ipsilateral ICA occlusion), and three were innominate artery thromboendarterectomies. Two remaining patients underwent bilateral ICA dilatation for bilateral amaurosis fugax secondary to ICA fibromuscular disease.

Results

Group I patients had no perioperative deaths (Table 21–4). Three patients sustained a perioperative stroke (4.2% stroke rate). One stroke was severe, requiring placement in a nursing home (this patient had associated TIAs in the ipsilateral hemisphere preoperatively). The second operative stroke resulted in a mild residual hemiparesis (the patient then remained asymptomatic for 12 years). The final operative stroke occurred in a patient who had a contralateral ICA occlusion and sustained a mild contralateral hemispheric stroke. This patient had only mild residual weakness 6 weeks postoperatively and was living independently at that time.

Two group I patients had perioperative myocardial infarctions (2.8%), and these events occurred in two of the three patients who sustained peri-

TABLE 21–4. Perioperative morbidity and mortality.

	Group I (66 Patients)		Group II (56 Patients)		Total (122 Patients)	
	No.	%	No.	%	No.	%
Death	0		0		0	
Stroke	3	4.2	1	1.6	4	3
Transient ischemic attack	0		2	3.2	2	1.5
Myocardial Infarction	2	2.8	1	1.6	3	2.2

operative strokes. Both patients recovered without any further cardiac complications.

No perioperative deaths occurred in group II patients (Table 21–4). One patient sustained a perioperative stroke (1.6%). This patient had had an ipsilateral hemispheric stroke 15 months before the operation. Recurrent ipsilateral hemispheric symptoms developed on postoperative day 10, and CT scan confirmed an increase in the area of old cerebral infarction. Postoperative TIAs occurred in two patients; one occurred shortly after the operation and the other on postoperative day 22. In both patients, carotid duplex scans showed patent reconstructions, and neither patient has had recurrent symptoms.

A single myocardial infarction occurred in group II in a patient undergoing innominate reconstruction. This patient completely recovered and has had no further cardiac problems.

Of the 66 group I patients, 49 (74%) were available for follow-up evaluation (Table 21–5). Thirty-three (67%) of these patients remained asymptomatic, with a mean follow-up of 97 months. Twenty-two were alive and asymptomatic at last contact (mean follow-up, 103 months), and 11 were asymptomatic until death (mean follow-up, 73 months). Of the 16 symptomatic patients, six had died at last follow-up (Table 21–6). Stroke and

TABLE 21–5. Follow-up data.

	Group I (66 patients)		Group II (56 patients)		Total	
	No.	%	No.	%	No.	%
Available for follow up	49	74	54	96	103	84
Neurologic status at last contact						
Asymptomatic	33	67	46	85	79	77
Ipsilateral stroke	2	4	1	2	3	3
Ipsilateral transient ischemic attack	2	4	1	2	3	3
Ipsilateral amaurosis fugax	9*	18	2	4	11	11
Contralateral stroke	1	2	2†	4	3	3
Contralateral transient ischemic attack	2	4	0		2	2
Contralateral amaurosis fugax	7‡	14	1	2	8	8
Stroke (site unknown)	4	8	0		4	4
Stroke	7	14	3	6	10	10

*One patient continued to have intermittent unilateral visual loss beginning 1 month after his operation; visual migraine has been diagnosed. A second patient remained asymptomatic for 8 years, at which time ipsilateral loss of vision developed. This visual loss was secondary to temporal arteritis. The patient was treated with steroids and improved. A third patient had an embolizing aortic valvular lesion responsible for both ipsilateral recurrent amaurosis fugax and the occurrence of contralateral amaurosis fugax.

†One of these was a retinal stroke.

‡One of the episodes was from an embolizing aortic valvular lesion (see above).

TABLE 21–6. Late mortality.

	Group I		Group II		Total	
	No.	%	No.	%	No.	%
Alive	32	65	49	91	81	79
Dead	17	35	5	9	22	21
Stroke deaths	8	47	0		8	36
Cardiovascular deaths	7	41	3	60	10	45
Death (other causes)	2	12	2	40	4	41

cardiovascular disease were responsible for 88% of the deaths; only two patients (12%) died from other causes. Of the patients who became symptomatic, many had more than one symptom.

Two patients had ipsilateral hemispheric strokes. One sustained a nonfatal stroke 51 months after the initial procedure and a subsequent fatal stroke 18 months later. In a second patient, asymptomatic restenosis developed 10.5 years after the initial procedure. Reoperative bifurcation surgery at another facility resulted in a fatal stroke.

Two patients had ipsilateral hemispheric TIAs at 1 and 10 years after their initial procedures. The first patient underwent reoperation and remained asymptomatic until death 5.5 years later. The second patient recently has had ipsilateral hemispheric TIAs and has noted ipsilateral transient visual dimming upon exposure to bright lights.

No ipsilateral retinal strokes occurred. Recurrent ipsilateral amaurosis fugax developed in nine patients (18%). Four patients underwent ipsilateral reoperation for recurrent ICA lesions causing amaurosis fugax at 2, 42, 70, and 124 months after their initial operations. Of the remaining five patients, one had recurrent ocular symptoms 1 month postoperatively, and these symptoms have reappeared at monthly intervals. His condition has been diagnosed as visual migraine, and these symptoms persist despite therapy. A second patient has had both ipsilateral and contralateral amaurosis fugax, and valvular aortic stenosis, not carotid disease, is thought to be responsible for these persistent ocular symptoms. In the third patient, frontal headaches and monocular visual loss developed 8 years after her initial operation, and temporal artery biopsy confirmed the presumptive diagnosis of temporal arteritis. The fourth patient with recurrent amaurosis had a patent carotid artery bifurcation with severe distal ICA disease on repeat angiography. The lesion was deemed inoperable, and this patient continues to experience visual dimming on exposure to bright lights. The fifth patient had three episodes of visual loss before having a fatal cardiac arrest 8 years after the initial procedure.

One contralateral hemispheric stroke occurred 2 months postoperatively (this patient had an associated contralateral ICA occlusion). Two patients sustained contralateral hemispheric TIAs. One of these patients had an appropriate carotid bifurcation thromboendarterectomy, and the other had no operation because of a distal ICA stenosis that was not reconstuctible.

Seven patients had contralateral amaurosis fugax. Two of these patients had contralateral carotid bifurcation thromboendarterectomies, and three patients had contralateral external carotid thromboendarterectomies because their ICA was occluded. The last two patients had an inaccessible distal ICA stenosis and an embolizing aortic valvular lesion (previously discussed). Of the overall group, 22 patients (33%) had an additional contralateral carotid bifurcation thromboendarterectomy for indications other than amaurosis fugax, reflecting the severity of their cerebrovascular disease.

Four patients sustained either a posterior circulation stroke or strokes for which the precise location could not be determined from follow-up data.

The overall group I late stroke rate was 14%; all of these patients died as a direct result of their stroke. One additional patient who sustained a perioperative stroke died 3 months postoperatively. Because his operative stroke was the proximate cause of his death, he is listed also as a stroke mortality (Table 21–6).

Of the 56 group II patients, 54 (96%) were available for follow-up evaluation (Table 21–5). Forty-six (85%) remained asymptomatic, with a mean follow-up of 22 months. Forty-one patients were alive and asymptomatic (mean follow-up, 23 months), and five patients were asymptomatic until death (mean follow-up, 19 months) (Table 21–5). Cardiovascular disease was responsible for three of the late deaths, and malignancy for the remaining two.

One ipsilateral stroke occurred 1 month postoperatively in a patient who had an ipsilateral ICA occlusion and an external carotid thromboendarterectomy. One patient had a single ipsilateral TIA 5 months postoperatively. Duplex scanning showed a patent reconstruction, and the patient was observed and had no further symptoms. Two patients (4%) had ipsilateral recurrent amaurosis fugax. The first patient had a single episode of amaurosis fugax 5 months postoperatively. The second patient had an initial external carotid thromboendarterectomy (the ICA was occluded) and recurrent ipsilateral amaurosis fugax developed 19 months later. An innominate thromboendarterectomy was performed then, without resolution of ocular symptoms.

Two patients had contralateral strokes. The first patient had a retinal stroke and has remained blind in the affected eye. The second patient had a cerebral stroke and was left with a mild residual hemiparesis.

No episodes of contralateral TIAs have occurred in group II. One patient had contralateral amaurosis fugax and was operated upon (previously described).

Overall, three late strokes have occurred in group II, two contralateral to the operated vessel and one ipsilateral; all three of these patients are alive with residual deficits.

Life-Table Analysis

Cox regression was used to determine whether the two groups differed with respect to the survival function describing the length of time until an ipsilateral ischemic event. No statistically significant difference in the survival function was found between these two groups for any of the end points considered (all *p*-values were greater than .2). Therefore, subsequent life-table analysis was performed by pooling the two study groups.

From the application of life-table analysis to our data, we estimated survival functions for each of four different ipsilateral events: hemispheric stroke, TIA, amaurosis fugax, and any ipsilateral ischemic event (Figs. 21–1 to 21–4). From this life-table analysis, we estimate that 96% of patients operated on for amaurosis fugax will remain free from an ipsilateral hemispheric stroke for at least 10 years (Fig. 21–1). Similarly, 98% of patients should be free from ipsilateral cerebral TIAs (Fig. 21–2) and 80% free from ipsilateral amaurosis fugax for at least 10 years (no ipsilateral retinal strokes occurred in the study group) (Fig. 21–3). Combining all ipsilateral ischemic events, 76% of patients undergoing operation for amaurosis fugax should be asymptomatic for at least 10 years (Fig. 21–4).

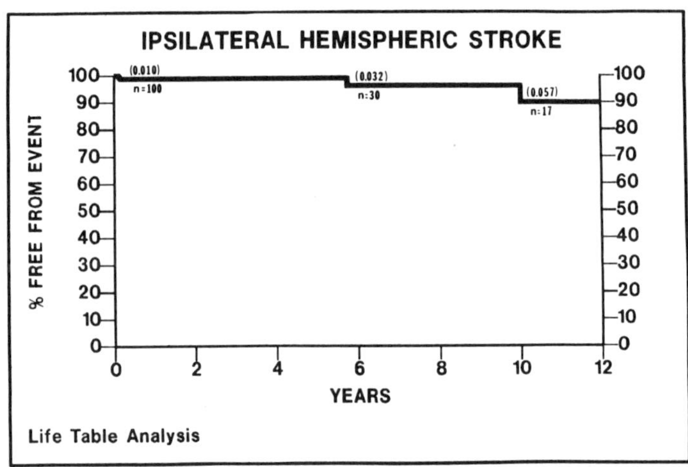

FIGURE 21–1. Estimated proportion of patients free from an ipsilateral hemispheric stroke after extracranial reconstruction for amaurosis fugax as a function of time (Kaplan-Meier). Values in parentheses indicate the standard error, and n, the number of patients available for analysis at each event occurrence.

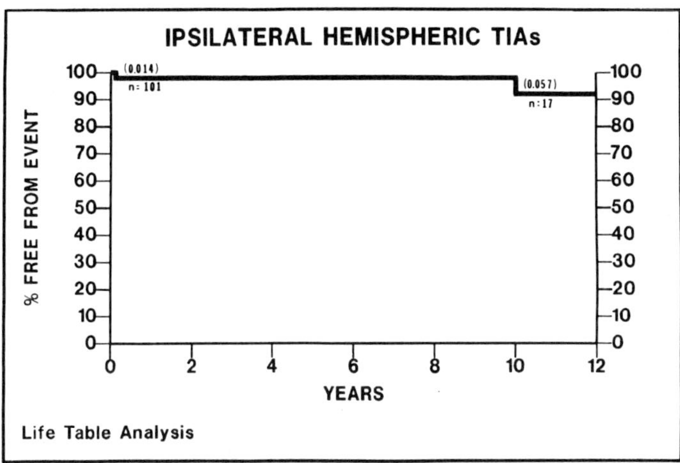

FIGURE 21–2. Estimated proportion of patients free from an ipsilateral transient ischemic attack after extracranial reconstruction for amaurosis fugax as a function of time (Kaplan-Meier). Values in parentheses indicate the standard error, and n, the number of patients available for analysis at each event occurrence.

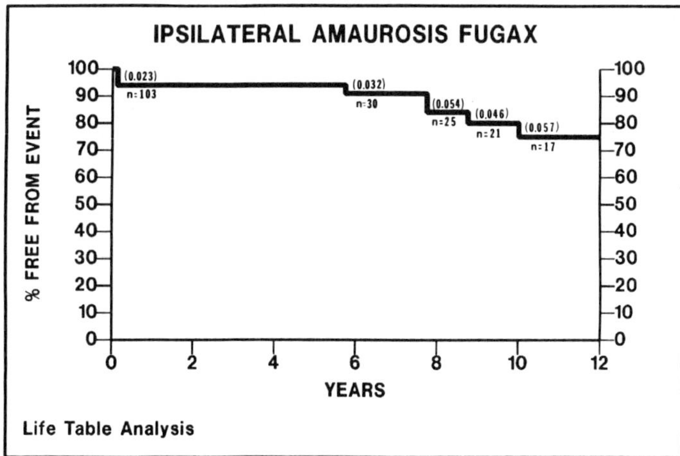

FIGURE 21–3. Estimated proportion of patients free from recurrent amaurosis fugax after extracranial reconstruction as a function of time (Kaplan-Meier). Values in parentheses indicate the standard error, and n, the number of patients available for analysis at each event occurrence.

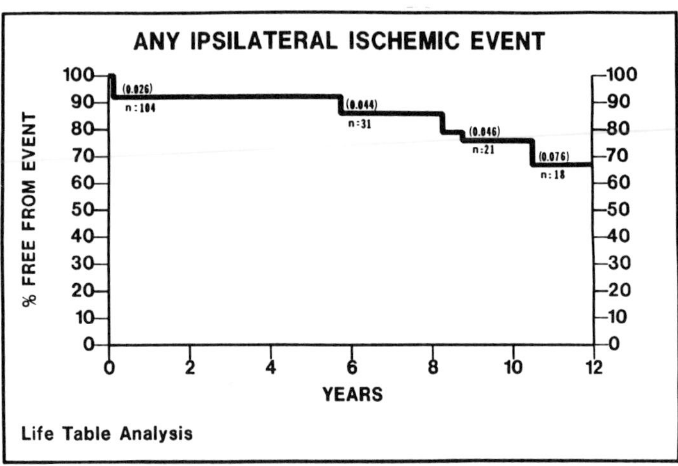

FIGURE 21–4. Estimated proportion of patients free from any ipsilateral ischemic event after extracranial reconstruction for amaurosis fugax as a function of time (Kaplan-Meier). Values in parentheses indicate the standard error, and n, the number of patients available for analysis at each event occurrence.

Discussion

Our results showed that ipsilateral amaurosis fugax recurred in a total of 11 patients (11%) (Table 21–5) who underwent cerebrovascular reconstruction for this indication. According to life-table analysis, 80% of patients undergoing cerebrovascular reconstruction should remain free of ipsilateral amaurosis fugax at 10 years. Three of the 11 recurrent episodes were caused by factors other than extracranial cerebrovascular disease. Previous publications (1,11,12) have noted the various causes for amaurosis fugax, and it remains encumbent upon the responsible physician to reasonably exclude these possibilities before subjecting the patient to cerebrovascular reconstruction. Stewart et al (10) noted 44 of 100 patients undergoing cerebrovascular reconstruction who had only ocular symptoms as the indication for operation. Of these 44 patients, only four (9%) had recurrent ocular symptoms after reconstruction (mean follow-up, 5.5 years). Bernstein and Dilley (13) noted seven episodes of recurrence (5%) in 131 patients undergoing cerebrovascular reconstruction for amaurosis fugax (mean follow-up, 36 months). The last two series combined with our results indicate that cerebrovascular reconstruction is successful in eliminating amaurosis fugax if careful preoperative assessment has excluded causes for this complaint other than extracranial cerebrovascular disease. Despite careful selection of patients, however, long-term follow-up will detect a small percentage of patients whose symptoms reappear because of recurrent extracranial cerebrovascular disease.

Ipsilateral retinal stroke did not occur in any of our patients after cerebrovascular reconstruction. Although it is unreasonable to suspect that this operation will have an absolute protective effect for subsequent retinal stroke, these excellent results compare favorably with the 11% prevalence of retinal stroke from nonoperative treatment reported by Marshall and Meadows (14).

Ipsilateral cerebral stroke occurred in only three patients after cerebrovascular reconstruction (Table 21–5), and our estimated 10-year ipsilateral stroke-free survival was 96%. Other series that have reported results of extracranial reconstruction have noted improved overall stroke-free survival in patients undergoing operation for amaurosis fugax (10,13). Bernstein and Dilley (13) found that the 5-year postoperative stroke-free survival of patients with amaurosis fugax was 94%. We conclude that cerebrovascular reconstruction performed in properly selected patients who have amaurosis fugax confers significant protection from long-term ipsilateral cerebral stroke and from overall cerebral stroke.

It is expected that patients undergoing extracranial cerebrovascular reconstruction will be protected from subsequent ipsilateral hemispheric or retinal ischemic events. However, because of cross-cerebral flow via the circle of Willis and other collateral pathways, additional protection to the contralateral hemisphere or retina may occur. When the patient has an associated ipsilateral ICA occlusion, collateral pathways become even more important in cerebral and retinal protection. In addition, when ipsilateral ICA occlusion is accompanied by disease involving the external carotid artery or the contralateral carotid bifurcation, these collateral pathways may be responsible for causing cerebral and retinal symptoms. Three patients with ICA occlusion associated with recurring ipsilateral amaurosis fugax were reported by Ehrenfeld and Lord in 1969 (16). All three patients had relief from their symptoms after appropriate extracranial reconstruction. A subsequent report by Burnbaum et al (17) described an additional three patients with amaurosis fugax and ipsilateral ICA occlusion. Brigham et al (18) described two patients with ICA occlusions who had amaurosis fugax only upon exposure to bright lights. These two patients had relief from their symptoms after external carotid thromboendarterectomy. In our present series, amaurosis fugax occurred in the presence of an associated ipsilateral ICA occlusion in 10 patients. Operations performed on these patients were designed to remove proximal obstructing lesions from either the ipsilateral external carotid artery or the contralateral carotid bifurcation. Of these 10 patients, nine have remained asymptomatic after cerebrovascular reconstruction (mean follow-up, 4.8 years). One patient has had recurrent amaurosis fugax but remains alive and stroke-free 2.5 years after the operation. These results support our continued recommendation for cerebrovascular reconstruction in symptomatic patients who have an ICA occlusion.

In those patients who have amaurosis fugax as a manifestation of extracranial cerebrovascular disease, appropriate cerebrovascular reconstruction offers protection from subsequent retinal or cerebral stroke and remains the treatment of choice.

Acknowledgment. Supported in part by the Pacific Vascular Research Foundation, San Francisco, California.

References

1. Fisher CM: Transient monocular blindness associated with hemiplegia. *Arch Ophthalmol* 1952;47:167–203.
2. DeWeese JA, Rob CG, Satran R, et al: Results of carotid endarterectomies for transient ischemic attacks: Five years later. *Ann Surg* 1973;178:258–264.
3. Thompson JE, Kartchner MM, Austin DJ, et al: Carotid endarterectomy for cerebrovascular insufficiency (stroke): Follow-up of 359 cases. *Ann Surg* 1966;163:751–763.
4. Fields WS, Maslenikov V, Meyer J: Joint study of extracranial arterial occlusions. *JAMA* 1970;211:1973–2003.
5. Browse NL, Ross Russell RW: Carotid endarterectomy and the Javid shunt: The early results of 215 consecutive operations for transient ischemic attacks. *Br J Surg* 1984;71:53–57.
6. Wylie EJ, Ehrenfeld WK: *Extracranial Occlusive cerebro-Vascular Disease: Diagnosis and Treatment*. Philadelphia, WB Saunders Co, 1970.
7. Hertzer NR, Arison R: Cumulative stroke and survival ten years after carotid endarterectomy. *J Vasc Surg* 1985;2:661–668.
8. Bernstein EF, Humber PB, Collins GM, et al: Life expectancy and stroke following carotid endarterectomy. *Ann Surg* 1983;198:80–86.
9. Whisnant JP, Sandok BA, Sundt TM: Carotid endarterectomy for unilateral carotid system transient cerebral ischemia. *Mayo Clinic Proc* 1983;58:171–175.
10. Stewart G, Ross Russell RW, Browse NL: The long-term results of carotid endarterectomy for transient ischemic attacks. *J Vasc Surg* 1986;4:600–605.
11. Cogan DG: Blackouts not obviously due to carotid occlusion. *Arch Ophthalmol* 1961;66:180–187.
12. Ross Russell RW: Transient cerebral ischemia, in *Vascular Disease of the Central Nervous System*. Edinburgh, Churchill Livingston, 1982, pp 204–272.
13. Bernstein EF, Dilley RB: Late results following carotid endarterectomy for amaurosis fugax. *J Vasc Surg* 1987 (submitted for publication).
14. Marshall J, Meadows S: The natural history of amaurosis fugax. *Brain* 1968;91:419–434.
15. Ehrenfeld WK, Hoyt WF, Wylie EJ: Embolization and transient blindness from carotid atheroma. *Arch Surg* 1966;93:787–794.
16. Ehrenfeld WK, Lord RSA: Transient monocular blindness through collateral pathways. *Surgery* 1969;65:911–915.

17. Burnbaum MD, Selhorst JB, Harbison JW, et al: Amaurosis fugax from disease of the external carotid artery. *Arch Neurol* 1977;34:532–555.
18. Brigham RA, Youkey JR, Clagett GP, et al: Bright-light amaurosis fugax: An unusual symptom of retinal hypoperfusion corrected by external carotid revascularization. *Surgery* 1985;97:363–367.

CHAPTER 22

Amaurosis Fugax (Transient Monocular Blindness): A Consensus Statement

The Amaurosis Fugax Study Group

(Henry J.M. Barnett, Eugene F. Bernstein, Allan D. Callow, Louis R. Caplan, John E. Carter, Donald J. Dalessio, Ralph B. Dilley, J. Donald Easton, William K. Ehrenfeld, William S. Fields, Jean-Claude Gautier, Laurence A. Harker, Michael J.G. Harrison, Sohan S. Hayreh, William F. Hoyt, Joseph B. Michelson, Jay P. Mohr, Andrew N. Nicolaides, Shirley M. Otis, Ralph W. Ross Russell, Péter J. Savino, Marjorie E. Seybold, Thoralf M. Sundt, Jr., James F. Toole, Shirley H. Wray)

New data and a fuller appreciation of the multiple etiologic and pathogenetic mechanisms involved have resulted in heightened interest in the symptom known as amaurosis fugax, fleeting blindness, or TMB. A symposium was held at the Scripps Clinic and Research Foundation in La Jolla, Calif, in March 1987, to discuss amaurosis fugax, and this Consensus Statement was prepared by the participants at its conclusion. It summarizes the current views of the authors, who represent the specialties of neurology, neuro-ophthalmology, neurosurgery, ophthalmology, hematology, and vascular surgery, on the pathogenesis, diagnostic evaluation, and currently preferred treatment plan for patients with TMB.

Pathophysiology

Definition and Description of the Phenomenon

Amaurosis fugax is defined herein as transient monocular visual loss secondary to ischemia or vascular insufficiency. Patients describe diminished or absent vision in one eye that progresses for a few seconds and lasts for seconds to a few minutes (1–3). The visual impairment progressively may involve the entire visual field, often impressing the patient that the loss of vision begins in the upper field, less frequently in the periphery, and rarely in the lower field (4). Patchy and sectoral loss may be described. Recurrent events tend to follow an identical pattern.

The majority of attacks occur without an obvious immediate precipitating factor. Uncommonly, the visual loss lasts for several hours, and yet full recovery occurs. Persistent visual loss after such an event is an indication of retinal or optic nerve infarction.

Etiology

Nonocular Conditions

Extracranial Cerebrovascular Disease

Thromboembolic

The visual disturbance in embolic amaurosis fugax is a sudden attack of partial or complete TMB that lasts seconds to minutes and is followed by complete recovery. The majority of attacks are due to thromboembolism into the ophthalmic circulation from the common carotid artery and its branches (internal or external carotid arteries or the occluded stump of either artery).

Amaurosis fugax is an important marker of generalized atherosclerotic disease. The carotid atherosclerotic lesion may be an occlusion, a stenosis, or an irregular, ulcerated lesion with or without stenosis (4–6). Stenosis of greater than 75% may be associated with thrombus formation in the poststenotic cul-de-sac. Irregular or ulcerated lesions also can be associated with retinal emboli. Other carotid pathology responsible for the episode may include fibromuscular dysplasia, spontaneous dissection, and aneurysm of the carotid bifurcation.

Material seen within the retinal arteries indicates embolism. Bright, yellowish, glinting lipid emboli, so-called Hollenhorst plaques, are the most common emboli seen in the eye (7–9). They most often are associated with atheromatous lesions of the ipsilateral carotid artery or, less frequently, atherosclerotic disease involving the aortic arch or the carotid siphon. It has been confirmed that this embolic material contains cholesterol (10). Some of the circulating microemboli that pass through the retinal arterioles, so-called pale or migrant emboli, are composed of fibrin and platelets (11). Calcific emboli, which are characteristically white and nonscintillating, may originate from the common carotid artery, more proximal arterial sites, or from calcific cardiac valvular disease (12,13). Amaurosis fugax associated with atherosclerotic occlusive disease may precede occlusion of the CRA or branch retinal arteries.

Hemodynamic

Amaurosis of a much less common type may occur in patients with extensive extracranial arterial occlusive disease, particularly disease involving the great vessels originating from the aortic arch. Visual loss under these circumstances is precipitated by a change in posture, exercise, or exposure to bright light and is due to retinal vascular insufficiency (14,15). The temporary episodes of hemodynamic monocular visual loss may be less rapid in onset than the brief transient attacks of embolic origin, with the visual loss developing over minutes rather than seconds and lasting slightly longer than embolic episodes. Recovery may take place more gradually. Symptoms of cerebral ischemia may coexist.

This pattern of attacks suggests a temporary failure of retinal circulation. These visual symptoms are due to retinal or choroidal ischemia. Compensation becomes inadequate when both the external and internal carotid arteries are stenotic or occluded. In the majority of patients with extensive occlusions of the major arteries arising from the aortic arch, the cause is severe atherosclerosis. In young women, the cause may be inflammatory arteritis (Takayasu's disease).

Other Nonocular Causes

Emboli of cardiac origin that reach the eye can originate from valvular disease, such as rheumatic disease, mitral valve prolapse, marantic or infectious endocarditis, or calcific valvular disease. Patients with intracardiac lesions, such as myxomas or mural thrombi (eg, associated with atrial fibrillation or myocardial infarction), usually have larger emboli that generally do not reach the eye. *Exogenous retinal emboli* from chronic IV drug abuse may produce transient monocular visual loss, and talc or other foreign intravascular material may be seen on ophthalmoscopy (16,17).

Hypoperfusion due to cardiac disease or acute hypovolemia may cause amaurosis fugax. Rarely, such visual loss is unilateral, and then often it is associated with preexisting asymmetric occlusive vascular disease. *Systemic diseases* can alter ocular blood flow and produce transient monocular visual loss by disturbing blood viscosity, cellular blood content, or blood coagulability. Rarely, patients have retinal *migraine* with transient visual loss thought to be due to vasospasm in the retinal arterial system (18–20).

Another group of patients with monocular blindness have no demonstrable ocular or systemic explanation for their symptoms. At present, the cause of this type must be considered *idiopathic*.

Ocular Vascular Diseases

Anterior ischemic optic neuropathy due to giant-cell arteritis affects persons 60 years or older and may be manifested as amaurosis fugax. The visual loss is caused by severe narrowing or occlusion of the PCA, with consequent acute ischemia of the optic nerve head (21,22).

Occlusion of the central retinal vein sometimes starts with attacks of amaurosis fugax due to transient slowing of the retinal arterial circulation produced by sudden occlusion of the central retinal vein. The funduscopic findings in this condition are characteristic and include engorged retinal veins and peripheral retinal hemorrhages (23).

Patients with *malignant arterial hypertension* sometimes may have amaurosis fugax due to ischemia of the optic nerve head (24). This always includes optic disk edema in addition to other fundus lesions characteristic of hypertension.

Conditions that Can Be Confused with Amaurosis Fugax

Nonvascular ophthalmic disorders may induce transient monocular visual loss. Among these conditions are transient changes in the media or in IOP, such as vitreous floaters, vitreous hemorrhage, hyphema, and glaucoma (25). Congenital anomalies of the optic disk, such as drusen or posterior staphyloma, also should be considered (26). Intraorbital masses also may produce gaze-dependent visual changes (27,28).

Neurologic disorders can cause temporary visual loss that patients localize to one eye or do not localize precisely. Brainstem, vestibular, and oculomotor lesions cause blurred vision, usually with rotation, oscillation of objects, or diplopia. Intraorbital tumors, optic neuritis, and compression of the optic nerve or optic chiasm by aneurysms or tumors usually cause more gradual and persistent monocular visual loss. Patients with papilledema from any cause note transient visual obscurations sometimes precipitated by maneuvers that increase ICP or IOP or decrease systemic blood pressure (29). Patients with multiple sclerosis and optic nerve damage may report transiently decreased vision in one or both eyes after exercise or exposure to heat. Neurologic lesions, such as migraine, that affect postchiasmal visual pathways cause homonymous defects in the visual field that the patient may describe erroneously as monocular. Sequential eye closure, tests for visual acuity, and examination of the visual field help localize the lesion. Scintillations, hallucinations, and the presence of other neurologic findings also identify a cerebral location. Visual loss also can be psychogenic.

Diagnostic Evaluation

Pace of the Evaluation

Because the evidence from several studies indicates a short interval between the transient event and a stroke or blindness from temporal arteritis, it is recommended that the workup for TMB be undertaken without delay. In the absence of temporal arteritis, the outlook for vision is good, but the risk of stroke approaches that for hemispheric TIA (30–35). Simultaneous evaluation of occult cardiac disease is justified by the high frequency of cardiac mortality in this group (36).

Algorithm

An algorithm for the workup has been proposed (Fig. 22–1). A detailed history should differentiate typical amaurosis fugax from those atypical visual spells due to a variety of mechanisms (37). Amaurosis fugax usually is transient, lasting minutes, but may be longer, lasting up to two hours.

Ophthalmic Examination

A complete ophthalmologic examination should seek evidence of unusual causes as well as those that support a diagnosis of embolic and retinal vascular disease (38). Unusual causes detectable by examination include narrow-angle glaucoma, hyphema, congenital anomaly of the optic disk, disk drusen, and the rare orbital tumor. Signs of ischemia include occlusion

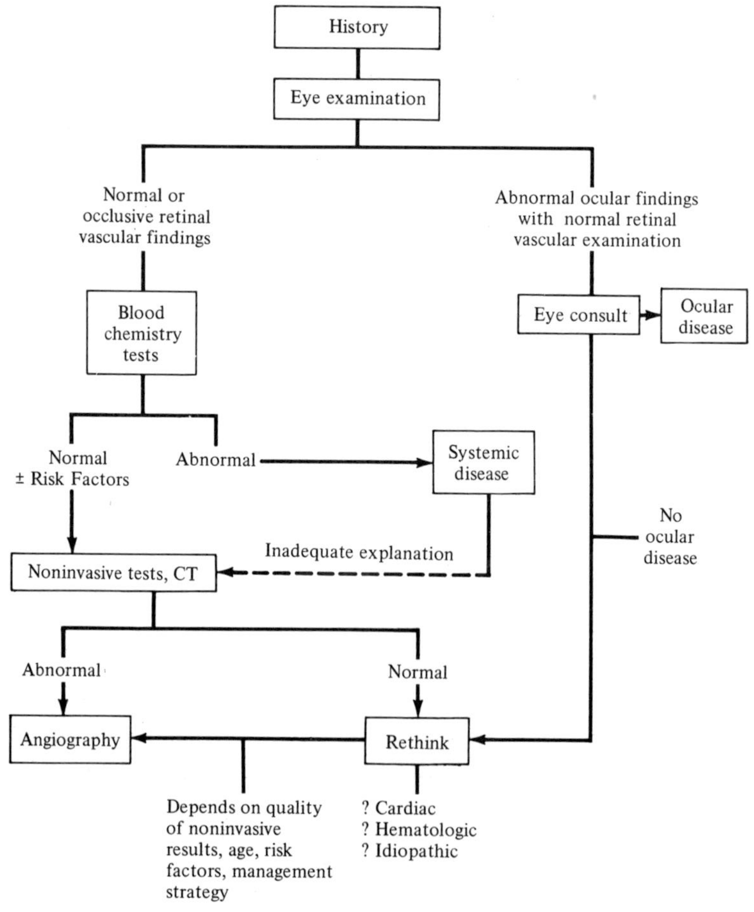

FIGURE 22–1. Scheme for workup of patients with amaurosis fugax.

of the branch retinal artery, regional retinal pallor, microinfarcts, and small hemorrhage(s) (2,3,9,39,40). Distended irregular veins and peripheral microaneurysms suggest retinal vascular insufficiency, for which fluorescein angiography may help in diagnosis.

Laboratory Studies

A limited battery of laboratory tests is recommended to detect associated systemic illnesses: A complete blood count for evidence of polycythemia or leukemia, platelet count for thrombocytosis, Westergren sedimentation rate for giant-cell arteritis, and screening for hyperlipidemia and diabetes (41–43). The value of a routine search for a prothrombotic state, with tests for lupus anticoagulant and for deficiencies in protein C, protein S, or antithrombin III, has not been established (44).

Noninvasive Carotid Artery Studies

High-quality duplex studies of the carotid artery are recommended strongly to identify occlusion, stenosis, or major ulceration at the carotid bifurcation and lesions of the proximal great vessels (5,45–47). If the results of the carotid duplex examination are normal, evidence of intracranial stenosis at the level of the carotid siphon should be sought by using pneumoplethysmography or ophthalmodynomometry or by using transcranial Doppler insonation of the siphon and circle of Willis. CT or MRI scans are recommended to obtain evidence of clinically silent cerebral embolism (48–51).

If the duplex and intracranial tests show no abnormalities, renewed diagnostic efforts must be made. A fluorescein angiogram is advisable to document previous embolic occlusion, microinfarction, ischemia in the PCA territory, or poor perfusion (52). Unfortunately, carotid angiography is usually inadequate to document ophthalmic artery disease (53).

The morbidity associated with angiography must be balanced both against the technique's low yield of the information and the low risk of stroke when the results of a high-quality duplex study are normal (54–56). Accordingly, routine carotid angiography is not recommended if the noninvasive studies are negative. Venous digital angiography is not indicated because of its low resolution (57). Other imaging approaches, such as thrombus-directed imaging procedures with low-density lipoproteins or labelled platelet studies and Doppler-documented plaque morphology to determine the activity of the carotid sinus mural thrombus, are not yet established (47,58). Ultrasonic documentation of plaque morphology also is promising, but its role has not been defined.

Amaurosis fugax is a marker of increased risk of death from myocardial infarction (36). Therefore, such patients should have a cardiac assessment both to identify cardiac sources of embolism and to detect those patients with ischemic heart disease (49,59,60).

At the end of the investigation, a minority, but frustratingly large, group of patients will be found in whom no cause is obvious (61). They most likely will be in the young age group, below 40. Invasive procedures are not warranted in these patients (62).

Treatment

General Issues

Some ocular vascular diseases and conditions that can be confused with amaurosis fugax have specific treatments. Especially important is the recognition and treatment of giant-cell arteritis and glaucoma. In addition, therapy is largely noncontroversial for the majority of other ocular vascular causes and the conditions that can be confused with amaurosis fugax. This Consensus Statement does not address them. Rather, emphasis is directed to those conditions associated with occlusive vascular disease resulting in TMB, partial or complete, for which treatment is controversial or unproven. This concerns, therefore, TMB secondary to ischemia affecting the retina, the choroid, or the optic nerve. Treatment is considered under the following headings: atherosclerosis, cardioembolism, and other.

Atherosclerosis

General Comments

The evidence for all forms of present therapy is less than compelling because of insufficient data, although certain trends are discernible. Several weaknesses of the available data are readily apparent. Most reports of therapy lump together amaurosis fugax and cerebral TIAs. Such a practice should be avoided because the natural history of the two conditions may be different. Additionally, a fundamental question is whether amaurosis fugax is being treated because of threat of blindness, threat of stroke, or both. The accepted primary implication is that amaurosis fugax caused by a carotid embolism is a precursor of hemispheric stroke (63,64). In a recent British study, the incidence of stroke in patients with this disorder was 2% per year (33). This was four times the expected annual rate in a matched population sample, but the expected stroke rate after a hemispheric TIA was substantially greater (65,66).

Several other problems are associated with the available data. In published reports of several categories of carotid disease, from minimal stenosis to occlusion, the numbers of patients in each subset are small. Angiographic or noninvasive evaluation of plaque characteristics and degree of stenosis are not always available. Few studies have been prospective and randomized. The variation from surgeon to surgeon in morbidity and mortality rates associated with carotid endarterectomy is important in any assessment of benefit and in comparison with other forms of treatment

(65,67). Additionally, data from aspirin trials are subject to different and occasionally conflicting interpretations. Treatment choice (ie, surgery *v* aspirin *v* no treatment) in many instances appears to be capricious and based on "intuition," "feelings," or "best case" judgment rather than on reliable data. This Consensus Statement reflects these uncertainties, and the recommendations for therapy are not well supported by data. In several instances, the recommendations represent current preferred practice by members of the Amaurosis Fugax Study Group. Some shifts in preference may evolve with more and better data acquisition in the next few years.

Considerable data from clinical trials show that aspirin reduces the prevalence of stroke plus death, and TIA, in patients with TIA (68–71). Although the reduction in stroke alone has not been statistically significant in most single studies, pooled data strongly suggest some benefit (72). Patients with amaurosis fugax have constituted about 15% of the patients studied in these trials, and it is *assumed* that the results apply to patients with amaurosis fugax in the trials as well as to patients with hemispheric TIAs.

Several substantial clinical trials (unstable angina (73,74), patency of saphenous vein grafts (75), TIA and minor stroke (76)) have shown no difference in the effect of low doses (300 to 325 mg daily) *v* high doses (900 to 1,300 mg daily) of aspirin, but a higher prevalence of side effects is associated with the higher dose. For this reason, all recommendations on aspirin are for 300 to 325 mg daily and pertain to both men and women.

Dipyridamole and sulfinpyrazone have not been shown to confer additional benefit over aspirin alone in trials involving patients with TIA and minor stroke (70,77). Other nonsteroidal antiinflammatory drugs or dipyridamole may have a place in the treatment of patients intolerant to aspirin. The combination of anticoagulant and dipyridamole is used widely in patients with prosthetic heart valves (78).

No conclusive evidence on the effect of anticoagulation in amaurosis fugax is available. Trials testing coumadin in stroke and TIA prevention in patients with TIA involved too few patients to be statistically significant (65,79–82).

Modifiable risk factors for stroke should be addressed, with particular attention to hypertension and smoking.

Type of Stenosis or Occlusion

The following classification is used in the discussion of treatment for the various carotid system atherosclerotic lesions that may be found associated with TMB.

Type of ICA stenosis or occlusion:

1. ICA occlusion
2. Greater than 75% stenosis (surgically inaccessible site)

3. Greater than 75% stenosis (surgically accessible site)
4. 50% to 75% stenosis
5. Less than 50% stenosis

The identification of plaque ulceration in any of the categories of carotid stenosis may lead to a more aggressive approach in therapy, inasmuch as many authorities agree that emboli of platelet-fibrin thrombi, atheromatous debris, and cholesterol crystals may be released from these ulcerated areas. Plaque appearance and composition (ie, degree of ulceration, hemorrhage, calcification, and lipid deposition) may have important clinical implications and may affect thinking about appropriate therapy.

Internal Carotid Artery Occlusion

Transient attacks, either ocular or cerebral, are less common in patients with occlusion of the ICA than in those with stenosis. Furthermore, TIAs may cease when a stenotic artery becomes occluded.

When a patient with amaurosis fugax is found to have a complete carotid occlusion, it is reasonable to treat the risk factors, give aspirin, and await developments. If amaurosis fugax or TIAs continue, the cause may be embolism, either from propagated thrombus in the carotid siphon or from embolism derived from the carotid stump traveling through external carotid collaterals. The cause also may be hemodynamic crises in a marginally perfused hemisphere or eye or giant-cell arteritis. Such attacks usually can be recognized by their clinical characteristics and provoking factors. Some of these lesions can be corrected by surgery (eg, external carotid ulceration or stenosis and ICA stump thrombosis with embolism).

Greater than 75% Stenosis (Surgically Inaccessible Site)

In some patients, especially those with severe hypertension or diabetes mellitus, carotid atheromas may be extensive throughout the artery. In others, stenosis may be localized at an inaccessible site (usually in the carotid artery siphon), with or without disease at the carotid bifurcation. In this group, aspirin therapy combined with general measures against underlying disease and risk factors is recommended. Some clinicians prefer anticoagulation.

Greater than 75% Stenosis (Surgically Accessible Site)

Some evidence suggests that high degrees of stenosis are associated with an increased risk of stroke. Intraluminal thrombi seen on angiography also may occur in this group, and the risk is substantial that a high-grade stenosis will proceed to occlusion.

Carotid endarterectomy is the treatment of choice when performed by a qualified surgeon on a patient with reasonable risk factors for surgery. It should be followed by treatment with aspirin and management of risk factors. If attacks continue after surgery, the patient should be reevaluated.

50% to 75% Stenosis

The risk of stroke in patients with amaurosis fugax and moderate ICA stenosis is thought to be lower than in the presence of a severe stenosis. Therapy for this category is particularly controversial, in part because of variability in techniques used for measurement of stenoses (eg, percentage of reduction in diameter or cross-sectional area). These variations prevent comparison of data across studies.

Patients with this degree of stenosis should be considered for carotid endarterectomy.

Aspirin therapy has been shown to reduce the risk of myocardial infarction and perhaps stroke as well.

Less than 50% Stenosis

Therapy for the group with less than 50% stenosis is controversial. Firm data are not available about the balance of risks and benefits of carotid surgery in this group. Pending such data, patients in this group should be treated with aspirin, with or without carotid endarterectomy. Factors favoring consideration of endarterectomy include crescendo amaurosis fugax, associated TIA or minor stroke, evidence of cerebral infarct on CT scan, retinal emboli observed on funduscopy, and ulceration of the carotid bulb. Failure of aspirin therapy in this category suggests the need for reconsideration of endarterectomy, particularly in the presence of ulceration.

Therapeutic Failure

Medical Failure:

Patients treated with aspirin may continue to have episodes of amaurosis fugax. In this case, reevaluation of the possibility that the atherosclerotic process has worsened is important. If the disease has progressed, surgical therapy may be indicated. If no change has occurred, continuation of aspirin or initiation of anticoagulation is indicated.

Surgical Failure:

If the episodes continue after endarterectomy, other possibilities must be considered, such as inadequate surgical removal of plaque, restenosis, or a tandem lesion that may be serving as a source of microemboli to the eye. Therapy must be individualized to suit the specific situation.

Cardioembolism

A cardiac cause requires the appropriate therapy: anticoagulation in the presence of mural thrombus, aspirin in mitral valve prolapse, or cardiac surgery as indicated after full cardiac assessment.

Other Causes

Giant-Cell Arteritis

Patients with amaurosis fugax alone or accompanied by other symptoms suggesting giant-cell arteritis should have a Westergren ESR determined immediately and should be placed on high doses of corticosteroids if the sedimentation rate is elevated. They then should be referred for a decision regarding further ocular evaluation and biopsy of the temporal artery. Further management should be based on the outcome of this evaluation.

Migraine

A few patients with migraine are stroke-prone. Generally, they are persons with complicated migraine or with uncomplicated migraine associated with atherosclerosis risk factors (eg, hypertension, hyperlipidemia, cigarette smoking) or other stroke risk factors (eg, use of oral contraceptives or the puerperium).

Patients under age 40 who have amaurosis fugax and uncomplicated migraine appear to require no treatment for the amaurosis fugax, but use of oral contraceptives should be avoided. Those patients who are over age 40, or who have complicated migraine or other stroke risk factors, should be treated with daily doses of 300 to 325 mg of aspirin, and vasoconstrictor agents should be avoided.

Idiopathic Causes

Patients under 40 years of age who have typical amaurosis fugax without any obvious cause appear to be at very low risk for subsequent stroke or permanent visual loss. They require no treatment, but a history of drug abuse should be sought. Those over age 40 are probably at higher risk and generally have been accepted as subjects in treatment trials for TIAs. They probably should be treated with daily doses of 300 to 325 mg of aspirin, and efforts should be made to modify their risk factors for atherosclerosis.

If their episodes of amaurosis fugax become frequent or prolonged, reconsideration of the diagnosis should be undertaken, and the need for further evaluation, particularly a search for a cardioembolic source, should be reconsidered.

Ethics

Almost every action we take in our daily lives has ethical considerations. This Consensus Statement is an impressive example. Many items in the statement have ethical overtones, some of minor importance, a few of major importance. For example, what are the ethical considerations engendered by recommendations for the management of patients with amaurosis fugax and carotid occlusive disease?

What is the optimal workup? Should all patients be referred to several specialists and be exposed to several technologies? Should all patients undergo noninvasive and angiographic evaluation despite known variations from place to place in both sophistication and reliability? Who is to say? What are the ethical implications in recommendations for therapy, for example, aspirin? What is the proper dose, and what is the proper frequency of administration if only 10% of normal platelets need be present to circumvent the aspirin effect?

What are the ethical issues related to carotid endarterectomy? For many surgeons, the operation is perceived as a good one and of durable result. Yet, the clinical community justifiably has questioned the overall nationwide results. What are the issues of importance to the patient? Although each of us would strive to acquaint the patient with the risks and hazards as well as the likelihood of benefit of the operation, in the light of insufficient data, this is very difficult to do. Experienced surgeons may feel compelled to recommend carotid endarterectomy in a given clinical situation because in their hands it is effective and safe.

If we admit a state of insufficient information, how ethical is any recommendation except one that seeks to enlarge our data base? Thus, further trials not only are needed but would seem to be directly helpful in solving the ethical issues.

In this Consensus Statement, it is impossible to give adequate and sufficient attention to the ethical issues and to the several constituencies: the patients, the third-party payers, the clergy, the legal profession, and many more. Although we do not have a statement that resolves these issues, we do recognize that for many practitioners and investigators the issues indeed may be large. For them, freedom of decision as to the best course for themselves and their patients according to their best judgment and their conscience is available. For others, choice of therapy—surgery or no surgery, aspirin or no aspirin—the ethical issues may be expressed differently. In their view, it may be unethical not to seek answers.

References

1. Ashby M, Oakley N, Lorentz I, et al: Recurrent transient monocular blindness. *Br Med J* 1963;2:894–897.
2. Fisher CM: Transient monocular blindness associated with hemiplegia. *Am Arch Ophthalmol* 1952;47:167–203.
3. Ross Russell RW: Observations on the retinal blood vessels in monocular blindness. *Lancet* 1961;2:1422–1428.
4. Wilson LA, Ross Russell RW: Amaurosis fugax and carotid artery disease: Indications for angiography. *Br Med J* 1977;2:435–437.
5. Pessin MD, Duncan GW, Mohr JP, et al: Clinical and angiographic features of carotid transient ischemic attacks. *N Engl J Med* 1977;296:358–362.

6. Parkins PJ, Kendall BD, Marshall J, et al: Amaurosis fugax: Some aspects of management. *J Neurol Neurosurg Psychiatry* 1982;45:1–6.
7. Hollenhorst RW: Significance of bright plaques in the retinal arterioles. *JAMA* 1961;178:123–129.
8. Hollenhorst RW: Vascular status of patients who have cholesterol emboli in the retina. *Am J Ophthalmol* 1966;81:1159–1165.
9. Ross Russell RW: Atheromatous retinal embolism. *Lancet* 1963;2:1354–1356.
10. David NJ, Klintworth GK, Frieberg SJ, et al: Fatal atheromatous cerebral embolism associated with bright plaques in the retinal arterioles. *Neurology* 1963;13:708–713.
11. Fisher CM: Observations of the fundus oculi in transient monocular blindness. *Neurology* 1959;9:333–347.
12. Arruga J, Sanders, MD: Ophthalmologic findings in seventy patients with evidence of retinal embolism. *Ophthalmology* 1982;89:1336–1347.
13. Brockmeier LB, Adolph RJ, Gustin BW, et al: Calcium emboli to the retinal artery in calcific aortic stenosis. *Am Heart J* 1981;101:32–37.
14. Ross Russell RW, Page NGR: Critical perfusion of brain and retina. *Brain* 1983;106:419–434.
15. Furlan AJ, Whisnant JP, Kessing J: Unilateral visual loss in bright light: An unusual symptom of carotid artery occlusive disease. *Arch Neurol* 1979;36:675–676.
16. Michelson, JB, Whitcher JP, Wilson S, et al: Foreign body granuloma of the retina associated with intravenous cocaine addiction. *Am J Ophthalmol* 1979;87:278–282.
17. Atlee WE: Talc and corn starch emboli in the eyes of drug abusers. *JAMA* 1972;219:49–51.
18. Carroll D: Retinal migraine. *Headache* 1970;10:9–13.
19. Krapin D: Occlusion of the central retinal artery in migraine. *N Engl J Med* 1964;270:359–360.
20. Coppetto JR, Lessell S, Sciarra R, et al: Vascular retinopathy in migraine. *Neurology* 1986;36:267–270.
21. Hayreh SS: Anterior ischaemic optic neuropathy: I. Terminology and pathogenesis. *Br J Ophthalmol* 1974;58:955–989.
22. Hayreh SS: *Anterior Ischemic Optic Neuropathy*. New York, Springer-Verlag, 1975.
23. Hayreh SS: So-called "central retinal vein occlusion": I. Pathogenesis, terminology, clinical features. *Ophthalmologica* (Basel) 1976;172:1–13.
24. Hayreh SS, Servais, GE, Virdi PS: Fundus lesions in malignant hypertension: V. hypertensive optic neuropathy. *Ophthalmology* 1986;93:74–87.
25. Ravitz J, Seybold ME: Transient monocular visual loss from narrow angle glaucoma. *Arch Neurol* 1984;41:991–993.
26. Seybold ME, Rosen PN: Peripillary staphyloma and amaurosis fugax. *Ann Ophthalmol* 1977;9:1139–1141.
27. Brown GC, Sheilds JA: Amaurosis fugax secondary to presumed cavernous hemangioma of the orbit. *Ann Ophthalmol* 1981;13:1205–1209.
28. Wilkes SR, Taoutmann JC, DeSanto LW, et al: Osteoma: An unusual cause of amaurosis fugax. *Mayo Clin Proc* 1979;54:258–260.
29. Hayreh, SS: Optic disc edema in raised intracranial pressure: IV. Associated visual disturbances and their pathogenesis. *Arch Opthalmol* 1977;95:1566–1579.

30. Marshall J, Meadows S: The natural history of amaurosis fugax. *Brain* 1968;91:419–434.
31. Hooshmand H, Vines FS, Lee HM, et al: Amaurosis fugax: Diagnostic and therapeutic aspects. *Stroke* 1974;5:643–647.
32. Pfaffenbach DD, Hollenhorst RW: Morbidity and survivorship of patients with embolic cholesterol crystals in the ocular fundus *Am J Ophthalmol* 1973;75:66–72.
33. Poole CJM, Ross Russell RW: Mortality and stroke after amaurosis fugax. *J Neurol Neurosurg Psychiatry* 1985;48:902–905.
34. Warlow CP: Transient ischemic attacks, in Matthews WB, Glaser GH (eds): *Recent Advances in Clinical Neurology*. Edinburgh, Churchill Livingstone, 1982, pp 191–214.
35. Hurwitz BJ, Heyman A, Wilkinson WE, et al: Comparison of amaurosis fugax and transient cerebral ischemia: A prospective study. *Ann Neurol* 1985;6:698–705.
36. Muuronen A, Kaste M: Outcome of 314 patients with transient ischemic attacks. *Stroke* 1982;13:24–31.
37. Hachinski VC, Porchawka J, Steel JC: Visual symptoms in the migraine syndrome. *Neurology* 1973;23:570–579.
38. Dyll DM, Margolis M, David NJ: Amaurosis fugax: Funduscopic and photographic observations during an attack. *Neurology* 1966;16:135–138.
39. Wolpow ER, Lupton RG: Transient vertical monocular hemianopia with anomalous retinal artery branching. *Stroke* 1981;12:691–692.
40. Gerstenfeld J: The fundus oculi in amaurosis fugax. *Am J Ophthalmol* 1964;58:198–205.
41. Levin J, Swanson PD: Idiopathic thrombocytosis: A treatable cause of transient ischemic attacks. *Neurology* 1968;18:711–713.
42. Wagener HP, Hollenhorst RW: The ocular lesions of temporal arteritis. *Am J Ophthalmol* 1958;45:617–630.
43. Dandona P, Bolger JP, Boag F, et al: Proliferative retinopathy and diabetes mellitus. *Lancet* 1984;1:1294.
44. Smith DB: Protein C deficiency: A cause of amaurosis fugax. *J Neurol Neurosurg Psychiatry* 1987;50:361–362.
45. Gaul J, Marks S, Weinberger J: Visual disturbance and carotid artery disease: 500 symptomatic patients studied by non-invasive carotid artery testing including B-mode ultrasonography. *Stroke* 1986;17:393–398.
46. Lees RS, Kistler JP, Sanders D: Duplex Doppler scanning and spectral bruit analysis for diagnosing carotid stenosis. *Circulation* 1982;66(suppl):102–105.
47. Wolverson MK, Bashiti HM, Peter GJ: Ultrasonic tissue characterization of atheromatous plaques using a high-resolution real-time scanner. *Ultrasound Med Biol* 1983;6:669–709.
48. Avad I, Modic M, Little J, et al: Focal parenchymal lesions in transient ischemic attacks: Correlation of computed tomography and magnetic resonance imaging. *Stroke* 1986;17:399–403.
49. DiBono DP, Warlow CP: Potential sources of emboli in patients with presumed transient cerebral or retinal ischemia. *Lancet* 1981;1:343–345.
50. Perrone P, Candelise L, Scott G, et al: CT evaluation in patients with transient ischemic attack: Correlation between clinical and angiographic findings. *Eur Neurol* 1979;18:217–221.

51. Sipponen JT, Kaste M, Sepponen RE, et al: Nuclear magnetic resonance imaging in reversible cerebral ischaemia. *Lancet* 1983;1:294–295.
52. Muci-Mendosa R, Arruga J, Edward WO, et al: Retinal fluorescein angiographic evidence for atheromatous microembolism. *Stroke* 1980;11:154–158.
53. Weinberger J, Bender AN, Yang WC: Amaurosis fugax associated with ophthalmic artery stenosis: Clinical simulation of carotid artery disease. *Stroke* 1980;11:290–292.
54. Earnest F, Forbes G, Sandbok BA, et al: Complications of cerebral angiography: Prospective assessment of risk. *AJNR* 1983;4:1191.
55. Edwards JH, Kricheff II, Riles T, et al: Angiographically undetected ulceration of the carotid bifurcation as a cause of embolic stroke. *Radiology* 1979;132:369–373.
56. Eikelboom B, Riles TR, Mintzer F, et al: Inaccuracy of angiography of the diagnosis of carotid ulceration. *Stroke* 1983;14:882–885.
57. Ludwig JW, Verhoeven LHJ, Engels PHC: Digital video subtraction angiography (DVSA) equipment: Angiographic technique in comparison with conventional angiography in different vascular areas. *Br J Radiol* 1982;55:545–553.
58. Lees RS, Lees AM, Strauss WH: External imaging of human atherosclerosis. *J Nucl Med* 1983;24:154–156.
59. Brockmeier LB, Adolph RJ, Gustin BW, et al: Calcium emboli to the retinal artery in calcifics aortic stenosis. *Am Heart J* 1981;101:32–37.
60. Caltrider ND, Irvine AR, Kline HJ, et al: Retinal embolism in patients with mitral valve prolapse. *Am J Ophthalmol* 1980;90:534–539.
61. Eadie MJ, Sutherland JM, Tyrer JH: Recurrent monocular blindness of uncertain cause. *Lancet* 1968;1:319–321.
62. Goodwin JA, Gorelick PB, Helgason CM: Symptoms of amaurosis fugax in atherosclerotic carotid artery disease. *Neurology* 1987;37:829–832.
63. Morax PV, Aron Rosa D, Gautier JC: Symptomes et signes ophtalmologique des stenoses et occlusions carotidiennes. *Bull Soc Ophthalmolog Fr* 1970, suppl 1, p 169.
64. Parkin PH, Kendall BE, Marshall J, et al: Amaurosis fugax: Some aspects of management. *J Neurol Neurosurg Psychiatry* 1982;45:1–6.
65. Easton JD, Hart RG, Sherman DH, et al: Diagnosis and management of ischemic stroke: Part I. Threatened stroke and its management. *Curr Probl Cardiol* 1983;8:1–76.
66. Whisnant JP, Matsumoto N, Elveback LR: Transient cerebral ischemic attacks in a community. *Mayo Clin Proc* 1973;48:194–198.
67. Fode NC, Sundt TM Jr, Robertson JT, et al: Multicenter retrospective review of results and complications of carotid endarterectomy in 1981. *Stroke* 1986;17:370–376.
68. Fields WS, Lemak NA, Frankowski RF, et al: Controlled trial of aspirin in cerebral ischemia. *Stroke* 1977;8:301–316.
69. Fields WS, Lemak NA, Frankowski RF, et al: Controlled trial of aspirin in cerebral ischemia: Part II. *Stroke* 1978;9:309–319.
70. The Canadian Cooperative Study Group: A randomized trial of aspirin and sulfinpyrazone in threatened stroke. *N Engl J Med* 1978;299:53–59.
71. Bousser MG, Eschwege E, Haguenau M, et al: "AICLA" controlled trial of aspirin and dipyridamole in the secondary prevention of atherothrombotic cerebral ischemia. *Stroke* 1983;14:5–14.

72. Antiplatelet Trialists Collaboration: Secondary prevention of vascular disease by prolonged antiplatelet therapy. *Br Med J* 1987 (in press).
73. Lewis HD Jr, David JW, Archibald DG, et al: Protective effects of aspirin against acute myocardial infarction and death in men with unstable angina: Results of a Veterans Administration cooperative study. *N Engl J Med* 1983;309:396–403.
74. Cairns JA, Gent M, Singer J, et al: Aspirin, sulfinpyrazone or both in unstable angina: Results of a Canadian multicenter trial. *N Engl J Med* 1985;313:1369–1375.
75. Lorenz RL, Weber M, Kotzur J, et al: Improved aorto-coronary bypass patency by low-dose aspirin (100 mg daily): Effects on platelet aggregation and thromboxane formation. *Lancet* 1984;1:1261–1264.
76. The UK-TIA Study Group: Design and protocol of the UK-TIA aspirin study, in, Tognoni G, Garattini S (eds): *Drug Treatment and Prevention in Cerebrovascular Disorders: Clinical Pharmacology and Drug Epidemiology*. Amsterdam, Elsevier, 1979, vol 2, pp 387–394.
77. American-Canadian Cooperative Study Group: Persantine aspirin trial in cerebral ischemia: Part II. Endpoint results. *Stroke* 1985;16:406–415.
78. Sullivan JM, Harken DE, Gorlin R: Pharmacologic control of thromboembolic complications of cardiac valve replacement. *N Engl J Med* 1971;284:1391–1394.
79. Report of the Veterans Administration Cooperative Study of Atherosclerosis, Neurology Section: An evaluation of anticoagulant therapy in the treatment of cerebrovascular disease. *Neurology* 1986;11:132–138.
80. Pearce JMS, Gubbay SS, Walton J: Long-term anticoagulant therapy in transient cerebral ischemic attacks. *Lancet* 1965;1:6–9.
81. Baker RN, Broward JA, Fang HC, et al: Anticoagulant therapy in cerebral infarction. *Neurology* 1962;12:823–835.
82. Baker RN, Schwartz W, Rose AS: Transient ischemic attacks: A report of a study of anticoagulant treatment. *Neurology* 1966;16:841–847.

Index